MW01054804

LEE A. DOERNTE, F...

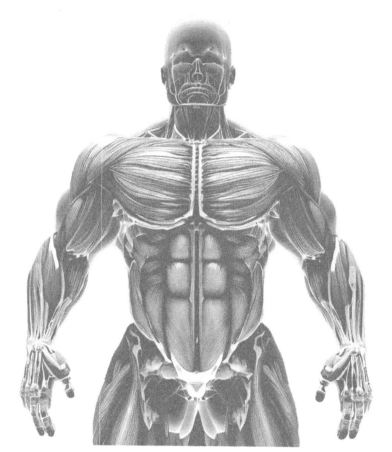

MUSCLE UNIVERSITY

AN IN-DEPTH GUIDE TO EXERCISE PHYSIOLOGY AND MAXIMIZING MUSCLE GROWTH

STRENGTH AND SIZE THROUGH SCIENCE

Copyright © 2023 by Lee A. Doernte, PhD

All rights reserved.

No part of this publication may be reproduced, distributed, or transmitted in any form or by any means, including photocopying, recording, or other electronic or mechanical methods, without the prior written permission of the publisher, except in the case of brief quotations embodied in critical reviews and certain other non-commercial uses permitted by copyright law.

TABLE OF CONTENTS

PREFACE

Welcome to **"Muscle University: An In-Depth Guide to Exercise Physiology and Maximizing Muscle Growth"**. Within the pages of this book, we embark on a journey through muscle physiology, exploring the mechanisms that govern muscle growth, function, and performance. Whether you are an athlete seeking to excel in your sport, a fitness enthusiast aiming to maintain a powerful physique, or simply an individual intrigued by the science behind muscle development, this book is your comprehensive guide to unlocking the full potential of your muscles.

At the heart of "Muscle University" lies a passion for understanding the complex interplay of factors that contribute to muscle growth and optimization. We aim to bridge the gap between scientific knowledge and practical application, providing you with evidence-based insights and strategies that you can implement in your training, nutrition, and recovery practices.

Whether you are an athlete striving to enhance your performance, a fitness enthusiast seeking to build strength and muscle, or a healthcare professional interested in expanding your knowledge, "Muscle University" has something to offer you. Each chapter is meticulously crafted to provide a comprehensive understanding of the topic at hand, supported by up-to-date research and practical examples.

Throughout this book, you will gain a deep appreciation for the intricate mechanisms that drive muscle function and growth. You will also uncover the science behind energy systems, nutrient metabolism, hormonal influences, periodization programming, and safe training practices. You will explore the interplay between the mind and muscles, as well as the critical role of recovery and injury prevention.

"Muscle University" aims to empower you with knowledge, enabling you to make informed decisions about your training, nutrition, and overall fitness journey. It serves as a guidebook, offering evidence-based strategies and practical tips for maximizing muscle growth, optimizing performance, and promoting healthy living.

In the preface, we lay the groundwork for the exciting journey ahead. We introduce the concept of Muscle University as a place of learning and exploration, where the mysteries of muscle physiology are unraveled, and the keys to maximizing muscle growth are unveiled.

We begin by clarifying the purpose and aim of this book – to provide you with a comprehensive understanding of exercise physiology principles and practical strategies for maximizing muscle growth. Whether you are a beginner or a seasoned fitness enthusiast, we believe that knowledge is power, and by understanding the science behind muscle function, you can optimize your training and achieve your desired results.

To assist you in navigating this educational journey, we guide you on how to effectively utilize this book. We also encourage you to approach each chapter with an open mind and a willingness to absorb the information presented. Take the time to reflect on how the concepts discussed can be applied to your own fitness journey, and consider how you can integrate the knowledge gained into your training, nutrition, and recovery practices.

We recognize that the pursuit of muscle growth is not a one-size-fits-all endeavor. Each individual has unique goals, preferences, and circumstances. Therefore, we strive to provide you with a wealth of knowledge and practical insights that can be geared toward your specific needs and applied in a way that aligns with your personal journey.

As you embark on this educational voyage, we encourage you to embrace the spirit of curiosity and discovery. Allow yourself to be captivated by the wonders of muscle physiology and the incredible potential that lies within your own body. Celebrate the journey of growth and transformation, knowing that with each step, you are moving closer to unlocking the true potential of your muscles.

We invite you to join us on this extraordinary expedition through "Muscle University." Together, let us match into the depths of exercise physiology, empower ourselves with knowledge, and unlock the door to muscle growth and performance.

Now, turn the page and let the journey begin.

Dr. Lee Doernte

CHAPTER 1

THE ANATOMY AND PHYSIOLOGY OF MUSCLES

The first chapter of "Muscle University" explores the anatomy of skeletal muscles. Anatomy is the foundation upon which our physiology is built. We gain valuable insights into how these remarkable tissues affect our athletic endeavors and our daily lives by delving into the intricacies of a muscle's structure.

Interestingly, skeletal muscles drive our every movement. They enable us to perform a wide range of activities, from simple gestures to athletic endeavors. Skeletal muscles are responsible for our physical strength, maintaining posture and stability, pumping blood through our veins, maintaining our body temperatures, protecting our organs, and stabilizing our joints.

At the macroscopic level, our body is a marvel of engineering. Muscles are intricately organized into distinct groups that function in a coordinated manner. These muscle groups are strategically located throughout the body, each serving a specific purpose and role in our daily movements and activities. These groups range from powerful quadriceps that propel us forward to the delicate muscles of our hands that allow for fine motor skills.

Each muscle group has its unique function, but they don't operate in isolation. Instead, they work together, synchronizing contractions and relaxations to generate powerful, efficient movement. For instance, when we lift an object, it's not just the biceps at work. The triceps, forearm, shoulder, and core muscles come into play, ensuring stability and strength. This collaborative effort between muscle groups ensures the body can handle a wide range of motions and tasks without undue strain on any single muscle group.

However, to truly appreciate the mechanisms of muscles, we must venture deeper into their microscopic structures. Within each muscle, we discover an intricate network of muscle fibers. These individual fibers are the building blocks of muscular tissue and generate force through contraction. Deeper into these fibers, we will explore the structure of fibers, including the arrangement of the contractile proteins and the importance of cellular components such as the sarcoplasmic reticulum and mitochondria. We will even explore what "the powerhouse of the cell" really means. Finally, we will examine the connective tissues that envelop and support the muscles, the tendons that attach muscles to bones, and the fascia that surrounds and separates muscle groups, aiding movement coordination and structural integrity.

As we explore muscle anatomy, we will encounter specialized terms and anatomical landmarks. Understanding these terms will enhance our ability to communicate and comprehend the intricate details of muscle structures. To aid this endeavor, a comprehensive glossary is provided at the end of the book, serving as a valuable reference tool.

Delving into the depths of muscle anatomy sets the stage for exploring muscle physiology, growth, and optimization. By studying muscle physiology, we will explore how muscle tissue types differ, function, adapt, and respond to stimuli. Through this knowledge, we can direct our training approaches, rehabilitation strategies, and overall fitness regimens to optimize our muscular health and performance.

So, let us embark on this journey into the world of muscles. It is time to uncover the intricacies of muscle structure and gain an appreciation for these remarkable tissues.

Anatomy Overview of a Muscle Fiber

The human body's ability to generate movement through muscle fibers is truly remarkable. These specialized cellular structures possess a unique shape that allows for effective sliding and synchronization, enabling them to work together seamlessly to produce motion. Composed of multiple cells that fuse together during development, muscle fibers contain multiple nuclei, adding to their complexity and intricacy. These structures are just one example of the amazing functions of the human body.

The sarcolemma, which serves as the muscle fiber's plasma membrane, is more than just a barrier. It actively conducts electrical impulses, known as action potentials that are essential for starting the contraction process. This active membrane has caveolae, small pockets that hold calcium ions, and ion channels that carefully manage the muscle cell's internal environment.

Inside the sarcolemma lies the sarcoplasm, a matrix rich in stored glycogen, serving as a primary energy source during short bursts of activity. This matrix also houses myoglobin, a protein that binds and stores oxygen, readying it for immediate use during muscle activity. The sarcoplasm facilitates many of the cell's metabolic reactions and provides the environment for the muscle's primary contractile elements, the myofibrils, to function.

Myofibrils, long contractile fibers running parallel within the muscle fiber, are predominantly made of proteins. They contain repeating units known as sarcomeres, which give the muscle its characteristic striated appearance. These sarcomeres are the smallest functional unit of a muscle. Each sarcomere is demarcated by Z-discs, anchoring the thin filaments and providing structural integrity. Within these sarcomeres, thick filaments made of myosin molecules interlace with thin filaments primarily composed of actin. The H-zone, located centrally, is where only thick filaments are present, and its size varies with muscle contraction. Titin, a colossal protein, spans half the sarcomere, connecting the Z-disc to the M-line, offering both structural support and elasticity.

Surrounding each myofibril is the sarcoplasmic reticulum (SR), a specialized endoplasmic reticulum. Its tubules and sacs are reservoirs of calcium ions. When an action potential strikes, voltage-sensitive channels in the SR release calcium into the sarcoplasm, setting the stage for contraction. The SR's terminal cisternae, reservoir-like structures, work closely with T-tubules to ensure rapid calcium release when signaled.

T-tubules, extensions of the sarcolemma, penetrate deep into the muscle cell. Their primary role is to carry action potentials into the muscle fiber's interior, ensuring a synchronized response to neural stimuli. These tubules are lined with a variety of ion channels and pumps, maintaining the internal ionic environment essential for muscle function.

Scattered throughout the sarcoplasm are mitochondria, the cell's "powerhouses". These double-membraned organelles produce ATP, which is especially vital during sustained muscle activity. Their inner membrane, with its folds called cristae, increases the surface area for ATP production.

Unlike most cells with a centrally located nucleus, muscle fibers have multiple nuclei situated just beneath the sarcolemma. These control centers house the cell's genetic material and direct the synthesis of proteins and enzymes essential for muscle function and repair.

Lastly, a globular protein, myoglobin, specific to muscle cells, temporarily stores oxygen, ensuring a rapid supply during the initial stages of muscle activity. Surrounding individual muscle fibers is the endomysium, a delicate layer of areolar connective tissue. It not only provides insulation and protection but also serves as a conduit for blood vessels and nerves.

Sarcomeres: The Heartbeat of Muscle Movement

In muscle tissue, the sarcomere stands out as a marvel of biological design. It's not just a structural unit; it's the very essence of muscle contraction. Nestled between two Z-discs in a muscle myofibril, the sarcomere is responsible for the characteristic striations we see in skeletal and cardiac muscles.

The Z-discs, those thin, dark lines, aren't just boundaries. They're anchors, holding the thin filaments in place and providing a foundation for the protein titin. As we move from the Z-discs inward, we encounter the thin filaments, primarily composed of the protein actin. But actin doesn't work alone. It's accompanied by the regulatory proteins, tropomyosin and troponin, which play a pivotal role in muscle contraction.

Centrally positioned within the sarcomere are the thick filaments of the protein myosin. Each myosin molecule is wonderfully designed, with a head that protrudes outward and a tail that forms the backbone of the filament. These heads are crucial players, reaching out and interacting with actin filaments during the contraction phase we call the "power stroke".

The sarcomere's landscape is defined by its bands. The A-band, a dark region, spans the entire length of the thick filaments and includes areas where thick and thin filaments overlap. Interestingly, whether the muscle is flexed in a contraction or relaxed, the A-band's length remains consistent. Contrasting with the A-band is the I-band, a lighter region containing only thin filaments. This band, bisected by the Z-disc, narrows during muscle contraction, showcasing the dynamic nature of the sarcomere.

Within the A-band lies the H-zone, a region where only thick filaments reside. As muscles contract, this zone shrinks, a testament to the sliding filament theory of muscle contraction. At the heart of the H-zone is the M-line, which not only holds the thick filaments in place but also anchors the colossal structural protein, titin.

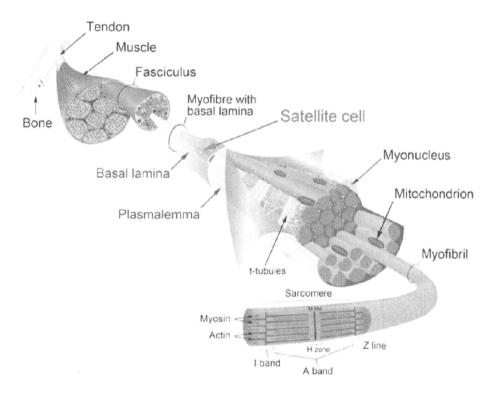

The dance of muscle contraction, orchestrated by the sarcomere, is a complex ballet of molecular interactions. When a muscle is signaled to contract, calcium ions flood the scene. These ions bind to troponin, instigating a change that reveals the myosin-binding sites on actin. The myosin heads, seizing this opportunity, attach to these sites, commencing the power stroke and pulling the actin filaments toward the center of the sarcomere. This action, driven by the energy molecule ATP, causes the sarcomere to shorten and the muscle to contract. The sarcomere's genius doesn't end with contraction. The protein titin ensures that after every powerful contraction, the muscle returns to its resting state. Titin's elasticity pulls the sarcomere back to its original length, preparing it for the next wave of contraction.

In muscle movement, sarcomere is the key player. Its design ensures efficient, coordinated contractions, while its adaptability to various stimuli underscores its pivotal role in muscle strength, endurance, and function.

Proteins of Muscle Fibers: The Building Blocks of Movement

Muscle fibers, the workhorses of movement and strength, owe their functionality to a complex interplay of proteins. These proteins give structure to the muscle and also drive the intricate processes of muscle contraction and relaxation.

Myosin

Myosin stands as the primary motor protein in muscle contraction, forming the very backbone of the thick filaments. Each myosin molecule is a marvel of biological engineering, comprising a head, a hinge-like neck, and a tail. The head, in particular, is crucial. It seeks out and binds to actin during contraction, pulling the thin filaments with a force that's powered by the energy molecule, ATP. This relationship between actin and myosin is at the heart of how our muscles contract.

Actin

Actin, often considered the star of the thin filaments in muscle fibers, plays a pivotal role in muscle contraction. Each individual actin molecule is meticulously designed with a binding site, designed for myosin. This site remains concealed, shielded by the protein tropomyosin when the muscle is in a relaxed state. However, the true magic happens during contraction. The binding sites become exposed, setting the stage for the myosin heads to bind and generate the force that powers our movements.

Troponin

Troponin, a complex protein with three distinct subunits, associates closely with actin. Its role is multifaceted: binding to actin, tropomyosin, and crucially, calcium ions. When calcium is present, troponin undergoes a transformation, a change in its shape that nudges tropomyosin away, revealing the myosin-binding sites on actin. This is a pivotal moment in the initiation of muscle contraction.

Tropomyosin

Tropomyosin, a regulatory sentinel, wraps itself around the actin filament with a specific mission: to cover the myosin-binding sites on actin when the muscle is at rest. But its role becomes even more crucial when calcium ions enter the scene. These ions bind to another protein, troponin, instigating a shift in tropomyosin. This shift reveals the binding sites, setting the stage for muscle contraction.

Titin

Titin, the largest protein known to science, is a marvel in muscle elasticity and structural support. Stretching from the Z-disc to the M-line within the sarcomere, titin behaves much like a spring. After the muscle contracts, titin ensures the muscle gracefully returns to its resting state. Beyond this, titin is deeply involved in muscle development and the assembly of the sarcomere, showcasing its multifaceted roles.

Nebulin

Nebulin, running parallel to actin, is believed to be a regulator, specifically of the length of actin filaments. This giant protein not only supports the thin filaments but also plays a role in maintaining their structural integrity, ensuring they function optimally during muscle contraction.

Dystrophin

Dystrophin serves as a bridge, connecting the internal muscle fiber cytoskeleton to the external matrix that surrounds cells. This connection is not just about structure; it's about support and stability. However, dystrophin's significance becomes even clearer when it's absent or malfunctioning. Genetic mutations in the dystrophin gene can lead to muscular dystrophies, disorders marked by progressive muscle weakness.

Myomesin and C-protein

Located in the heart of the sarcomere, the M-line, both myomesin and C-protein have the vital task of holding the thick filaments in place. Their presence ensures the sarcomere retains its structural integrity, allowing for efficient muscle contraction.

α-Actinin

α-Actinin, found at the Z-disc, has the crucial role of anchoring the thin filaments in place. By maintaining the organized structure of the sarcomere, α-actinin ensures that the actin filaments are perfectly aligned, and ready for the next wave of contraction.

In muscle movement, these proteins are the threads that create a masterpiece of strength, movement, and endurance. Each protein, with its unique role, contributes to muscle contraction, allowing us to move, dance, lift, and even breathe.

Muscle Fiber Types: Type I, Type IIa, and Type IIb

Introduction to Muscle Fiber Types

Within human physiology, muscles emerge as awe-inspiring masterpieces of biological engineering. They are the silent force that fuels our every action, from the faintest flutter of an eyelash to the dynamic burst of a sprinter launching off the blocks. These muscles, with their intricate structures and dynamic capabilities, are not just functional entities; they are a testament to nature's unparalleled design prowess.

Central to this muscular dynamism is an intricate array of fiber types, each meticulously designed to serve specific roles and respond to varied demands. These fibers, systematically classified as Type I, Type IIa, and Type IIb, might not be the stars of the show when we think of our physical feats, but they are indeed crucial. They are the foundation upon which our every motion is built, influencing not only the raw power and speed of our movements but also the stamina and resilience with which we execute them.

Each of these fiber types is wonderfully designed in its own right:

- **Type I fibers** are the endurance stalwarts, designed for activities that require sustained effort over extended periods. They are the workhorses, ensuring we can walk, stand, or even maintain posture for hours on end without succumbing to fatigue.

- **Type IIa fibers** are the versatile all-rounders, adept at both power and endurance. They bridge the gap between raw strength and lasting stamina, making them invaluable in activities that demand a blend of both.

- **Type IIb fibers** are the powerhouses, built for short, high-intensity bursts of activity. They come into play when we need to summon strength quickly, be it in lifting a heavy object or sprinting to catch a bus.

But the story doesn't end with just categorizing these fibers. Each type boasts a unique metabolic profile, structural design, and enzymatic activity that dictates its function, performance capabilities, and adaptability. By delving deeper into muscle fiber types, we embark on a journey of discovery. We'll explore the intricate science underpinning their roles, the factors that influence their distribution, and the training strategies that can optimize their potential. This knowledge is pivotal for athletes, trainers, and anyone keen on understanding the mechanics of human movement, ensuring that they can harness the full potential of their muscles and achieve their desired athletic outcomes. So, let us dive into the intricacies of each fiber type.

Type I Muscle Fibers (Slow-Twitch or Oxidative Fibers)

Type I muscle fibers, often termed "endurance fibers", are a testament to nature's precision engineering. These fibers are intricately designed to support sustained activities, revealing a complex interplay of biochemistry, cellular biology, and physiology.

Sarcomere Structure

- **Actin and Myosin Arrangement:** The sarcomeres in Type I fibers have a unique arrangement of actin and myosin filaments. This alignment is optimized for slow, controlled contractions, ensuring efficient force production over extended periods.

- **Z-lines:** The Z-lines in Type I fibers are closer together than in fast-twitch fibers, resulting in shorter sarcomeres. This structural difference contributes to their slower contraction speed.

- **Sarcoplasmic Reticulum (SR):** The SR in Type I fibers releases calcium ions more slowly during muscle contraction, leading to a slower contraction response. This controlled release is crucial for maintaining prolonged contractions.

- **T-Tubules:** Type I fibers have narrower T-tubules, which are channels that help transmit electrical signals deep into the muscle cell. This structure aids in the synchronized contraction of the fiber.

Biochemical Properties and Metabolism

- **Enzymatic Profile:** Type I fibers have a high concentration of enzymes geared towards aerobic metabolism, particularly those involved in the Krebs cycle and the electron transport chain. This enzymatic profile ensures efficient ATP production over extended periods.

- **Lipid Droplets:** These fibers contain more lipid droplets than their fast-twitch counterparts. These droplets store fats, which serve as a significant energy source during prolonged activities.

- **Glycogen Stores:** While they do store glycogen, Type I fibers have relatively lower glycogen content compared to fast-twitch fibers. They rely more on fats and glucose from the bloodstream for energy.

Physiological Characteristics and Functional Implications

- **Oxygen Utilization:** The high myoglobin content, combined with a dense capillary network surrounding each fiber, ensures optimal oxygen delivery and utilization. This setup supports the fiber's reliance on aerobic metabolism.

- **Thermal Output:** Type I fibers produce less heat per ATP generated, a crucial adaptation for endurance. This efficient energy production reduces the risk of overheating during prolonged activities.

- **Neural Innervation:** The motor units (a motor neuron and the muscle fibers it controls) associated with Type I fibers are smaller. This allows for finer control and more prolonged, sustained contractions.

Training Adaptations and Potential

- **Hypertrophy versus Endurance:** While Type I fibers can increase in size with resistance training, their primary adaptation to training is enhanced endurance. This is achieved through increased mitochondrial density, enhanced capillarization, and improved oxygen utilization.

- **Fatigue Resistance:** Over time, with consistent endurance training, Type I fibers can further enhance their fatigue resistance. This is achieved through a combination of increased fuel stores, improved metabolic efficiency, and enhanced waste product removal.

Type I muscle fibers are a wonder of evolutionary adaptation, showcasing how cellular structure and function can meet specific demands. Every component, from the sarcomere's design to the enzymatic profile, is designed for endurance. A granular understanding of these fibers provides invaluable insights for athletes, trainers, and physiologists aiming to optimize endurance and performance.

Type IIa Muscle Fibers (Fast-Twitch Oxidative Fibers): A Granular Examination

Type IIa muscle fibers, often termed "fast-twitch oxidative fibers", represent a unique blend of speed and endurance within the muscular system. These fibers are adept at handling both short bursts of intense activity and moderately prolonged efforts, making them versatile players in various physical endeavors.

Sarcomere Structure

- **Actin and Myosin Arrangement:** The sarcomeres in Type IIa fibers have an arrangement of actin and myosin filaments that allows for faster contractions than Type I fibers but slower than Type IIb fibers. This intermediate arrangement provides them with their unique functional characteristics.

- **Z-lines:** The Z-lines in Type IIa fibers are spaced in a manner that allows for rapid contraction while still maintaining some level of endurance.

- **Sarcoplasmic Reticulum (SR):** The SR in Type IIa fibers releases calcium ions more rapidly than in Type I fibers but not as quickly as in Type IIb fibers. This balance ensures a faster contraction response while still allowing for some sustained activity.

- **T-Tubules:** Type IIa fibers have T-tubules that are broader than Type I fibers, which facilitate the transmission of electrical signals throughout the muscle cell, leading to quicker contraction responses.

Biochemical Properties and Metabolism:

- **Enzymatic Profile:** Type IIa fibers possess enzymes that support both aerobic and anaerobic metabolism. This dual enzymatic profile allows them to produce ATP quickly during short bursts of activity and maintain ATP production during longer activities.

- **Lipid Droplets:** Type IIa fibers contain lipid droplets, though not as densely as Type I fibers. These droplets provide an energy reserve, especially during prolonged activities.

- **Glycogen Stores:** These fibers have a substantial glycogen content, allowing them to generate energy quickly during high-intensity activities.

Physiological Characteristics and Functional Implications:

- **Oxygen Utilization:** While they don't have as high a myoglobin content as Type I fibers, Type IIa fibers still maintain a decent oxygen storage capacity. Their capillary network, though less dense than Type I fibers, ensures adequate oxygen delivery for their metabolic needs.

- **Thermal Output:** Type IIa fibers produce more heat per ATP generated than Type I fibers, reflecting their faster, more intense energy production during short bursts of activity.

- **Neural Innervation:** The motor units associated with Type IIa fibers are larger than those of Type I fibers but smaller than Type IIb fibers. This intermediate size allows for rapid, forceful contractions while still maintaining some level of control.

Training Adaptations and Potential:

- **Hypertrophy versus Endurance:** Type IIa fibers respond well to both strength and endurance training. Resistance training can lead to hypertrophy, increasing their size and force output. Endurance training can enhance their oxidative capacity, improving their stamina.

- **Fatigue Resistance:** While they fatigue faster than Type I fibers, Type IIa fibers have a moderate resistance to fatigue, especially when compared to Type IIb fibers. Training can enhance this resistance, allowing for better performance in activities that require both power and endurance.

Type IIa muscle fibers are a testament to the body's adaptability, bridging the gap between pure endurance (Type I) and pure power (Type IIb). Their unique structural and functional characteristics make them invaluable in a range of physical activities, from middle-distance running to weightlifting. A granular understanding of these fibers offers insights for optimizing training regimens and enhancing athletic performance.

Type IIb Muscle Fibers (Fast-Twitch Glycolytic Fibers): A Granular Examination

Type IIb muscle fibers, often termed "fast-twitch glycolytic fibers", are the epitome of rapid force generation in the muscular system. These fibers excel in short, explosive activities, making them the go-to for actions requiring immediate power generation.

Sarcomere Structure

- **Actin and Myosin Arrangement:** The sarcomeres in Type IIb fibers are designed for rapid force production. Their actin and myosin filaments are arranged to facilitate the fastest contractions among all muscle fiber types.

- **Z-lines:** The Z-lines in Type IIb fibers are spaced to allow for the quickest and most forceful contractions, reflecting their primary role in high-intensity, short-duration activities.

- **Sarcoplasmic Reticulum (SR):** The SR in Type IIb fibers is adept at releasing calcium ions at an incredibly rapid rate, ensuring instantaneous muscle contractions.

- **T-Tubules:** Type IIb fibers possess the broadest T-tubules among muscle fiber types, ensuring that electrical signals are transmitted swiftly and effectively throughout the muscle cell.

Biochemical Properties and Metabolism:

- **Enzymatic Profile:** Type IIb fibers are rich in enzymes that support anaerobic metabolism, particularly those involved in the glycolytic pathway. This allows them to produce ATP at an extremely rapid rate, albeit for short durations.

- **Lipid Droplets:** Type IIb fibers have fewer lipid droplets compared to Type I and Type IIa fibers, which indicates their primary reliance on glycogen as an energy source.
- **Glycogen Stores:** These fibers are densely packed with glycogen, providing a ready source of glucose for quick energy production during high-intensity activities.

Physiological Characteristics and Functional Implications

- **Oxygen Utilization:** Type IIb fibers have a lower myoglobin content compared to other fiber types, as their primary energy production doesn't rely heavily on oxygen. Their capillary network is also less dense, reflecting their anaerobic energy production preference.
- **Thermal Output:** Due to their rapid ATP production via glycolysis, Type IIb fibers generate a significant amount of heat in a short time, which can be a limiting factor in their duration of activity.
- **Neural Innervation:** The motor units associated with Type IIb fibers are the largest among muscle fiber types. This allows for the most forceful contractions, suitable for high-intensity activities like sprinting or heavy weightlifting.

Training Adaptations and Potential

- **Hypertrophy versus Endurance:** Type IIb fibers are highly responsive to resistance training, leading to significant hypertrophy. Their size and force output can be increased with targeted strength training.
- **Fatigue Resistance:** Type IIb fibers fatigue rapidly due to their reliance on anaerobic metabolism. However, with training, their anaerobic capacity can be enhanced, allowing for slightly longer durations of high-intensity activity.

Type IIb muscle fibers are nature's answer to activities that demand rapid, forceful contractions. From sprinters exploding off the starting blocks to weightlifters lifting heavy loads, these fibers are at the heart of high-intensity, short-duration activities. A granular understanding of Type IIb fibers is crucial for athletes and trainers aiming to maximize power and speed in their respective disciplines.

The Muscle Fibers: Decoding Athletic Potential and Performance

Every human body is a masterpiece, intricately designed through millions of years of evolution. One of the most fascinating aspects of this design is the distribution of muscle fiber types, which plays a central role in determining our physical strengths and weaknesses.

When we talk about athletic abilities, the balance between endurance and power comes into focus. Individuals with a higher proportion of Type I fibers, for instance, are naturally inclined towards activities that require sustained energy output, such as long-distance running, cycling, or certain dance forms. In contrast, those with a dominance of Type II fibers, especially Type IIb, are built for quick, explosive actions. These individuals might do well in sports like weightlifting or sprinting.

The nuances of sports specialization further highlight the importance of muscle fiber composition. In athletics, the muscle composition of a 400m runner, who requires both speed and endurance, will differ from that of a marathoner, who relies primarily on sustained energy output. Similarly, in team sports like basketball or football, different positions might favor different muscle compositions. For instance, a basketball player positioned near the hoop might benefit from the explosive power of Type II fibers for jumping, while a football midfielder, covering vast distances during a match, might predominantly utilize Type I fibers.

Again, our genetic lineage plays a significant role in determining our muscle fiber composition. The lifestyles of our ancestors, whether they were hunters or farmers, can influence our muscle makeup. Modern sports science is even exploring the potential of genetic testing to predict athletic potential, analyzing genes associated with muscle composition to forecast an individual's suitability for specific sports.

Training and external stimuli can fine-tune our muscle fibers. Endurance activities, for example, can enhance the aerobic capacity of Type I fibers, making them more efficient in using oxygen. On the other hand, strength training exercises can stimulate Type II fibers, enhancing their anaerobic energy production. Environmental factors, such as training at high altitudes where oxygen is less available, can push Type I fibers to become even more efficient. Additionally, our diet, especially carbohydrate intake, can influence the energy storage capabilities of our muscle fibers.

While training can induce adaptations in muscle fibers, it's essential to understand the difference between adaptation and alteration. We can't change a Type I fiber into a Type II fiber, but there's evidence suggesting that Type IIa fibers can exhibit characteristics of either Type I or Type IIb fibers based on specific training regimens. However, every individual has a limit to how much their muscle fibers can adapt, and recognizing this limit is crucial to ensure effective training without risking injuries.

The insights gained from understanding muscle fiber composition are invaluable for trainers and athletes. Training plans designed with an individual's unique muscle composition in mind can ensure optimal results from every workout. Moreover, understanding the different recovery needs of various muscle fiber types can help in designing effective rest and recovery schedules.

As we progress through "Muscle University", we will explore training methods and strategies that can maximize the potential of different muscle fiber types. By harnessing the specific strengths and capabilities of each fiber type, we can push our limits, unlock our athletic potential, and achieve remarkable results.

Continue to the next section as we unlock the secrets of the sliding filament theory of muscle contraction, the mechanism behind the remarkable ability of muscles to generate force and enable movement.

The Sliding Filament Theory of Muscle Contraction: A Deep Dive into Muscular Dynamics

The muscle physiology stands as a testament to nature's intricate design and precision. Central to this marvel is the sliding filament theory, a concept that has reshaped our comprehension of muscular dynamics. Conceived by the visionary Huxleys in the mid-20th century, this theory offers a granular perspective into the microscopic choreography that underpins muscle contraction, revealing the intricate processes that transform a neural signal into tangible movement.

Actin and Myosin: The Dynamic Powerhouses of Muscle Contraction

At the heart of the sliding filament theory are the proteins actin and myosin. They are not just molecular structures but are dynamic entities that coordinate muscle contraction. Nestled within the sarcomere, the fundamental contractile unit of muscle fibers, these proteins await their cue to spring into action. The sarcomere, with its repeating units along the length of a muscle fiber, is a hotbed of activity, with actin and myosin at its epicenter. Their interaction, governed by a series of biochemical reactions, is the essence of muscle movement.

Resting Phase: The Calm Before the Storm

In a muscular state, actin and myosin maintain a specific spatial relationship, akin to dancers awaiting the first notes of a song. They overlap, but not fully, in a meticulously maintained arrangement that ensures rapid response when the contraction signal arrives. This overlap is not random; it's a product of precise biological engineering, ensuring that when the signal for contraction arrives, the transition from rest to activity is seamless and efficient. This poised state is a testament to the muscle's readiness, always to respond to the body's many demands.

21

MUSCLE UNIVERSITY

1. **Signal Reception:** The initiation is marked by an action potential, an electrical impulse that sweeps across the muscle fiber. This isn't a mere surface event. The impulse penetrates the muscle fiber's depths through a labyrinthine network of T-tubules. These tubules are like highways, ensuring the signal's rapid dissemination to the remotest corners of the muscle cell, preparing every part for the impending contraction.

2. **The Calcium Surge:** The action potential has a significant ally in the sarcoplasmic reticulum, a specialized organelle within the muscle cell. Upon sensing the electrical disturbance, the sarcoplasmic reticulum releases a deluge of calcium ions (Ca2+) into the sarcoplasm. This calcium influx is akin to a conductor raising his baton, signaling the start of the actin-myosin interaction.

3. **Decoding the Molecular Lock:** Calcium ions have a specific target: the protein troponin. Upon binding, they induce a conformational change in troponin, which in turn nudges its partner protein, tropomyosin, to shift its position. This molecular interaction exposes the myosin-binding sites on actin filaments, setting the stage for the main event.

4. **Cross-Bridge Formation:** The stage is set, and the myosin heads, energized by ATP, eagerly bind to the now-accessible sites on actin. This binding forms cross-bridges, marking the onset of a synchronized molecular level.

5. **The Power Stroke's Majesty:** The myosin heads, anchored firmly to actin, execute a powerful pivot. This motion pulls the actin filaments toward the sarcomere's center. It's a forceful, yet precise movement, culminating in the muscle contraction we perceive.

6. **Decoupling and Recalibration:** The dance isn't eternal. A fresh ATP molecule binds to the myosin head, prompting it to release its grip on the actin filament. This ATP isn't just a detachment signal; it provides the energy to reposition the myosin head, priming it for the next cycle of binding and force generation.

7. **The Perpetual Dance:** The cycle isn't a one-off event. As long as the sarcoplasm is awash with calcium ions and there's a steady supply of ATP, the binding, power stroke, release, and reset cycle perpetuates, causing sustained muscle contraction.

8. **The Graceful Finale:** Every performance has its curtain call. As the action potential wanes, specialized pumps in the sarcoplasmic reticulum swing into action, actively transporting calcium ions back into their storage. With the decline in calcium

concentration, the troponin-tropomyosin complex resumes its resting stance, obscuring the myosin-binding sites. The muscle, having completed its task, returns to a state of relaxation.

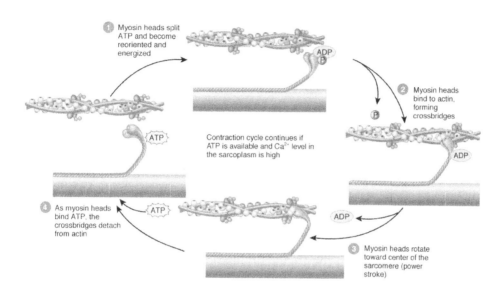

Implications and Practical Applications

The sliding filament theory is more than a mere academic concept; it's a foundational pillar in the fields of sports science, physical therapy, and athletic training. By understanding muscle contraction at the microscopic level, trainers, therapists, and athletes can channel their training regimens to optimize strength, enhance power, and accelerate muscle development.

In essence, the sliding filament theory offers a window into muscle physiology. It showcases the delicate interplay of proteins, ions, and energy molecules, all working in harmony to power the vast range of movements, from the subtlest twitch to the most explosive burst of strength.

As we continue our journey through "Muscle University", we will explore the factors that influence muscle contraction, such as motor unit activation, force generation, and the role of energy systems. By delving into the intricacies of muscle contraction, we gain insights that guide our training approaches, help prevent injuries, and unlock our full potential for muscular performance.

With the foundation of muscle anatomy and an understanding of the sliding filament theory, we are equipped to delve even further into the depths of muscle physiology. In the subsequent chapters, we will explore energy systems, muscle growth mechanisms, nutritional foundations, exercise programming, recovery strategies, injury prevention, and real-world case studies. Each chapter builds upon the previous, empowering us with the knowledge needed to optimize our muscle growth and achieve remarkable results.

Summary of Muscle contraction steps:

1. Action potential (AP) starts in the brain.

2. AP arrives at the axon terminal, and releases acetylcholine (ACh).

3. ACh crosses synapse, and binds to ACh receptors on plasmalemma.

4. AP travels down plasmalemma and T-tubules.

5. Triggers Ca2+ release from the sarcoplasmic reticulum (SR).

6. Ca2+ binds to troponin on the thin actin filament.

7. The troponin -Ca2+ complex moves tropomyosin revealing a connecting point for myosin head.

8. Myosin head connects to actin and pulls actin toward the sarcomere center (the power stroke).

9. After the power stroke ends, Myosin detaches from the active site, the head rotates back to its original position, and then attaches to another active site farther down the actin chain.

10. The process continues until Z-disk reaches myosin filaments or AP stops and Ca2+ gets pumped back into SR.

Continue to Chapter 2 as we unlock the mysteries of energy systems and their vital role in muscle function. Prepare to dive into ATP, anaerobic glycolysis, and aerobic respiration, and discover how these energy pathways fuel our muscles' incredible abilities.

CHAPTER 2

ENERGY SYSTEMS AND MUSCLE FUNCTION

The human body, a masterpiece of evolutionary design, is a complex web of systems and processes. Each heartbeat, every breath, and all our movements, conscious or reflexive, are underpinned by a ceaseless demand for energy. This energy, both the spark of life and the power to function, is the cornerstone of our existence. But where does this energy come from? How is it harnessed, stored, and utilized? And what happens when we push our bodies to the limit, demanding optimal performance and endurance?

At a glance, we might perceive our actions as simple outcomes of will and intent. Yet, beneath the surface, a network of biochemical reactions is at play. These reactions ensure that our muscles contract, our heart beats, and our brain processes information. Central to this biochemical reaction is the molecule adenosine triphosphate (ATP), often termed the 'energy currency' of life. But ATP doesn't act alone. Its generation, utilization, and recycling involve a series of energy systems, each with its unique characteristics, advantages, and limitations.

In this chapter, we will examine the microscopic world of our cells, exploring the intricacies of energy production and consumption. We'll uncover the secrets of ATP, revealing its pivotal role in sustaining life and activity. We'll delve into the fast-paced realm of anaerobic glycolysis, where energy is rapidly generated for short, intense bursts of activity. And we'll navigate the more measured and sustainable pathways of aerobic respiration, which powers our body during prolonged periods of exertion.

But this exploration isn't just about understanding the 'how'. It's about appreciating the 'why'. Why does an athlete's performance vary between a 100-meter sprint and a marathon? Why do we feel that burning sensation in our muscles after an intense workout? And how can knowledge of our energy systems inform our training, nutrition, and recovery strategies?

By the end of this chapter, you won't just understand the science; you will also appreciate the art of the human body, in its relentless pursuit of balance, efficiency, and survival. Armed with this knowledge, you will be better equipped to harness your body's potential, optimize your performance, and embark on a journey of health, fitness, and discovery.

Certainly! Let's craft this together into a more narrative, book-style format.

ATP: The Cellular Powerhouse

In cellular biology, adenosine triphosphate, more commonly known as ATP commands attention with every step. While textbooks and lectures often relegate it to the role of the cell's 'energy currency', such a description barely scratches the surface of its significance. ATP is not just a molecule; it's a life's energy, a maestro commanding many cellular reactions that underpin our very existence.

In fact, a world without ATP is like a world where the heart doesn't beat, where thoughts don't form, and where muscles don't contract. It's a world devoid of movement, of life. Such is the importance of this molecule. Every blink of an eye, every whisper of a thought, and every beat of the heart – they all hinge on the energy released from ATP.

But what gives ATP this unparalleled significance? ATP is a molecule designed for energy storage and transfer. Its structure, comprising an adenosine base and three phosphate groups, is a biological engineering. The bonds between these phosphate groups are like coiled springs, packed with potential energy. When the cell needs power, these bonds are broken in a controlled manner, releasing the stored energy to fuel countless cellular processes.

Yet, ATP's role isn't just about providing energy. It's also a communicator, a signaler. It helps cells understand their energy status, guiding them in making decisions about growth, repair, and response to their environment. In a way, ATP is the cell's barometer, its gauge of energy wealth or poverty.

As we study these cellular processes, from the splitting of glucose in glycolysis to the intricate steps of the Krebs cycle, ATP is our constant companion. It's the product of our cellular respiration, the goal of our metabolic pathways, and the ingredient for our cellular activities.

In the narrative of life, ATP emerges as a protagonist, a molecule that encapsulates the essence of life's energy. It bridges the gap between the abstract world of biochemistry and the tangible realities of our daily existence. Every movement, every thought, every breath is a testament to the power and significance of ATP, the true cellular powerhouse.

The Structure of ATP

In biology, where countless molecules play intricate roles, ATP stands out in its design and function. Its structure, a testament to nature's ingenuity, is perfectly directed to its monumental role as the primary energy carrier within all living organisms.

ATP is a nucleotide, a foundational unit that many might recall from discussions about the building blocks of DNA and RNA. This connection to our genetic material isn't just a footnote; it's a profound reflection of ATP's deep-seated role in the tapestry of life. The molecule's foundational unit, adenosine, is a harmonious combination of adenine, a nitrogenous base, and ribose, a five-carbon sugar. This duo provides a stable platform, preparing the molecule's true powerhouses: the trio of phosphate groups.

These phosphate groups, each carrying a negative charge, are like three siblings in close quarters, their mutual repulsion creating a palpable tension. It's this tension, this stored potential that gives ATP its might. When the bond between the second and third phosphate groups is severed, energy is unleashed, ready to be harnessed by the cell.

But ATP's story is cyclical. Once it has given up its energy, it transforms into ADP, a molecule that's just one phosphate short of its former glory. Yet, with the right conditions and a dash of cellular magic, ADP can be reinvigorated, reclaiming a phosphate group and rising once more as ATP.

Nestled within our cells, the mitochondria, often hailed as the cell's powerhouses, play a pivotal role in this rebirth. They work tirelessly, ensuring that ATP is continually regenerated, supporting the journey of life.

As we study cellular energy, the intricate design and profound significance of ATP become ever clearer. It's not just a molecule; it's a testament to the beauty and complexity of life itself.

ATP in Action

Within the cell, ATP stands as a beacon of energy and function. It's not merely a molecule; it's a dynamic force, driving countless processes and ensuring the harmonious operation of life at the cellular level.

Every twitch of a muscle fiber, every fleeting thought that crosses through our neurons, finds its energetic roots in ATP. This molecule often likened to the currency of the cell, facilitates vital energy transactions. Just as money powers our economies, ATP powers the cellular world, ensuring that life's many processes unfold seamlessly.

But the life of an ATP molecule is fleeting. In moments of intense activity, such as during a sprint or a heavy lift, our muscle cells can exhaust their ATP reserves almost instantly. Yet, remarkably, these stores are rapidly replenished, a testament to the cell's incredible efficiency and the pivotal role of ATP. This rapid turnover, this ceaseless cycle of expenditure and regeneration, underscores ATP's central role in meeting the cell's ever-changing energy demands.

Beyond its famed role as an energy donor, ATP wears many hats. It's a key player in cellular signaling, acting as a messenger that helps cells communicate, adapt, and respond to their ever-changing environment. It's also instrumental in the synthesis of our genetic blueprints, DNA, and RNA, ensuring that the story of life is faithfully transcribed and passed down through generations.

Yet, one of ATP's most crucial roles often goes unnoticed. It serves as the primary power source for the pumps that maintain the delicate balance of ions across cell membranes. These pumps, vital for cellular health and function, rely on ATP to operate. Without it, they would falter, and the intricate balance upon which cellular life hinges would be thrown into disarray.

As we examine deeper the cellular energy, the profound significance of ATP becomes increasingly clear. It's not just an energy molecule; it's the very essence of cellular life.

ATP-PCr Cycle: Immediate Energy Reservoir

The intricacies of human physiology are vast and complex, with each system playing a pivotal role in ensuring optimal function. Among these systems, the energy pathways stand out for their crucial role in powering every movement, from the subtlest gestures to the most strenuous exertions. The ATP-PCr cycle, in particular, serves as a testament to the body's ingenious mechanisms for meeting immediate energy demands.

The Essence of Energy in the Human Body

Every action, whether it's blinking an eye, taking a step, or sprinting to catch a bus, requires energy. This energy is stored in the form of adenosine triphosphate (ATP), often termed the 'energy currency' of the cell. However, the body's storage of ATP is limited, enough only for a few seconds of intense activity. This is where the ATP-PCr cycle comes into play.

The ATP-PCr Cycle: A Brief Overview

The ATP-PCr cycle, also known as the phosphagen system, is one of the body's primary anaerobic energy pathways. "Anaerobic" means it operates without the need for oxygen, allowing it to produce energy rapidly. This system is particularly active during the initial stages of high-intensity activities, providing the immediate energy required.

Phosphocreatine: The Body's Energy Reservoir

Phosphocreatine (PCr) acts as a reserve of high-energy phosphate. When the body engages in sudden, intense activity and ATP stores are quickly used up, PCr comes to the rescue. It donates its phosphate group to the depleted adenosine diphosphate (ADP), regenerating ATP almost instantaneously. This process is facilitated by the enzyme creatine kinase, ensuring a rapid response to energy demands.

The Role of the ATP-PCr System in Physical Activities

Imagine a weightlifter attempting a maximum lift, a sprinter exploding off the starting blocks, or a basketball player making a jump shot. In all these scenarios, the body doesn't have the luxury of time to produce energy through slower, aerobic pathways. The ATP-PCr system is perfectly suited for these moments, delivering the necessary energy almost instantly.

However, the rapidity of the ATP-PCr system comes at a cost: its duration is limited. Within about 10 seconds, the reserves of PCr are depleted, and the body must transition to other energy systems to continue the activity.

The ATP-PCr cycle is a testament to the body's adaptability and precision. It underscores the body's ability to cater to diverse energy needs, ensuring that we can respond to various physical challenges effectively. Whether we're aware of it or not, every explosive movement we make is powered, at least in part, by this remarkable energy system. It's a reminder of the intricate processes that occur within us, enabling us to move, play, and live with vitality.

Nature of the ATP-PCr Cycle

Location: Cytoplasm and Muscle Cells

Deep within the intricate cellular architecture of our body lies the ATP-PCr energy system, a vital component in our physiological toolkit. Nestled primarily within the cytoplasm, this system is especially prominent in muscle cells. The strategic placement of the ATP-PCr system within these cells is no mere coincidence. By residing so close to the heart of the action, it is perfectly positioned to respond to the body's energy demands with remarkable speed.

Imagine a well-oiled machine, with every cog and wheel placed just where it needs to be for maximum efficiency. The ATP-PCr system is much like that crucial cog, situated precisely where it can make the most difference. Its location within the cytoplasm of muscle cells ensures that, when the body calls for a sudden burst of energy, the ATP-PCr system can deliver immediately. It's akin to having a rapid-response team always on standby, ready to spring into action at a moment's notice, ensuring that our muscles have the energy they need to perform optimally.

Immediate Source of Energy for Short Bursts of Activity

In our body's energy systems, the ATP-PCr cycle stands out as the soloist, ready to take center stage when a swift and powerful performance is required. Think of those moments when an athlete explodes off the starting blocks, a weightlifter hoists a massive weight overhead, or when you sprint to catch a bus. These short, intense bursts of activity demand energy at a rate that other systems simply can't match in real-time.

Many of our body's energy systems are like marathon runners, built for endurance and sustainability. They rely on intricate biochemical reactions, methodically converting fuel sources into usable energy. While efficient and essential for prolonged activities, these processes are not designed for speed. They're the steady, enduring engines that keep us going during prolonged exertion.

Enter the ATP-PCr cycle, the sprinter among the marathoners. It doesn't rely on lengthy, complex pathways to produce energy. Instead, it taps into its reservoir of phosphocreatine (PCr) to quickly regenerate ATP, the primary energy currency of cells. This rapid conversion is akin to having a turbocharger in a car. Just as a turbocharger can provide an immediate surge of power to a vehicle, the ATP-PCr cycle delivers an instantaneous boost of energy to our muscles. The ATP-PCr cycle produces ATP at a 1:1 ratio (1 ATP for every 1 creatine). It's the body's natural nitrous system, propelling us forward with incredible force, even if just for a few precious seconds.

However, like all turbo boosts, this surge is fleeting. The ATP-PCr cycle is not designed for duration but for intensity. It's our body's way of ensuring that when we need a sudden, powerful burst of energy, we have a system in place that's primed and ready to deliver.

Mechanism of the ATP-PCr Cycle

When we look deeper into our body's energy systems, the ATP-PCr cycle emerges as a masterclass in efficiency and speed. But how does this system work its magic, especially when the spotlight is on and the pressure is high?

Utilization of Stored Phosphocreatine (PCr) to Regenerate ATP

The intricacy of energy within our cells is a testament to nature's brilliance. Central to it is ATP (adenosine triphosphate), often likened to a rechargeable battery. When it is fully ready to go, it's ATP. But as it powers our cellular functions, it releases energy and transforms into ADP (adenosine diphosphate), similar to a battery running low on charge.

Now, imagine being in the middle of an intense workout or sprinting towards a finish line. Your cells are working overtime, and the demand for ATP is immense. But there's a catch: the body's direct storage of ATP is limited and can run out quickly under such strenuous conditions. Just when it seems like the energy might run out, phosphocreatine (PCr) makes its entrance.

Residing within our muscle cells, PCr is like an emergency backup generator. It's not always running, but when the primary power source (ATP) is running low, PCr is ready to jump into action. As ATP levels dwindle, PCr donates its phosphate group to the energy-depleted ADP, effectively recharging it back into ATP. This transformation isn't a slow, drawn-out process; it's rapid, ensuring that our muscles have a near-constant supply of energy, especially during those moments when every second counts.

This dynamic between ATP and PCr is akin to a perfectly choreographed dance. As one partner tires, the other seamlessly steps in, ensuring the performance continues flawlessly. It's this harmonious interplay, happening at the microscopic level within our cells that allows us to push our physical boundaries, time and time again.

Rapid Provision of Energy for Activities Lasting Up to 10 Seconds

Every superhero, no matter how powerful, has an Achilles' heel, and the ATP-PCr system is no exception. Think of it as the Usain Bolt of our cellular energy systems: unmatched in speed, unparalleled in power, but limited in endurance. It's the system our body calls upon when we need a sudden, explosive burst of energy. Like a drag racer shooting off the starting line with a roar, the ATP-PCr system delivers an incredible surge of power, but it's a short-lived spectacle.

Picture this: a matchstick that burns with an intense flame but is consumed within moments. That's the ATP-PCr system for you. It can propel us to sprint at full tilt, leap to catch a ball, or lift a weight we've never lifted before. But just as quickly as it flares to life, it's spent, lasting a mere 10 seconds at its peak.

But nature, in its infinite wisdom, has equipped us with backup systems. As the ATP-PCr system's energy dwindles, it's like a relay runner passing the baton to the next athlete in line. Our body seamlessly transitions to other energy sources, like the glycolytic or the oxidative system. While these systems might not have the rapid-fire energy release of the ATP-PCr system, they are the endurance athletes, capable of supporting longer durations of effort.

It's this intricate choreography of energy systems, each taking the lead when its strength is needed most that allows us to adapt and perform across a vast spectrum of activities. Whether we're going for gold in a 100-meter dash, running a marathon, or just enjoying a leisurely walk in the park, our body's energy systems work in harmony, ensuring we have the energy to see us through.

Applications and Limitations

The ATP-PCr system is akin to the nitrous oxide boost in a race car. When activated, it provides an immediate surge of power, propelling the vehicle forward with incredible speed. But just as the nitrous boost is finite and runs out after a few moments, so does the energy from the ATP-PCr system.

The Body's Turbocharger for High-Octane Activities

Imagine the starting buzzer of a 100m race. As the athlete runs off the blocks, every muscle fiber is firing at maximum capacity. Or picture a weightlifter, muscles bulging, as they attempt a one-rep max lift. In both scenarios, the body demands a sudden and intense burst of energy, and the ATP-PCr system answers the call immediately. It's the body's go-to for those moments when we push our limits, when every millisecond counts, and when there's no room for delay. It's not just about speed; it's about raw, unbridled power.

A Brilliant Flash, But Not a Sustained Flame

However, every strength comes with a trade-off. The ATP-PCr system is like a firework: a spectacular display of energy, but one that's over in a flash. Our muscles have a limited reserve of phosphocreatine, and once it's used up, the ATP-PCr system's contribution dwindles. That's why sprinters, no matter how fit, can't maintain their top speed for an extended period. After that initial burst, the body starts to transition to other energy systems, which are more enduring but less explosive in their output.

Harnessing the Power and Recognizing the Limits

For athletes, coaches, and fitness enthusiasts, understanding the ATP-PCr system's capabilities and constraints is crucial. It can inform training regimens, recovery periods, and competition strategies. For instance, a sprinter might focus on maximizing their ATP-PCr output for a race, while a long-distance runner would train their body to efficiently transition from the ATP-PCr system to the aerobic system.

In essence, the ATP-PCr system is a testament to the body's incredible adaptability and specialization. It's a reminder that we're equipped not just for endurance or strength alone, but for a dynamic blend of both, ready to meet the diverse challenges we encounter.

Anaerobic Glycolysis: The Sprinter of Energy Systems

In cellular energy production, where processes are met with precision and purpose, anaerobic glycolysis stands out as the sprinter on the track, always ready for the gunshot. Among the many metabolic pathways, it's the one that doesn't wait for steady oxygenated breaths. Instead, it dashes forward, responding to the urgent call of muscles that scream for immediate energy.

Imagine, for a moment, the world's most elite sprinters lining up for the 100-meter dash. The stadium is silent, and the tension is palpable. As the gunshot pierces the air, these athletes explode off the blocks, every fiber of their being focused on the finish line mere seconds away. There's no time for pacing or strategy; it's all about raw, unbridled speed. This is the essence of anaerobic glycolysis. It's not the marathon runner, pacing itself for the long haul, nor the middle-distance runner, balancing speed with endurance. It's the sprinter, all power and intensity, demanding energy here and now.

But why does our body need such a rapid response? Life, in all its unpredictability, often throws situations that demand immediate action. Whether it's the sudden sprint to catch a bus, the explosive power needed to lift a heavy object, or the rapid response in a fight-or-flight situation, our body requires an energy system that can deliver fast. Oxygen, as vital as it is, can sometimes lag behind, especially during these sudden bursts of activity. That's where anaerobic glycolysis steps in, ensuring that our cells have the energy they need, even when oxygen is momentarily in short supply.

In cellular processes, anaerobic glycolysis is the bold stroke of color, the dash of intensity. It's a testament to nature's foresight, ensuring that we're equipped to handle the unexpected, the urgent, and the intense.

Anaerobic Glycolysis: The Swift Responder of Cellular Metabolism

In cellular biology, where processes are as varied as they are vital, anaerobic glycolysis stands out as a rapid responder, a system designed for immediacy. The anaerobic cycle produces ATP at a 2 or 3:1 ratio (2 or 3 ATP for every 1 glucose). But to truly appreciate its role, we must first journey into its nature, its locale, and its unique independence from oxygen.

The Cytoplasm: A Bustling Cellular Neighborhood

Imagine, if you will, a sprawling city. Skyscrapers touch the sky, roads weave in intricate patterns, and every corner is alive with activity. This city is the cell, and within it, various districts or neighborhoods each have their unique roles. One such district, the cytoplasm, is akin to the city's downtown area. It's where the action is palpable, where processes happen at a breakneck pace, and where anaerobic glycolysis has set up shop.

The cytoplasm, with its gel-like consistency, fills the cell, cradling organelles and providing a medium for countless reactions. It's here, away from the structured confines of the mitochondria, that anaerobic glycolysis thrives. The very location of this process speaks to its nature. It's not tucked away in some cellular suburb; it's right in the heart of the action, ready to spring into motion when called upon.

Breathing Without Air: The Oxygen-Independent Maestro

The very name "anaerobic glycolysis" carries with it a hint of its defining characteristic. "Anaerobic", derived from the Greek words meaning "without air", paints a picture of a process that has learned to operate without the life-giving molecule of oxygen. But why would a process evolve to function without oxygen, especially when so many cellular processes rely on it?

The answer lies in the unpredictable nature of life. There are moments, fleeting yet intense when our bodies demand energy at a rate that outpaces the oxygen supply. Imagine the final stretch of a 100-meter dash, the climactic lift of a weightlifting competition, or the sudden sprint when one's life is in danger. It's in these moments, when every second counts, that anaerobic glycolysis shines.

By operating independently of oxygen, anaerobic glycolysis ensures that our cells never find themselves energy-strapped in critical moments. It's a backup system, a safety net, ensuring that even when the regular channels of energy production are overwhelmed, the cell can still produce the ATP it needs to function.

In cellular metabolism, however, anaerobic glycolysis emerges as a hero of sorts. It's not the most efficient pathway, nor is it the one the cell would choose under normal circumstances. But in those crucial moments, when the stakes are high and time is of the essence, anaerobic glycolysis steps up, ensuring that the cellular city never experiences a blackout.

Steps and Products of Anaerobic Glycolysis: From Glucose to Energy and Beyond

In cellular reactions, anaerobic glycolysis operates like a seasoned street vendor, swiftly converting raw materials into valuable products. This rapid energy-producing process, though seemingly straightforward, is a masterclass in biochemical efficiency. Let's go through its steps and the products it yields.

The Breakdown of Glucose: The Starting Point

At the heart of anaerobic glycolysis is glucose, the simple sugar that acts as the primary fuel. Think of glucose as the raw gold that's about to be refined. It can be sourced directly from the bloodstream, where it's transported after we consume carbohydrate-rich foods. Alternatively, during times of heightened energy demand, our muscles can tap into their glycogen reserves, breaking down this stored form of glucose to fuel the process.

Once glucose has been earmarked for anaerobic glycolysis, it undergoes a series of enzymatic reactions. Each step is meticulously orchestrated, ensuring that energy is harnessed at every possible turn. As enzymes act on glucose, cleaving its bonds and rearranging its atoms, the molecule is transformed, releasing energy that the cell can harness.

ATP Production and the Emergence of Lactic Acid

The peak of anaerobic glycolysis is the production of ATP. In this high-stakes game of energy provision, the cell cannot afford to be lackadaisical. And so, anaerobic glycolysis delivers, generating ATP with a speed that few other processes can match. But, as with any rapid production line, there are byproducts.

Then, enters lactic acid. As glucose is diligently broken down, there's an accumulation of hydrogen ions. These ions, eager to bond, associate with pyruvate, a key intermediate in glycolysis, leading to the formation of lactic acid. For many, lactic acid is synonymous with the burning sensation felt during an intense workout, that fiery reminder of muscles pushed to their limit. But beyond this, lactic acid is more than just a byproduct; it's a testament to the cell's adaptability. In certain conditions, lactic acid can be shuttled to the liver, where it's converted back to glucose in a process known as the Cori cycle, showcasing the body's remarkable ability to recycle and repurpose.

In cellular metabolism, anaerobic glycolysis emerges as a swift and efficient craftsman, taking the raw material of glucose and skillfully converting it into the precious currency of ATP, all while going through the challenges of byproduct management.

Applications and Limitations of Anaerobic Glycolysis: The Sprinter's Strength and Shortcoming

In metabolic processes, anaerobic glycolysis stands as a sprinter, poised and ready to go at a moment's notice. Its role is both vital and specialized, catering to specific demands of the body. But like every sprinter who can't maintain their top speed for a marathon, anaerobic glycolysis, too, has its strengths and limitations.

The Ideal Responder to Explosive Demands

Imagine the final moments of a 100-meter dash. The crowd is roaring, the finish line is in sight, and every muscle fiber is firing in unison, propelling the athlete forward. In these critical seconds, the body doesn't have the time to rely on slower, more sustained energy systems. It needs power, and it needs it now. This is where anaerobic glycolysis shines.

Anaerobic glycolysis is the body's rapid response team. It's the system that kicks into overdrive when there's a sudden, explosive demand for energy. Whether it's that final push in a race, the high jump's apex, or the split-second decisions and reflexes in a fast-paced game, anaerobic glycolysis ensures that the muscles are well-supplied with the ATP they need to excel. It's the body's turbocharger that provides that extra boost when it matters most.

The Trade-offs of Speed

But, as with all things in biology, there's a trade-off. The very strength of anaerobic glycolysis – its speed is also the root of its limitation. Just as a sports car might guzzle fuel at high speeds, anaerobic glycolysis, too, has a voracious appetite for glucose, and its reserves are limited.

While it can produce ATP at an astonishing rate, it can't maintain this production indefinitely. The system's ATP yield is limited, and as it operates, there's an accumulation of byproducts, most notably lactic acid. This acid can be a double-edged sword while adapting the body's capabilities. As it accumulates, it can lead to a drop in the pH level within the muscle. This increased acidity can affect the muscle's ability to contract efficiently, leading to the familiar sensation of muscle burn and fatigue.

Furthermore, the rapid consumption of glucose can deplete local reserves, necessitating a switch to other energy systems or a period of recovery to replenish these stores.

A Balancing Act

In metabolic processes, anaerobic glycolysis is the exhilarating crescendo, a burst of energy and power. But like any crescendo, it's followed by a softer, more sustained melody. The body, in its infinite wisdom, balances the explosive power of anaerobic glycolysis with the sustained energy production of other systems, ensuring that we're equipped for both the sprints and marathons of life.

Aerobic Respiration: The Marathon Runner's Pathway

In the energy systems, where each pathway has its unique role, aerobic respiration stands out as the marathon runner, gracefully pacing itself mile after mile. While anaerobic glycolysis dashes ahead, fueled by the thrill of the sprint, aerobic respiration embodies endurance and persistence. It's not about the rush or the explosive burst; it's about the journey, the long stretches of road, and the steady breaths and heartbeats. This is the system our bodies lean on when the finish line is not a few seconds away but miles ahead. The aerobic cycle produces ATP at a 33-36:1 ratio (33 to 36 ATP for every 1 glucose). It ensures that even as the miles add up, our muscles receive a consistent, sustainable supply of energy, allowing us to go the distance.

As we delve deeper into aerobic respiration, we'll uncover the intricacies of this remarkable pathway, understanding how it fuels our most prolonged endeavors and why it's pivotal to our endurance and stamina.

Nature of Aerobic Respiration: The Cell's Powerhouses

Deep within the bustling cityscape of the cell, nestled among various structures and organelles, lies the mitochondria. Often hailed as the "powerhouses" of the cell, these organelles are not just energy producers; they are the grand stages where aerobic respiration unfolds.

The Mitochondrial Stage

The mitochondria, with their unique double-membraned structure, are architectural marvels. Their inner membrane is intricately folded into structures known as cristae.

These folds aren't merely aesthetic features; they are strategic designs that maximize the surface area, providing ample space for the many enzymes and molecules involved in aerobic metabolism. It's within these folds that the cell's most efficient energy-producing reactions occur.

Imagine, if you will, a grand theater. The stage is set, the actors are in place, and the performance is about to begin. In the above scenario, glucose, and fatty acids are the lead actors, and oxygen plays a pivotal supporting role. Together, under the meticulous direction of various enzymes, they perform a harmonious function, each meant to produce the most coveted molecule: ATP.

The Role of Oxygen: The Breath of Life

The term "aerobic" is derived from the Greek word 'aero' meaning 'air'. It's a fitting name, for this pathway is wholly reliant on oxygen. But why is oxygen so crucial? The answer lies in the chemistry of life. Oxygen acts as the final electron acceptor in the electron transport chain, a series of reactions that culminate in the production of ATP. Without oxygen, this chain would come to a halt, and the efficient extraction of energy from glucose and fatty acids would be compromised.

Aerobic respiration is a testament to the body's incredible efficiency. By utilizing oxygen, the body can extract a significant amount of energy from each glucose molecule, far surpassing what anaerobic pathways can achieve. It's a slow burn, a methodical process that ensures our muscles and organs receive a steady supply of energy during prolonged activities.

In energy production, aerobic respiration stands as a methodical maestro, orchestrating a complex series of reactions to harness the maximum energy possible. It's a reminder of the body's remarkable ability to adapt and optimize, ensuring we're equipped for both the sprints and the marathons of life.

Steps and Products of Aerobic Respiration: The Methodical Unraveling of Energy

In cellular processes, aerobic respiration stands as a magnum opus, a series of intricate steps that methodically extract energy from our primary fuels: glucose and fatty acids. This process is not a hasty affair; it's a deliberate, multi-stage process that maximizes the energy yield from each molecule. Let's delve into the stages of this remarkable pathway and the bounty it produces.

The Glycolysis

Every grand performance begins with an overture, setting the stage for what's to come. In aerobic respiration, this overture is glycolysis. Located in the cytoplasm, glycolysis is a series of reactions that break down glucose into pyruvate. This process, interestingly, is shared with anaerobic glycolysis. However, while anaerobic glycolysis might end with the formation of lactic acid, in the presence of oxygen, the story takes a different turn. The pyruvate molecules, rather than becoming lactic acid, are ushered into the mitochondria, the cell's energy-producing centers, setting the stage for the next act.

The Mitochondrial Marvel: Krebs Cycle and Electron Transport Chain

Within the mitochondria's confines, pyruvate transforms, entering the Krebs cycle (also known as the citric acid cycle). This cycle is a series of chemical reactions that further break down pyruvate, releasing energy and transferring it to molecules like NADH and FADH2. These molecules, laden with energy, then feed into the electron transport chain, reactions that pump out ATP with remarkable efficiency.

But glucose isn't the only star of this show. Fatty acids, the long chains of carbon and hydrogen that store vast amounts of energy, also play a pivotal role. These fatty acids undergo a process called beta-oxidation within the mitochondria. This process methodically cleaves the fatty acid chains, producing fragments that can feed directly into the Krebs cycle. What's the result? With an even greater yield of energy-rich molecules are ready to contribute to ATP production.

The ATP Production and the Creation of Water

Aerobic respiration's climax is nothing short of spectacular. For every glucose molecule that enters this pathway, up to 36 ATP molecules can be produced. This remarkable yield showcases the efficiency and prowess of aerobic respiration. But ATP isn't the only product. As glucose and fatty acids are fully oxidized, they produce carbon dioxide, which we exhale, and water. This water isn't just a byproduct; it's a testament to the body's incredible chemistry, turning oxygen and the remnants of glucose and fatty acids into a molecule essential for life.

In the narrative of energy production, aerobic respiration emerges as a master storyteller, weaving together complex reactions to harness energy from our primary fuels. It's a testament to the body's adaptability and efficiency, ensuring we have the energy we need for life's many marathons.

Beta-Oxidation and Fat Metabolism: The Slow Burn of Endurance

During energy production, while carbohydrates often take center stage, fats play an equally pivotal role, especially during prolonged activities. Fats, with their dense energy stores, are like the slow-burning logs in a fireplace, providing sustained energy long after the quick-burning kindling (glucose) has been consumed. Central to the metabolism of fats is a process known as beta-oxidation. The beta-oxidation cycle produces ATP at a 100+:1 ratio (at least 100 ATP for every 1 free fatty acid). Let's delve deep into this pathway and understand how it contributes to our energy landscape.

The Intricacies of the Beta-Oxidation Cycle

Beta-oxidation is a methodical process, a series of enzymatic reactions that methodically cleave fatty acids, producing fragments that can feed directly into the Krebs cycle. But where does this process occur? Its occurrence is within the mitochondria, the cell's energy-producing centers. Here, long chains of fatty acids are broken down, step by step, two carbons at a time. These two-carbon fragments, known as acetyl-CoA, are then ready to enter the Krebs cycle, further contributing to ATP production.

Imagine a long rope being gradually unraveled, strand by strand. Each segment of the rope can be thought of as a segment of the fatty acid chain, and as each segment is separated, it's repurposed, and transformed into energy. This is the essence of beta-oxidation: the systematic breakdown of fatty acids, converting them into usable energy.

Fatty Acids: The Heroes of ATP Production

While glucose is often hailed as the primary fuel for our cells, fatty acids are equally crucial, especially during prolonged activities. Why? This is because they store more than twice the energy of carbohydrates. When our immediate glucose stores are depleted, and the body needs to maintain a steady supply of energy, it turns to its fat reserves.

As fatty acids undergo beta-oxidation and feed into the Krebs cycle, they produce a significant amount of NADH and FADH2, molecules that play a pivotal role in the electron transport chain. The result? A bounty of ATP. In fact, the complete oxidation of a single fatty acid can produce many more ATP molecules than a glucose molecule, showcasing the efficiency and importance of fat metabolism.

In energy production, while carbohydrates might be the sprinters, fats are the marathon runners. They ensure that even during the most extended endeavors, our muscles have a steady, reliable source of energy. Beta-oxidation stands as a testament to the body's incredible ability to harness energy from various sources, ensuring we're equipped for both the sprints and the marathons of life.

Applications and Limitations of Aerobic Respiration: The Long-Distance Runner's Trusty Companion

In energy systems, each pathway has its unique strengths, geared toward specific demands and scenarios. Aerobic respiration, with its methodical and sustained energy production, is perfectly suited for the long haul. But like every system, it has its nuances, its strengths, and its limitations.

The Trusty Steed for Endurance

Imagine a long-distance runner, each step measured, each breath synchronized. Or picture a cyclist, steadily pedaling through winding roads, the landscape changing, but the pace remaining consistent. These scenarios epitomize where aerobic respiration shines brightest. It's the energy system that powers prolonged activities, whether it's a marathon, an extended cycling session, or even a leisurely, yet brisk, walk through nature's trails.

Aerobic respiration ensures that our muscles never run out of ATP during these endeavors. It provides a consistent, steady stream of energy, allowing us to maintain our pace, keep pushing, to go the distance without faltering. It's the trusty steed that endurance athletes, and indeed all of us, rely on when the journey is long and the path requires persistence.

The Oxygen Lifeline

However, even the most reliable systems have their constraints. The essence of aerobic respiration, its very lifeblood, is oxygen. Every step of the process, from the Krebs cycle to the electron transport chain, hinges on the presence of oxygen. It's what allows for the complete breakdown of glucose and fatty acids, maximizing ATP production.

But what happens when the demand for oxygen suddenly spikes, outpacing its supply? Imagine that long-distance runner again, this time deciding to sprint midway through the race. The body's oxygen needs to surge, and for a brief moment, aerobic respiration can't keep up. In these scenarios, the body, in its infinite wisdom, reverts to its rapid responder: anaerobic glycolysis. It's a temporary shift, a backup plan, ensuring that the muscles don't run out of energy even when oxygen is momentarily in short supply.

This interplay, this dance between aerobic and anaerobic systems, is a testament to the body's adaptability. It showcases how our energy systems aren't isolated pathways but interconnected networks, each stepping in when needed, each filling a specific niche.

In metabolic pathways, aerobic respiration stands as a testament to endurance and adaptability. It's a reminder that our bodies are marvels of engineering, capable of sustaining prolonged efforts and adapting to ever-changing demands.

Conclusion: The Harmony of Energy Systems

The human body, in all its complexity, is a marvel of nature. As we've journeyed through this chapter, we've delved deep into the intricate energy systems that power our every move, every thought, and every heartbeat. From the immediate burst of energy provided by anaerobic glycolysis to the sustained, enduring power of aerobic respiration, our bodies have evolved a sophisticated array of mechanisms to ensure we always have the energy we need, precisely when we need it.

Energy system	Oxygen necessary?	Overall chemical reaction	Relative rate of ATP formed per second	ATP formed per molecule of substrate	Available capacity
ATP-PCr	No	PCr to Cr	10	1	<15 s
Glycolysis (anaerobic glycolysis)	No	Glucose or glycogen	5	2-3	~1 min
Oxidative from Carbohydrates (aerobic glycolysis)	Yes	Glucose or glycogen to CO_2 and H_2O	2.5	36-39	~90 min
Oxidative from fats (beta oxidation)	Yes	FFA or triglycerides to CO_2 and H_2O	1.5	>100	Days

Recap of Our Journey

We began our exploration with ATP, the cellular powerhouse. This molecule, with its adenosine base and three phosphate groups, is the embodiment of cellular energy. It's the bridge between the microscopic cellular reactions and the tangible experiences of our daily activities, from lifting a weight to sprinting to catch a bus.

Our journey then took us to the world of anaerobic glycolysis, the sprinter of energy systems. Located within the bustling metropolis of the cell's cytoplasm, this system operates independently of oxygen, providing rapid energy during short, high-intensity activities. However, its swift response comes with limitations, including a limited ATP yield and the potential for muscle fatigue due to lactic acid accumulation.

From the sprints, we moved to the marathons with aerobic respiration. This system, operating within the mitochondria, is the marathon runner of energy systems. It relies on oxygen to extract energy from glucose and fatty acids, producing a bounty of ATP. We again delved into the intricacies of glucose oxidation and the role of beta-oxidation in fat metabolism, appreciating the adaptability of this system in using various fuels based on activity duration and intensity.

The Intersection of Knowledge, Training, and Nutrition

In fitness and health, knowledge is the foundation upon which we build our strategies, routines, and habits. As we've journeyed through the intricate pathways of energy systems, a recurring theme emerges: the profound impact of ensuring that our training and nutrition align with these systems.

Training with Purpose

Every athlete, whether amateur or professional, has specific goals. Some aim for explosive power, others for sustained endurance, and many seek a balance between the two. Understanding the energy systems at play allows us to train with purpose and precision.

For those targeting short, explosive activities, emphasizing workouts that challenge the anaerobic glycolysis system can lead to significant gains. High-intensity interval training (HIIT), plyometrics, and heavy weightlifting sets are prime examples. By pushing the limits of this system, we not only enhance its efficiency but also improve our body's ability to manage and buffer the lactic acid produced, delaying the onset of fatigue.

Conversely, endurance athletes, such as marathon runners or long-distance cyclists, benefit immensely from training regimens that predominantly tap into the aerobic respiration system. Long, steady-state cardio sessions, tempo runs, and even certain resistance training circuits can enhance the efficiency of this system, improving oxygen delivery and utilization, and increasing the body's ability to tap into fat reserves for energy.

Nutrition: Fueling the Machine

But training is just one piece of the puzzle. Nutrition plays an equally, if not more, critical role. By understanding which energy system is predominantly at play during various activities, we can channel our nutrition to support and optimize that system.

For activities relying heavily on anaerobic glycolysis, ensuring adequate carbohydrate intake becomes paramount. Carbohydrates replenish muscle glycogen stores, providing the necessary fuel for short, intense bursts of activity. Post-workout recovery meals rich in carbohydrates can accelerate glycogen replenishment, ensuring the muscles are primed and ready for the next session.

On the other hand, endurance activities that lean on aerobic respiration benefit from a balanced intake of carbohydrates and fats. While carbohydrates provide a quick source of energy, fats, especially during prolonged activities, become a vital energy reserve. Ensuring a diet rich in healthy fats can optimize the body's ability to tap into these reserves when needed.

The Power of Informed Choices

The knowledge of our body's energy systems isn't just academic; it's profoundly practical. It empowers us to make informed choices, both in our training and our nutrition. By aligning our strategies with the underlying physiology, we not only optimize performance but also ensure that our bodies are nourished, supported, and primed for every challenge ahead.

CHAPTER 3

NUTRITIONAL FOUNDATIONS FOR MUSCLE GROWTH

Every bite of food, every sip of a drink, is not merely an act of satiating hunger or quenching a momentary thirst. It's a directive, toward the effective growth of our muscles and tissues. This special bite is made up of amino acids, sugars, fatty acids, vitamins, and minerals. Interestingly, our muscles understand, respond to, and thrive upon these supplies for optimal performance.

The Central Role of Nutrition in the Muscle Saga

Muscles, in their ceaseless contraction and relaxation, are more than just the machinery of movement. They are dynamic entities, constantly evolving, growing, repairing, and adapting. Nutrition is the maestro that conducts this activity. It provides the basis for muscle growth, the time for repair, and the ground for optimal function.

Imagine a construction site, bustling with activity. The raw materials – bricks, cement, and steel are analogous to the nutrients we consume. Without these materials, the magnificent structure – in this case, our muscular system cannot take shape. Nutrition, thus, is not just about calories; it's about providing muscles with the right quality and quantity of materials they need to function, grow, and excel.

Macronutrients: The Triumvirate of Muscle Nutrition

In nutrition, while every nutrient has its significance, it's the macronutrients such as proteins, carbohydrates, and fats that stand as the pillars supporting the muscle health.

> **Proteins:** Often termed the building blocks of the body, proteins are indispensable for muscle health. They are the raw materials that repair the wear and tear muscles undergo during physical activity. They provide the amino acids that are the precursors for muscle growth.

- **Carbohydrates:** These are the primary energy providers, the fuel that muscles burn to perform every action, from the most mundane to the most strenuous.

- **Fats:** Often misunderstood and maligned, fats play several crucial roles in muscle health. They provide energy, especially during prolonged activities, support cellular function, and are vital for the production of certain hormones that influence muscle growth.

The Symbiotic Relationship Between Nutrition and Muscles

Muscles: More Than Just Powerhouses

When we think of muscles, we often visualize bulging biceps or chiseled abs, symbolizing strength and athleticism. However, muscles are more than just powerhouses of movement. They are living, dynamic tissues, constantly adapting and evolving in response to the stresses we place upon them. Whether it's the strain of lifting a heavy weight, the endurance required for a long run, or the flexibility needed for a yoga pose, our muscles respond, adapt, and grow.

The Role of Nutrition: Fueling and Building

Nutrition helps in muscle growth and development. Every morsel of food we consume, every sip of a protein shake, or bite of a lean steak, is broken down into its constituent nutrients. These nutrients, once absorbed, embark on a journey through our bloodstream, eventually reaching the very heart of our muscles.

Proteins provide the building blocks, aiding in the repair of muscle fibers that have been subjected to the wear and tear of exercise. Carbohydrates offer the fuel, replenishing glycogen stores and ensuring that muscles have the energy they need for their next activity. Fats, often overlooked, play a crucial role in hormone production and cellular function, both of which are vital for muscle health.

Diet: The Architect of Muscle Development

But it's not just about the macronutrients. Vitamins and minerals, those micronutrients that often take a backseat in dietary discussions, are equally crucial. They serve as co-factors in countless metabolic reactions, ensuring that the processes of muscle repair, growth, and function proceed smoothly.

In essence, our diet acts as the architect of our muscular development. It lays the foundation, provides the building blocks, and ensures that the construction process, the growth, and repair of muscle tissue, proceed without a hitch.

Muscles and nutrition engage in a delicate dance, each influencing and being influenced by the other. As we challenge our muscles through physical activity, our nutritional needs evolve. Conversely, the quality and quantity of our nutrition directly impact our muscle health, growth, and function. Recognizing and respecting this symbiotic relationship is key to achieving optimal muscle development and overall physical well-being.

Distinct Roles of Macronutrients in Energy, Muscle Repair, and Physiological Processes

Proteins: Often known as the building blocks of the body, proteins are central to muscle health. Comprising chains of amino acids, proteins are essential for repairing muscle tissue damaged during exercise. They support the synthesis of new muscle fibers, aiding in muscle growth and strength gains. Beyond muscles, proteins play a role in nearly every physiological process, from enzyme function to hormone production.

Carbohydrates: Carbohydrates are the primary fuel source for many of our body's activities; they are crucial for energy generation. Once ingested, they are broken down into simpler sugars like glucose, which is then either used immediately for energy or stored in the muscles and liver as glycogen. During intense physical activity, these glycogen stores become the primary energy reservoir, underscoring the importance of adequate carbohydrate intake for athletes and active individuals. Moreover, carbohydrates play a protective role, preventing the body from using proteins as a primary energy source, thereby ensuring proteins can focus on their primary role in repair and growth.

Fats: While often misunderstood, fats are indispensable for optimal health. They serve as a dense source of energy, especially vital during prolonged, low-intensity activities where carbohydrate reserves might run low. Fats also play a pivotal role in the absorption of certain vitamins, the production of vital hormones, and the insulation and protection of organs. Essential fatty acids, a subset of fats, are crucial for brain health, inflammation regulation, and overall cellular function.

In human health and performance, understanding the roles of these macronutrients is paramount. They are the threads that weave the fabric of our physiological well-being, each playing its part, each indispensable. As we delve deeper into nutrition and muscle function, we'll uncover the nuances of these macronutrients, exploring how to optimize their intake for muscle growth, athletic performance, and overall health.

Proteins: The Building Blocks of Muscular Might

Role as the Building Blocks of Muscles

Muscles, in all their dynamic glory, are more than just tissues that enable movement. They are intricate tapestries woven from countless protein threads. Each muscle fiber, sinew, and tendon in our body is a testament to the architectural marvel that proteins represent.

Imagine for a moment the vast complexity of a single muscle fiber. Within it, there's a labyrinthine network of proteins, each with a specific role, each contributing to the muscle's overall function. These proteins aren't just passive structures; they're dynamic, constantly interacting, changing, and adapting based on the demands placed upon them.

The strength we feel when lifting a heavy object, the elasticity that allows our muscles to stretch and then return to their original shape, the endurance that lets us run mile after mile - all these attributes are conferred by proteins. Myosin, actin, troponin, and tropomyosin are just a few of the key players in this activity, working in harmony to facilitate muscle contraction and relaxation.

But proteins don't just give muscles their physical attributes. They are the translators, the intermediaries that convert neural impulses into tangible action. When our brain sends a command to lift an arm, it's the proteins in our biceps and triceps that heed the call, contracting and relaxing to produce movement.

Furthermore, the scaffolding role of proteins cannot be understated. Beyond their functional roles in contraction, proteins provide the structural integrity to muscles. They are the framework, the beams, and the pillars that hold our muscles together, ensuring they remain robust and resilient against daily wear and tear.

In essence, to understand muscles is to appreciate the multifaceted roles of proteins. Protein works to ensure that every leap, sprint, and lift is executed with precision. As we examine muscle physiology, the central theme that emerges is the importance of proteins in shaping our muscular narrative.

Importance in Muscle Repair, Growth, and Maintenance: The Regenerative Power of Proteins

The human body is a marvel of adaptability and resilience, and our muscles are a prime example of this. Every time we engage in physical activity, especially the strenuous exertion of resistance training or high-intensity workouts, we're not just building strength or endurance. We're also causing minute disruptions in the muscle fibers, creating microscopic tears that might seem detrimental at first glance. However, these tiny injuries are the precursors to muscle growth, and proteins are the diligent workers behind this transformative process.

Imagine the muscle fiber as a wall made of bricks. With every heavy lift or intense sprint, some of these bricks crack or dislodge. Now, if left unattended, these cracks could weaken the wall. But our body has an efficient repair crew in the form of proteins. They rush to the site of damage, patching up the cracks, and often adding more bricks than were originally present. This addition is what we recognize as muscle growth or hypertrophy. The muscle becomes denser, stronger, and more capable of handling future stresses. It's a beautiful cycle of breakdown, repair, and enhancement, all made possible by proteins.

But the role of proteins doesn't stop at repairing exercise-induced damage. Even as we go about our daily routines, with no deliberate physical stress imposed on our muscles, they remain in a state of flux. Muscles aren't static entities; they're dynamic tissues, always in a state of turnover. Think of it as a constant renovation project. Old, worn-out proteins (bricks that have weathered many storms) are methodically replaced with new ones. This turnover is crucial. It ensures that our muscles don't become complacent. They remain ever-vigilant, ready to respond to any demand, any challenge that life throws at them.

In essence, proteins are the guardians of muscle integrity. They ensure that our muscles not only recover from the stresses of exercise but also evolve, becoming better with each passing challenge. Moreover, they maintain the day-to-day health and functionality of our muscles, ensuring longevity and peak performance throughout our lives.

Composition and Significance of Amino Acids: The Fundamental Units of Proteins

At the heart of every protein, from the tiniest enzyme to the most complex structural component of our muscles, lies amino acids. These compounds often likened to beads on a string or links in a chain, are the foundational units from which proteins are constructed. Their significance in biology and human physiology cannot be overstated.

Imagine a vast library, each book is unique with its own story and message. Now, consider that every book in this library is written using just 20 letters. This is the marvel of proteins and amino acids. From just 20 amino acids, our bodies can craft an astonishing array of proteins, each with a distinct role and function.

Each amino acid, with its specific chemical structure and properties, contributes uniquely to the protein's final shape and function. It's like a jigsaw puzzle where each piece, though different, fits perfectly to create a coherent picture. Among these 20 amino acids, nine hold a special status – they are 'essential'. Our bodies, for all their complexity, cannot synthesize these nine amino acids. This means that our diet must supply them. They are indispensable, and any deficiency can disrupt the delicate balance of protein synthesis.

The sequence of amino acids in a protein is not random. It's a meticulously coded message, a blueprint that determines the protein's shape, properties, and function. Just as changing the order of words in a sentence can alter its meaning, even a slight change in the sequence of amino acids can profoundly affect a protein's function. Some sequences give rise to the proteins that allow our muscles to contract and relax. Others form the enzymes that catalyze countless chemical reactions in our bodies, the antibodies that defend us against invaders, or the hormones that regulate myriad physiological processes.

This incredible versatility of proteins, all stemming from the diverse combinations of amino acids, highlights the importance of nutrition. A diet that provides a rich array of amino acids ensures that our bodies have the necessary tools to construct the proteins we need. Whether it's for muscle growth, immune defense, or metabolic regulation, these amino acids are the raw materials from which our body crafts its molecular machinery.

Therefore, amino acids are more than just building blocks. They are the keystones of life's processes, the fundamental units from which life is composed.

Effects of Resistance Training on Protein Synthesis

The beauty of the human body is the ability to adapt to changes. When subjected to challenges, it responds, adjusts, and strengthens. One of the most potent stimuli that triggers such a response is resistance training. This form of exercise, encompassing activities like weightlifting, bodyweight exercises, and resistance band workouts, has profound implications for protein synthesis and breakdown within our muscles.

Imagine the muscle as a dynamic construction site. Under normal conditions, there's a balance between the building (protein synthesis) and the tearing down (protein breakdown). However, when resistance training is introduced into the mix, this construction site becomes a hive of accelerated activity.

During an intense workout, as weights are lifted and muscles contract against resistance, the muscle fibers experience microscopic damage. This isn't a cause for alarm; it's a natural outcome of pushing the muscles beyond their usual limits. This damage, these tiny tears in the muscle fibers, set off myriads of events. The immediate aftermath of the workout sees an uptick in protein breakdown. The body is responding to the stress, breaking down older proteins, and making way for new construction.

But the real magic happens in the recovery phase. In the hours, days, and even weeks post-workout, there's a significant surge in protein synthesis. The body, recognizing the inflicted damage, goes into overdrive to repair, rebuild, and reinforce. This heightened state of protein synthesis, when it outpaces protein breakdown, is the foundation of muscle growth. Over time, consistent training and adequate recovery lead to visible muscle growth and increased strength.

But there's another layer to this anabolic response. Resistance training doesn't just stimulate the muscles; it also primes them to respond more effectively to dietary protein. After a workout, the muscles are like sponges, eager and ready to soak up nutrients. This period often termed the 'anabolic window', represents a time when the muscle's sensitivity to amino acids is at its peak. Consuming protein-rich foods or supplements during this window ensures rapid delivery of amino acids to the recovering muscles, further enhancing the protein synthesis machinery.

In essence, resistance training and protein synthesis share a symbiotic relationship. The physical stress of lifting weights provides the trigger, setting off a chain reaction of muscle repair and growth. In response, the body's protein synthesis machinery kicks into high gear, using dietary amino acids as the raw materials to construct stronger, more resilient muscle fibers.

Recommended Protein Intake

The Intricacies of Protein in Nutrition

Within the vast spectrum of nutrients that our bodies require, protein holds a unique and indispensable position. It's not just another item on the nutritional checklist; it's the very foundation of our muscular system, the fuel for repair, and the catalyst for growth. As we delve deeper into the world of nutrition, we find that protein isn't a one-size-fits-all kind of nutrient. Its requirements are as varied as the activities we engage in and the goals we set for ourselves.

The Dynamic Role of Protein in Physical Activity

Every time we engage in physical activity, from the simplest stretch to the most grueling marathon, we're essentially putting our muscles to work. These muscles, composed primarily of protein, undergo wear and tear, especially during intense workouts. This wear and tear, while a natural part of the muscle-building process, necessitates repair. And the primary agent for this repair is protein.

Imagine a brick wall representing a muscle. Over time, with stress and strain, some bricks might get cracked or chipped. Protein acts like the mason who diligently replaces or repairs these bricks, ensuring the wall remains strong and intact. But the mason needs a steady supply of bricks to do his job. And in our analogy, these bricks are the protein we consume.

The Spectrum of Physical Activities and Protein Needs

Different physical activities exert varying levels of stress on our muscles. A casual walk in the park, while beneficial for overall health, doesn't strain the muscles as much as a heavy weightlifting session or a high-intensity interval training (HIIT) workout. Consequently, the protein requirements for these activities differ.

- **Weightlifting and Strength Training:** These activities focus on muscle growth, which is the process of increasing the size of muscle cells. The micro-tears caused by lifting heavy weights signal the body to repair and build the muscles back stronger. This rebuilding process is protein-intensive, often requiring higher protein intake to support optimal muscle growth.

- **Endurance Sports:** Marathon runners, cyclists, and swimmers, while not focusing on muscle size, still place significant demands on their muscles. The prolonged nature of these activities means that muscles are in use for extended periods, leading to wear and tear. Adequate protein intake ensures that these endurance athletes recover efficiently and maintain muscle health.

- **High-Intensity Interval Training (HIIT):** This form of exercise, characterized by short bursts of intense activity followed by rest periods, places acute stress on muscles in a short time frame. The rapid on-off nature of HIIT means that muscles need to recover quickly, and a robust protein intake can support this rapid recovery.

Individualizing Protein Intake

While general guidelines provide a starting point, it's crucial to recognize that individual needs can vary. Factors like age, metabolic rate, gender, and specific fitness goals play a role in determining optimal protein intake. For instance, a young male bodybuilder might have different protein requirements than a middle-aged woman training for her first marathon.

Moreover, it's not just about quantity but also quality. The source of protein, its amino acid profile, and its bioavailability can influence its effectiveness in supporting muscle health.

In conclusion, as we go through fitness and nutrition, understanding protein intake becomes essential. We can ensure that our muscles have the support they need to function, recover, and thrive by channeling our protein consumption to our specific needs and activities.

The Baseline: Sedentary Individuals

Understanding Sedentary Lifestyles

In today's modern world, many find themselves leading sedentary lifestyles. Whether it's due to desk-bound jobs, technological conveniences, or other factors, prolonged periods of inactivity have become commonplace. But even in the absence of strenuous physical activity, our bodies continue to function, grow, repair, and maintain themselves. Interestingly, the heart of these processes lies in protein.

Why Protein is Still Essential

While it might be tempting to think that sedentary individuals require minimal protein, this isn't the case. Every day, our bodies undergo many processes that rely on protein. Skin cells are regenerated, hair grows, enzymes facilitate countless biochemical reactions, and even our immune system, which relies on protein-based antibodies, remains on constant alert. All these processes, though they might not be as evident as muscle contractions during a workout, necessitate a steady supply of protein.

Determining the Baseline

For those not engaging in regular physical activity, the baseline protein requirement is set at approximately 0.8 grams per kilogram of body weight. This recommendation is derived from extensive research and is designed to meet the protein needs of about 97-98% of healthy sedentary adults. It ensures that the body has enough protein to support essential physiological functions without the added demands of exercise-induced muscle repair and growth.

For instance, consider a sedentary individual weighing 70 kilograms (about 154 pounds). Their daily protein requirement would be around 56 grams. This amount can be easily met through a balanced diet that includes sources like dairy, lean meats, legumes, and grains.

The Risks of Inadequate Protein Intake

Even for sedentary individuals, consistently consuming protein below the recommended levels can have consequences. Protein deficiencies might manifest as muscle wasting, weakened immunity, hair loss, and even hormonal imbalances. It's a testament to the fact that, regardless of our activity levels, protein remains a cornerstone of health.

While sedentary lifestyles might not place overt demands on our muscles in the way that regular exercise does, the importance of protein remains non-negotiable. It's the silent workhorse, facilitating countless processes that keep us alive, functional, and healthy. Recognizing and meeting the protein needs of sedentary individuals is crucial in ensuring overall well-being and preventing potential health issues.

Elevated Needs: The Active and the Athletic

The Dynamic World of the Physically Active

In human activity, there exists a group whose daily routines push the boundaries of physical exertion. These are the athletes, the fitness enthusiasts, the marathoners, and even the weekend warriors. Their commitment to physical excellence doesn't just shape their bodies; it reshapes their nutritional needs, especially when it comes to protein.

Why More Activity Demands More Protein

Muscles are not static entities. They adapt, grow, and change in response to the stresses placed upon them. Every squat, every sprint, and every lifted weight imposes a demand on muscle fibers, causing tiny micro tears. While this might sound alarming, it's a natural and essential part of muscle development. These micro tears signal the body to rush in with resources for repair. And the primary resource it uses is protein.

The process of repairing and rebuilding muscle tissue is protein-intensive. The body needs to break down dietary protein into its constituent amino acids, which are then used to repair damaged muscle fibers and build new ones. This cycle of damage, repair, and growth is what leads to muscle strengthening and growth over time.

Channeling Protein Intake to Activity Levels

For those who've made physical activity a cornerstone of their lives, generic protein recommendations won't suffice. Their elevated exertion levels necessitate an elevated protein intake. Research suggests that individuals engaged in regular intense physical activity may require protein intakes ranging from 1.2 to 2.0 grams per kilogram of body weight.

The specific amount within this range depends on several factors:

1. **Nature of Activity:** A long-distance runner might have different protein needs compared to a weightlifter. While both activities are demanding, they stress the muscles in different ways and thus have varied protein requirements for optimal recovery and performance.

2. **Intensity and Duration:** An individual engaging in high-intensity interval training (HIIT) for short durations might have different protein needs than someone doing moderate-intensity steady-state cardio for longer periods.

3. **Goals:** Someone aiming for muscle growth would likely benefit from protein intake on the higher end of the recommended range. In contrast, an individual focusing on endurance might find their needs adequately met with a slightly lower intake.

Practical Implications

Consider a 75-kilogram individual who's a dedicated bodybuilder. Aiming for muscle size and strength, they might target a protein intake of around 150 grams per day (2 grams per kilogram). Conversely, a person of the same weight who enjoys daily jogs might aim for closer to 90 grams of protein daily.

Physical activity, in its many forms, imposes unique demands on the body. Meeting these demands, especially when it comes to protein intake, is crucial for optimal performance, recovery, and health. By understanding and channeling protein intake to individual needs and goals, active individuals can ensure they're fueling their bodies for success.

Fine-Tuning Your Intake

The Individuality of Protein Needs

Dive into any nutrition guide, and you'll be met with a barrage of numbers, percentages, and recommended daily intakes. While these figures provide a valuable starting point, they are, at best, general guidelines. When it comes to protein intake, especially for the active individual, a one-size-fits-all approach simply doesn't work.

Every person is a unique blend of genetics, lifestyle, and goals. Factors such as age can influence protein metabolism, with older adults potentially requiring more protein to combat age-related muscle loss. Gender differences, too, can play a role, with variations in muscle mass and hormonal profiles influencing protein needs. Then there's the metabolic rate, which can vary widely among individuals, affecting how efficiently the body utilizes dietary protein.

Quality Over Quantity

While the quantity of protein is undeniably important, the quality of protein sources consumed can't be overlooked. Not all proteins are created equal. Different foods contain different profiles of amino acids, with some being richer in certain essential amino acids than others.

For instance, animal-based proteins like meat, poultry, and dairy are considered 'complete' proteins because they provide all nine essential amino acids in adequate amounts. Plant-based proteins, on the other hand, might be deficient in one or more essential amino acids. However, by consuming a diverse range of plant-based protein sources, such as combining beans with rice, one can ensure a comprehensive amino acid profile.

Adjusting to Your Goals

Your training goals can also dictate your protein needs. Are you aiming for muscle growth? Or is endurance your primary focus? Perhaps you're training for flexibility and balance. Each goal places distinct demands on the muscles and, by extension, on protein requirements. Someone aiming for muscle size might prioritize protein-rich post-workout meals to maximize muscle protein synthesis, while an endurance athlete might focus on a balanced intake of protein, carbs, and fats for sustained energy.

The Art and Science of Protein Intake

Understanding protein needs is both an art and a science. The science provides the baseline, and the general guidelines to start from. The art comes in fine-tuning these recommendations, adjusting based on personal experiences, recovery rates, and specific goals.

In the end, protein stands as a pillar of nutrition, especially for the active individual. It's not just about hitting a number but about understanding the nuances, and the interplay of factors that dictate individual needs. By embracing both the art and science of protein intake, one can pave the way for optimal muscle health, recovery, and athletic prowess.

Carbohydrates

The Essence of Carbohydrates in Human Physiology

Carbohydrates, often simply referred to as 'carbs', hold a special place in nutrition, especially when it comes to physical activity. While proteins are celebrated for their role in muscle repair and fats for their long-term energy storage, carbohydrates stand out as the immediate go-to source of energy, especially during exercise.

The Immediate Energy Reservoir

Imagine the body as a complex machine. Just as a car needs gasoline to run, our bodies require fuel to function, and carbohydrates serve as this primary fuel. When we consume foods rich in carbohydrates, such as grains, fruits, and vegetables, our digestive system breaks them down into simpler sugars, primarily glucose. This glucose then enters the bloodstream, ready to be delivered to cells throughout the body.

Muscle cells, in particular, are voracious consumers of glucose, especially during exercise. As we engage in physical activity, the demand for immediate energy increases. Carbohydrates, stored in the muscles and liver as glycogen, are quickly mobilized. Through a process called glycolysis, glycogen is broken down, releasing glucose which is then used to produce ATP, the molecule that powers muscle contractions.

Intensity Matters: The Shift in Carbohydrate Utilization

The role of carbohydrates becomes even more pronounced during high-intensity activities. Think of sprinting, high-intensity interval training, or heavy weight lifting. In these scenarios, the body doesn't have the luxury of time to tap into fat stores for energy. Instead, it relies heavily on the rapid breakdown of carbohydrates to meet the immediate energy demands.

However, it's worth noting that as exercise intensity decreases and duration increases, the body begins to utilize a mix of carbohydrates and fats. For instance, during a marathon, while carbohydrates are essential, especially in the latter stages of the race, fats also contribute significantly to energy production.

The Indispensable Role of Carbohydrates

Carbohydrates are not just another component of our diet; they are the primary energy currency for our muscles during exercise. Ensuring adequate carbohydrate intake, especially before and after workouts, can optimize performance, delay the onset of fatigue, and support recovery. In exercise and sports, carbohydrates truly reign supreme as the premier fuel source.

Replenishing Muscle Glycogen: The Key to Recovery and Performance

Understanding Muscle Glycogen

To appreciate the significance of replenishing muscle glycogen, one must first grasp the concept of glycogen itself. Glycogen is the primary storage form of glucose in our bodies. Think of it as a densely packed cluster of glucose molecules, stored primarily in our muscles and liver. While the liver's glycogen serves as a reserve to maintain blood sugar levels, muscle glycogen directly fuels muscular activity.

The Depletion Dilemma

During exercise, especially prolonged or high-intensity activities, our muscles tap into these glycogen reserves. As the exercise progresses, these stores gradually deplete. It's this depletion that often leads to the familiar sensations of fatigue, reduced energy output, and even the 'hitting the wall' phenomenon experienced by endurance athletes.

The more intense and prolonged the activity, the greater the depletion. For instance, a marathon runner or a cyclist participating in a long race might exhaust a significant portion, if not all, of their muscle glycogen stores.

Replenishing: Not Just Recovery, But Preparation

After exercise, one of the body's primary objectives is to restore these depleted glycogen stores. Consuming carbohydrates after a workout triggers a surge in insulin, a hormone that facilitates the uptake of glucose into muscle cells and its conversion into glycogen.

But why is this replenishment so crucial? Firstly, it's about recovery. Restoring glycogen ensures that muscles are 'refueled' and ready for the next activity. It aids in reducing muscle soreness and accelerates the overall recovery process.

Secondly, it's about preparation. For athletes or individuals who train frequently, perhaps multiple times a day or over consecutive days, replenishing glycogen is essential. Without adequate restoration, performance in subsequent workouts or competitions can be severely compromised.

The Timing and Type Matter

While consuming carbohydrates post-exercise is beneficial, the timing can optimize the replenishment rate. The initial hours post-exercise, often termed the 'glycogen window' witness an enhanced rate of glycogen synthesis. Consuming carbohydrates, especially high-glycemic ones that lead to a rapid rise in blood sugar, during this window can significantly accelerate the replenishment process.

The Symbiotic Relationship of Exercise and Carbohydrates

The relationship between exercise and carbohydrates is symbiotic. While physical activity utilizes carbohydrate stores, the post-exercise nutritional strategy, centered on carbohydrate consumption, ensures the restoration of these vital energy reserves. In exercise physiology, the importance of replenishing muscle glycogen stands out as a testament to the intricate balance of exertion and recovery.

Recommended Carbohydrate Intake

Carbohydrates, often the center of many dietary debates, remain an indispensable source of energy for the human body. They fuel our brains, support our workouts, and provide the energy we need for our daily activities. However, the question that often arises is: How much should one consume? The answer, as with many aspects of nutrition, is not one-size-fits-all. It varies based on individual goals, activity levels, and metabolic health.

Understanding Carbohydrate Needs

Basic Energy Requirements: The Foundation of Carbohydrate Intake

Carbohydrates, often viewed through energy provision, play a multifaceted role in our physiology. Beyond merely fueling our workouts or daily activities, they are integral to the very fabric of our bodily functions. Let's delve deeper into the foundational carbohydrate needs of the human body.

The Brain: A Glucose-Hungry Organ

The human brain, a marvel of nature, is incredibly energy-intensive. Despite accounting for only about 2% of an adult's body weight, the brain consumes approximately 20% of the body's energy. Glucose, derived primarily from carbohydrates, is its preferred fuel source. In situations where glucose is scarce, the brain can adapt to use ketones, but glucose remains its primary and preferred energy source.

Cellular Processes and Maintenance

Every cell in our body, from the ones that make up our skin to those in our internal organs, requires energy to function. This energy, in the form of ATP, is often derived from glucose. Cellular processes, such as protein synthesis, DNA replication, and cellular repair, all hinge on the energy provided by carbohydrates.

Blood Glucose Levels

Maintaining blood glucose levels within a narrow range is crucial for our health and well-being. Blood glucose serves as a readily available energy source, ensuring that organs, especially those that can't store energy like the brain, always have access to energy. When we consume carbohydrates, they are broken down into glucose, which then enters the bloodstream. Insulin, a hormone produced by the pancreas, facilitates the uptake of this glucose into cells, ensuring that blood glucose levels remain stable.

The Baseline Requirement

Given the myriad roles carbohydrates play, it's no surprise that even in the absence of physical activity, our bodies require a significant amount of them. Dietary guidelines suggest a baseline requirement of around 130 grams of carbohydrates per day for adults. This figure is derived from the minimum amount of glucose used by the brain and other organs in a day. It's worth noting that while this is a general recommendation, individual needs can vary based on factors like metabolic health, age, and specific physiological conditions.

In Conclusion

The 130 grams per day recommendation serves as a foundational guideline, ensuring that our most basic physiological processes are supported. However, as we'll explore further, physical activity, health goals, and individual variations can influence our optimal carbohydrate intake.

Activity-Driven Needs

Physical activity, in its many forms, places unique demands on our bodies. Whether it's a long-distance run, a weightlifting session, or the agility of a dance routine, our muscles are hard at work, contracting and relaxing in response to our every command. And at the heart of this muscular activity lies a crucial energy source: carbohydrates.

Glycogen: The Muscle's Energy Reserve

Within our muscles, carbohydrates are stored as glycogen, a branched polymer of glucose. Think of glycogen as a densely packed energy reserve, ready to be mobilized the moment our muscles spring into action. When we embark on a physical endeavor, the body begins to break down glycogen back into glucose, which is then used to produce ATP, the cellular currency of energy.

Aerobic versus Anaerobic

The reliance on glycogen varies depending on the nature of the activity. During aerobic exercises, such as jogging or swimming, the body uses a mix of fats and glycogen as source energy. However, as the intensity of the activity increases, the balance shifts more towards glycogen. This is because glycogen can be broken down more rapidly than fats, providing the quick energy bursts required for high-intensity activities.

In contrast, during anaerobic activities like sprinting or heavy weightlifting, the body relies almost exclusively on glycogen. These activities are characterized by short, intense bursts of effort, and the body needs an immediate energy source to meet these demands.

Depletion and Replenishment

Given the heavy reliance on glycogen during physical activity, it's possible, especially during prolonged or high-intensity workouts, to deplete these stores. Have you ever hit 'the wall' during a marathon or felt completely drained after an intense gym session? That's often a sign that your glycogen stores are running low.

During post-exercise, it's crucial to replenish these depleted glycogen stores. Consuming carbohydrates after a workout ensures that the muscles are restocked and ready for the next activity. This replenishment is not just about preparing for the next workout; it's also about aiding recovery and minimizing muscle soreness.

The intricate relationship between physical activity and carbohydrate needs underscores the importance of tailoring one's diet to their activity level. While the baseline carbohydrate requirement supports our basic physiological functions, those who lead an active lifestyle must be mindful of their increased carbohydrate needs, ensuring optimal performance, recovery, and overall muscle health.

Channeling Intake to Lifestyle: Sedentary Lifestyle

Understanding Carbohydrate Needs for the Sedentary

While it might seem counterintuitive, even those who are largely inactive have a notable requirement for carbohydrates. This is because, irrespective of physical activity, our bodies have a baseline energy demand. Our organs, especially the brain, rely heavily on glucose, a form of carbohydrate, to function optimally. Additionally, basic activities like breathing, maintaining body temperature, and even the act of thinking, all consume energy.

For individuals leading a sedentary lifestyle, the recommended carbohydrate intake is geared towards meeting these foundational energy needs without promoting excessive calorie consumption, which could lead to weight gain.

Breaking Down the Numbers

Dietary guidelines suggest that carbohydrates should constitute about 45-50% of the total daily caloric intake for sedentary individuals. Let's put this into perspective with some simple math:

Imagine someone who consumes a total of 2000 calories each day. If 45% of these calories come from carbohydrates, that's 900 calories. Since each gram of carbohydrate provides 4 calories, this translates to 225 grams of carbohydrates. On the higher end, at 50%, it would be 1000 calories from carbohydrates, or 250 grams.

Choosing Quality Carbohydrates

While meeting this target is essential, the source of these carbohydrates also matters. Even for those who aren't physically active, opting for whole grains, fruits, and vegetables ensures a steady release of energy and provides essential nutrients and fiber. In contrast, refined sugars and processed foods can lead to energy spikes and crashes, and over time, can contribute to various health issues.

Leading a sedentary lifestyle doesn't negate the need for carbohydrates. It merely adjusts the quantity. By understanding and meeting these needs with quality sources, even those who are less active can support their body's fundamental functions and promote overall well-being.

Moderately Active: Balancing Energy for Light Activity

In physical activity, many individuals fall into the category of being 'moderately active'. This doesn't necessarily mean they're hitting the gym daily or running marathons. Instead, it encompasses those who incorporate light to moderate physical activities into their daily routine. This could be a brisk walk in the park, cycling to work, gardening, or even the hustle and bustle of daily household chores.

Carbohydrate Needs for the Moderately Active

The energy demands for someone who is moderately active are notably higher than those leading a sedentary lifestyle. The body burns more calories during these activities, and as such, requires a more substantial fuel source. Carbohydrates, being the primary energy source, play a pivotal role in meeting these demands.

When we engage in activities like walking or light chores, our muscles tap into their glycogen stores, a form of stored carbohydrate, to generate energy. To ensure these glycogen stores are replenished and that there's a steady supply of energy for these activities, a moderately active individual's diet should be adequately rich in carbohydrates.

The Numbers Game

For the moderately active, dietary guidelines suggest that carbohydrates should constitute about 50-55% of their total daily caloric intake. For example:

Consider an individual consuming 2200 calories daily, which is slightly higher than the sedentary intake due to increased activity. At 50% carbohydrate intake, this amounts to 1100 calories from carbohydrates, translating to 275 grams. If they lean towards the higher end, at 55%, they'd be consuming 1210 calories from carbohydrates, or about 302.5 grams.

Prioritizing Nutrient-Dense Carbohydrates

While the quantity of carbohydrates is essential, the quality remains paramount. Moderately active individuals should focus on nutrient-dense carbohydrate sources. Whole grains, legumes, fruits, and vegetables not only provide the necessary energy but also come packed with vitamins, minerals, and fiber. These nutrients support overall health, enhance digestion, and ensure sustained energy release, preventing those dreaded mid-day slumps.

Being moderately active brings with it a unique set of dietary needs. By understanding the importance of carbohydrates in fueling light to moderate activities and choosing high-quality sources, individuals can ensure they're adequately powered for their daily endeavors while also reaping the broader health benefits of a balanced diet.

Highly Active and Athletes

In physical exertion, there's a marked difference between those who are moderately active and those who push their bodies to the limits. Whether it's the professional athlete training for their next competition, the marathon runner clocking in miles every day, or the construction worker laboring under the sun, the energy demands are immense. For these individuals, carbohydrates aren't just a part of their diet; they are the linchpin holding their energy levels together.

The Elevated Carbohydrate Needs

The reason behind the heightened carbohydrate requirement for highly active athletes is straightforward: intense physical activity depletes glycogen stores at a rapid rate.

Glycogen, stored in the muscles and liver, is the body's primary fuel source during high-intensity activities. Once these reserves start running low, performance can decline, and fatigue sets in.

To prevent hitting this 'wall' and to ensure that the body has ample reserves to tap into, a diet rich in carbohydrates is crucial. For the highly active, dietary guidelines suggest that carbohydrates should make up about 55-65% of their total daily caloric intake.

Endurance Athletes

Endurance sports, like long-distance running, cycling, or triathlons, place unique demands on the body. Not only is the duration of the activity extended, but the energy expenditure is also consistently high. During heavy training phases or in the lead-up to a competition, endurance athletes might find that their carbohydrate needs are even more elevated. For them, carbohydrates might need to constitute up to 70% of their total daily calories.

Let's break this down with an example:

Consider an endurance athlete consuming 3000 calories daily during a heavy training phase. At 70% carbohydrate intake, this translates to 2100 calories from carbohydrates, which is a whopping 525 grams.

Choosing the Right Carbohydrates

While the focus is on quantity, the quality of carbohydrates remains paramount. Highly active individuals and athletes should prioritize complex carbohydrates like whole grains, starchy vegetables, and legumes. These not only provide sustained energy but also ensure a steady release of glucose into the bloodstream, preventing energy spikes and crashes. Additionally, incorporating fruits, rich in simple sugars, can offer quick energy boosts, especially post-workout, aiding in rapid glycogen replenishment.

For those pushing their bodies to extremes, understanding the pivotal role of carbohydrates is essential. By tailoring their carbohydrate intake to their activity levels and choosing nutrient-dense sources, they can ensure optimal performance, rapid recovery, and overall well-being.

Special Considerations: Navigating the Complex World of Carbohydrate Intake

In nutrition, where trends and new diets emerge regularly, carbohydrates often find themselves at the center of many debates. While the general guidelines emphasize the importance of carbohydrates, especially for active individuals, some specific diets and considerations challenge this norm. One such approach that has gained significant traction in recent years is the low-carb and ketogenic diet.

Low-Carb and Ketogenic Diets: A Brief Overview

At its core, a low-carb diet is precisely what it sounds like: a dietary approach that reduces carbohydrate intake significantly below typical dietary recommendations. The ketogenic diet, a subset of low-carb diets, takes this a step further. It drastically reduces carbohydrate intake, usually to less than 50 grams per day, and increases fat intake. The goal is to shift the body's primary energy source from glucose to ketones, compounds produced when the body burns fat for energy in the absence of sufficient carbohydrates.

Potential Benefits and Applications

The ketogenic diet, originally developed as a treatment for epilepsy, has shown promise in various health contexts. Some individuals find success with weight loss, improved blood sugar control, and even enhanced mental clarity on this diet. Moreover, there's emerging research suggesting potential benefits for conditions like Alzheimer's disease, certain cancers, and even brain injuries.

The Athletic Perspective

For athletes, the ketogenic diet presents a conundrum. On the one hand, becoming "fat-adapted" might offer a vast reservoir of energy, given the body's extensive fat stores compared to limited glycogen reserves. On the other hand, the diet might limit optimal performance during high-intensity activities that primarily rely on glycogen.

Proceed with Caution

While the potential benefits of low-carb and ketogenic diets are intriguing, they aren't without challenges. Transitioning to such a diet can come with side effects, often termed the "keto flu", which includes symptoms like fatigue, headaches, and mood swings. Moreover, the long-term effects of these diets, especially in the context of high-intensity athletic performance, are still under research.

Given these considerations, it's paramount for anyone considering a significant shift in carbohydrate intake, especially athletes, to consult with a nutritionist or healthcare provider. Personalized guidance can ensure that the diet aligns with individual goals, health conditions, and activity levels.

Metabolic Health: Navigating Carbohydrate Intake Amidst Medical Conditions

In human health, metabolism plays a central role, in governing how our bodies utilize the nutrients we consume. For most, the body's handling of carbohydrates is a seamless process, converting them into glucose, which then fuels our cells. However, for individuals with metabolic conditions like diabetes or insulin resistance, this process becomes more complex, necessitating a careful approach to carbohydrate consumption.

Understanding the Metabolic Challenge

At the heart of metabolic conditions like diabetes is a disruption in the body's ability to manage blood sugar levels. Under typical circumstances, the hormone insulin facilitates the uptake of glucose into cells. However, in conditions like type 2 diabetes, the body's response to insulin is diminished, leading to elevated blood sugar levels. Over time, consistently high blood sugar can result in many health complications, from cardiovascular diseases to nerve damage.

Carbohydrates and Blood Sugar Management

Given that carbohydrates directly influence blood sugar levels, individuals with metabolic conditions must approach their intake with precision. It's not just about the quantity, but also the quality and timing:

- **Quality Matters:** All carbohydrates aren't created equal when it comes to their impact on blood sugar. Fiber-rich sources like whole grains, legumes, and vegetables lead to a slower, more controlled rise in blood sugar compared to refined carbohydrates like white bread or sugary beverages.

- **Timing is Crucial:** Distributing carbohydrate intake evenly throughout the day can prevent drastic spikes and drops in blood sugar. For those on insulin or certain medications, aligning carbohydrate consumption with medication doses is vital.

Personalized Approach to Carbohydrate Intake

While general guidelines provide a starting point, metabolic health is deeply individual. Factors like the type and severity of the condition, concurrent medications, activity levels, and even stress can influence carbohydrate needs and tolerance. As such, a personalized approach, often designed with the guidance of a registered dietitian or endocrinologist, is paramount.

Lifestyle and Metabolic Health

While carbohydrate management is a cornerstone of metabolic health, it's just one piece of the puzzle. Regular physical activity, stress management, adequate sleep, and other dietary considerations play integral roles in managing and potentially improving metabolic conditions.

While carbohydrates are a fundamental aspect of our diet, their role takes on heightened significance for those with metabolic conditions. An individualized approach to intake can pave the way for better health outcomes and improved quality of life.

Age and Gender: The Factors Influencing Carbohydrate Needs

In nutrition, understanding individual needs is paramount. While we often focus on activity levels or specific health conditions when determining dietary requirements, two fundamental factors – age and gender play pivotal roles in shaping our carbohydrate needs. Delving into these aspects provides a clearer picture of how our bodies' demand for this essential macronutrient evolves throughout life.

The Growing Years: Children and Teenagers

Childhood and adolescence are periods of rapid growth and development. The body is not just maintaining its functions but is in a continuous state of expansion and maturation.

- **Fueling Growth:** Carbohydrates serve as a primary energy source, supporting the heightened metabolic rates seen in children and teenagers. This energy supports everything from brain development to the physical growth spurts typical of the teenage years.

- **Supporting Activity:** Younger individuals are often more active, with play, sports, and general exploration demanding significant energy. Carbohydrates provide the quick and efficient fuel to support these bursts of activity.

Gender Differences: Beyond the Binary

While it's essential to avoid over-generalizations, there are some physiological differences between male and female bodies that can influence carbohydrate needs.

- **Muscle Mass:** Men typically have a higher muscle mass compared to women. Muscles store glucose in the form of glycogen, which means that individuals with more muscle might have slightly increased carbohydrate needs, especially if they're active.

- **Hormonal Variations:** The menstrual cycle in women can influence carbohydrate metabolism. Some women might experience changes in blood sugar levels or insulin sensitivity at different points in their cycle, which can affect their carbohydrate needs and tolerance.

- **Life Phases:** Specific periods, such as pregnancy or menopause, come with unique nutritional requirements. For instance, during pregnancy, there's an increased demand for energy, partly met by carbohydrates, to support the growing fetus.

Adapting to Life's Changes

As we navigate the different stages of life, our nutritional needs evolve too. It's crucial to adapt our diets accordingly, ensuring we provide our bodies with the right diet in the right amounts. Regular check-ins with healthcare professionals or nutritionists can help modify our diets to our changing needs.

In sum, age and gender are foundational elements that shape our carbohydrate requirements. Recognizing and respecting these factors ensures that our nutritional strategies are aligned with our bodies' unique demands at every life stage.

The Balancing Act

Navigating the world of nutrition, particularly the domain of carbohydrates, is akin to mastering a delicate dance. Each step, each choice, is a move towards achieving harmony between what we consume and what our bodies truly need.

Carbohydrates, often vilified in popular media, are, in reality, a cornerstone of our energy metabolism. They fuel our daily activities, from the mundane to the strenuous, and support essential bodily functions. But like any aspect of nutrition, the key lies in balance and understanding.

- **Knowledge as Power:** The first step in mastering this balance is education. By understanding the role of carbohydrates, their sources, and their impact on our bodies, we can make informed decisions. This knowledge empowers us to choose the right type and amount of carbohydrates that align with our unique lifestyles and health goals.

- **Tuning In:** Beyond external knowledge, it's crucial to cultivate an internal awareness. Listening to our bodies, recognizing the signals they send post-consumption of certain foods, and understanding our energy levels can provide invaluable insights. This self-awareness allows us to fine-tune our carbohydrate intake, ensuring it aligns with our body's feedback.

- **The Trial and Error Journey:** Nutrition is not a one-size-fits-all domain. What works for one individual might not work for another. Therefore, it's essential to approach carbohydrate intake with an open mind, ready to experiment, assess, and adjust.

This iterative process, over time, helps pinpoint the optimal carbohydrate balance for an individual.

- **Holistic Health:** Carbohydrates are just one piece of the nutritional puzzle. While they play a significant role, it's essential to view them within the broader context of a balanced diet, rich in proteins, fats, vitamins, and minerals. Achieving this balance ensures that our bodies receive all the nutrients they need to function optimally.

In health and well-being, carbohydrates are vibrant threads, weaving energy and vitality into our lives. By approaching their intake with knowledge, awareness, and adaptability, we can ensure that this energy source serves us in the best possible way, fueling our journeys toward optimal health and vitality.

Fats: The Heroes of Physiological Harmony

In nutrition, fats often find themselves cloaked in mystery, sometimes even maligned. Yet, these molecules, diverse in their structures and functions, are pivotal to life. They are not merely sources of energy but play intricate roles, ensuring the body's harmonious functioning.

The Multifaceted Roles of Fats

At a glance, fats might seem like simple energy reservoirs, but delve deeper, and their myriad functions begin to unfold.

1. **Energy Reservoirs:** Indeed, fats are dense energy stores. Gram for gram, they provide more than double the energy compared to proteins and carbohydrates. This energy is especially crucial during prolonged activities when glycogen stores deplete, and the body seeks alternative energy sources.

2. **Cellular Function and Integrity:** Every cell in our body is enveloped in a lipid bilayer, a protective membrane primarily composed of fats. This membrane not only provides structural integrity to the cell but also plays a role in nutrient transport, signaling, and cellular interactions.

3. **Hormone Production:** Fats are precursors to several hormones, especially the steroid hormones like cortisol, estrogen, and testosterone. These hormones play pivotal roles in metabolism, growth, stress response, and reproductive functions.

4. **Absorption of Fat-Soluble Vitamins:** Vitamins A, D, E, and K are fat-soluble, meaning they require fats for their absorption in the gut. Without adequate dietary fats, the body's ability to absorb and utilize these vitamins diminishes, potentially leading to deficiencies.

5. **Thermal Insulation and Organ Protection:** Adipose tissue, primarily composed of stored fats, acts as an insulator, helping maintain body temperature. Additionally, fats cushion vital organs, protecting them from physical shocks and injuries.

6. **Brain Health and Function:** The human brain is, by weight, nearly 60% fat. Essential fatty acids, like omega-3s, play a crucial role in cognitive functions, memory, and mood regulation.

In the narrative of human physiology, fats emerge not as mere side characters but as protagonists, ensuring the story unfolds seamlessly. They are the heroes, working tirelessly behind the scenes, orchestrating a multitude of processes that keep us healthy, energetic, and vibrant.

Fats: The Pillars of Health and Performance

In human physiology and athletic prowess, fats stand tall as silent pillars, underpinning many of the processes that keep us alive, thriving, and performing at our best. Their role, often overshadowed by the more vocal debates around carbohydrates and proteins, is profound, influencing everything from our cellular membranes to our marathon times.

The Dual Role of Fats in Health and Performance

- **Guardians of Cellular Integrity:** Every cell in our body is encased in a lipid bilayer, a protective barrier that determines what enters and exits the cell. This lipid bilayer is primarily composed of fats. They ensure the cell's structural integrity, its responsiveness to external signals, and its ability to communicate with neighboring cells. In essence, fats are the sentinels that guard the very units of life.

- **Masters of Metabolic Efficiency:** Fats are energy-dense, packing more than double the calories per gram compared to carbohydrates or proteins. This energy density is not just a numerical quirk; it's a testament to fats' role as the body's primary energy reservoir. In endurance sports, where glycogen stores can be quickly depleted, the body taps into its fat reserves, ensuring a steady energy supply for prolonged durations.

- **Custodians of Cognitive Health:** The brain, that intricate organ in charge of our thoughts, emotions, and actions, is predominantly fat. Essential fatty acids, especially omega-3s, play a pivotal role in cognitive functions, mood regulation, and even mental resilience. A diet rich in these fats can be the cornerstone of optimal brain health, warding off cognitive decline and enhancing mental sharpness.

- **Regulators of Hormonal Harmony:** Fats are the precursors to a multitude of hormones, those chemical messengers that regulate everything from our mood to our muscle growth. Steroid hormones, responsible for our stress response, reproductive health, and even our metabolic rate, are synthesized from cholesterol, a lipid molecule. A balanced intake of fats ensures this hormonal orchestra plays in harmony, influencing our health and performance.

- **Protectors Against Inflammation:** Chronic inflammation, the silent undercurrent behind many modern ailments, can be mitigated by certain fats. Omega-3 fatty acids found abundantly in fish oils, have potent anti-inflammatory properties. For athletes, this means faster recovery times, reduced muscle soreness, and enhanced readiness for the next training session.

- **Sculptors of Body Composition:** Beyond their role as an energy source, fats influence body composition. They induce satiety, potentially reducing overall calorie consumption. Moreover, a diet balanced in healthy fats can optimize fat metabolism, promoting a leaner physique and better muscle definition.

In the grand narrative of health and performance, fats emerge not as mere background players but as protagonists. They shape our health from the cellular level, influence our athletic performance, and play a pivotal role in our overall well-being. Embracing fats, understanding their multifaceted roles, and integrating them judiciously into our diets sets the stage for a life of vitality, strength, and optimal performance.

Fats: The Essential Guide to Optimal Intake

In nutrition, is essential for both health and performance. But how much fat should one consume? The answer, like many things in nutrition, is influenced by individual goals, activity levels, and health considerations.

Decoding Fat Intake: From Basics to Individual Needs

The Foundational Requirement

In nutrition, each thread, each nutrient, plays its part. Among these, dietary fats stand out, not just as a source of energy but as vital contributors to a multitude of physiological processes that keep us functioning optimally.

Every cell in our body, from the neurons firing in our brain to the muscle cells contracting in our legs, is enveloped in a membrane rich in fats. This lipid bilayer is crucial for cellular function, acting as a barrier, a gateway, and a communication hub. Fats, in this context, are not just structural elements but dynamic entities that influence how cells interact, respond, and adapt.

Beyond the cellular realm, fats play a pivotal role in hormone production. Steroid hormones, which include sex hormones like estrogen and testosterone, as well as hormones like cortisol, are derived from cholesterol, a type of lipid. These hormones orchestrate many physiological responses, from reproductive functions to stress responses.

Then there's the realm of vitamins, essential micronutrients that our bodies require in small amounts. Among these, the fat-soluble vitamins - A, D, E, and K deserve special mention. As the name suggests, these vitamins are soluble in fats and oils, and dietary fats aid in their absorption in the gut. Vitamin A, crucial for vision; Vitamin D, the sunshine vitamin essential for bone health; Vitamin E, a potent antioxidant; and Vitamin K, vital for blood clotting, all rely on dietary fats for optimal absorption and function.

Given these multifaceted roles of fats, it's no surprise that they are an essential component of our diet. For the average adult, fats should make up about 20-35% of our total daily caloric intake. This range ensures that we reap the benefits of fats, from energy provision to physiological support, while maintaining a balanced intake of other macronutrients.

In essence, while the world of nutrition is vast and varied, the foundational requirement for fats remains consistent. They are not just a footnote in our dietary story but a central character, influencing chapters of health, growth, and vitality.

Activity Levels and Fat Intake: The Hero of Endurance

In the theater of nutrition and exercise, carbohydrates often play the leading role, especially when the discussion turns to quick bursts of energy and rapid recovery. They're the immediate fuel, the sprinters in the marathon of metabolism. But behind the scenes, working diligently and consistently, are fats, the heroes, especially when the journey is long and the pace is steady.

Imagine the body as a hybrid car. Carbohydrates are the electric charge, great for quick starts and short distances. Fats, on the other hand, are the traditional fuel, perfect for long drives on the open road. During prolonged, low to moderate-intensity exercises, when the immediate reserves of carbohydrates begin to deplete, fats step into the limelight. They break down to release energy, ensuring that the muscles continue to function efficiently, even hours into an activity.

Endurance athletes, those who run marathons, cycle long distances, or engage in triathlons, have a unique relationship with fats. For them, fats are not just a backup energy source; they are primary fuel, especially during the later stages of their events. As they push past the first few hours, with glycogen stores dwindling, the body taps into its fat reserves, breaking them down to keep the legs moving, the heart pumping, and the spirit racing.

However, this reliance on fats for energy doesn't necessarily translate to a drastically different fat intake for endurance athletes compared to the general population. The foundational principles remain the same, with fats constituting about 20-35% of their daily caloric intake. What changes, however, is the strategy: the timing of fat consumption, and the types of fats chosen for optimizing performance and recovery.

For instance, in the days leading up to a big race, an athlete might focus on carbohydrate loading to maximize glycogen stores. But in their regular training diet, healthy fats from sources like avocados, nuts, seeds, and fatty fish find prominence. Post-training, the emphasis might shift to a balance of proteins and carbohydrates to aid muscle recovery, but fats still play a role in supporting overall nutrient absorption and reducing inflammation.

In conclusion, while carbohydrates might steal the show when it comes to sports nutrition, fats play a consistent, crucial role, especially in the world of endurance. They remind us that in the marathon of life and sport, it's not just about the quick sprints but the sustained pace, the resilience, and the long haul.

Age, Gender, and Metabolic Considerations: Tailoring Fat Intake to Life's Seasons

Nutrition is a dynamic science, evolving and adapting to the unique needs of an individual. It's not a one-size-fits-all approach but rather a designed plan that considers various factors, including age, gender, and metabolic rate. Among the macronutrients, fats, with their diverse roles in the body, require special attention when determining optimal intake based on these considerations.

The Aging Metabolism: As the sands of time flow, our bodies undergo numerous changes. One of the most significant shifts is in our metabolic rate. With age, the body's basal metabolic rate – the energy expended while at rest tends to decrease. This decline means that as we grow older, we might not require as many calories as we did in our youth.

Consequently, the absolute amount of fats we need might decrease. However, the quality of fats becomes even more crucial. Older adults benefit from omega-3 fatty acids, found in fatty fish and flaxseeds, which can support cognitive function and reduce inflammation.

The Hormones: Gender plays a pivotal role in nutrition, and fats are no exception. Men and women have different hormonal profiles, which can influence how they metabolize and utilize fats. For instance, estrogen, predominant in women, can affect fat storage and breakdown. Before menopause, women might find that they store fats more in the hips and thighs, while men, influenced by testosterone, might store them in the abdominal region.

During post-menopause, as estrogen levels drop, women might notice a shift in fat distribution, moving more towards the abdominal area. This change can also influence their overall fat requirements. Post-menopausal women might benefit from a slightly increased intake of healthy fats, especially those rich in omega-3s, to support heart health and bone density.

Muscle Mass and Fat: Another factor to consider is muscle mass. Muscles, being metabolically active, influence our daily energy requirements. Men, typically having a higher muscle mass than women, might have a slightly elevated metabolic rate. This difference means that their caloric needs, and by extension, their fat requirements, might be higher. However, it's essential to balance this with physical activity levels, as a sedentary lifestyle can offset the metabolic advantages of higher muscle mass.

In nutrition, however, understanding the interplay of age, gender, and metabolism is crucial. It reminds us that our dietary needs are fluid, changing with life's seasons. By tuning into these changes and adjusting our fat intake accordingly, we can support our bodies in every phase, ensuring optimal health and vitality.

Special Dietary Approaches

In nutrition, various dietary approaches have emerged, each with its unique philosophy and macronutrient distribution. Among these, high-fat diets, particularly the ketogenic approach, have garnered significant attention in recent years. But what drives these diets, and how do they reshape the body's energy dynamics?

The Ketogenic Paradigm: The ketogenic diet is a radical departure from traditional macronutrient distributions. Instead of relying on carbohydrates as the primary energy source, this approach emphasizes fats, pushing them to constitute a staggering 70-80% of daily caloric intake. What is then the rationale? It is simply to shift the body's metabolic machinery from burning glucose, derived from carbohydrates, to burning ketones, produced from the breakdown of fats. This state, known as ketosis, transforms the body into a fat-burning machine.

The Metabolic Shift: The human body is remarkably adaptable. When carbohydrates are scarce, as they are in a ketogenic diet, the liver begins converting fats into ketones, molecules that can serve as an alternative fuel for the brain and muscles. This shift is not just a mere metabolic switch but a profound transformation in how the body sources and utilizes energy. It's akin to changing the primary fuel of a car from gasoline to electric power.

Potential Benefits and Considerations: The ketogenic diet has shown promise in managing specific metabolic conditions, notably epilepsy in children and, to some extent, type 2 diabetes. Some individuals also turn to this approach for weight loss, given its appetite-suppressing effects and the potential for rapid fat loss. However, it's not without its challenges. The initial phase of the diet can be accompanied by the "keto flu", a collection of symptoms including fatigue, dizziness, and irritability, as the body adjusts to its new energy source.

Moreover, the long-term effects of such a high-fat intake remain a topic of ongoing research. Concerns have been raised about potential impacts on heart health, given the diet's emphasis on saturated fats. There's also the challenge of nutrient balance, as the severe restriction of carbohydrates can limit the intake of fiber-rich foods, essential vitamins, and minerals.

Proceeding with Caution: Given the complexities and potential challenges of the ketogenic diet, it's not a journey to embark on lightly. Professional guidance is paramount. Consulting with a nutritionist or healthcare provider can ensure that the diet meets individual needs, balancing the potential benefits with any risks. Regular monitoring, both of metabolic markers and overall well-being, can help fine-tune the approach, ensuring it remains aligned with health goals.

In dietary approaches, the ketogenic diet stands out as a testament to the body's adaptability. While it offers potential benefits, it underscores the importance of individualized nutrition, reminding us that what works for one person might not necessarily work for another.

Quality Over Quantity: While determining the right amount of fat is essential, the quality of fat sources is paramount. Unsaturated fats, found in foods like avocados, nuts, seeds, and olive oil, are heart-healthy and anti-inflammatory. Omega-3 fatty acids, especially from fatty fish, offer numerous health benefits. On the other hand, trans fats and excessive saturated fats, often found in processed foods and certain animal products, should be limited.

Choose Quality Over Quantity

In nutrition, fats often find themselves at the center of heated debates. Are they friends or foes? Beneficial or detrimental? While the quantity of fats consumed is undeniably important, the quality of these fats can significantly influence overall health and well-being. Let's examine fats deeper, distinguishing the beneficial from the potentially harmful, and understand why the source of our fats matters just as much as the amount.

Beneficial Unsaturated Fats: When we speak of heart-healthy fats, unsaturated fats often take the spotlight. These fats, characterized by their liquid state at room temperature, are predominantly found in plant-based sources. Think of the rich, green flesh of avocados, the crunchy delight of nuts, the aromatic allure of olive oil, and the tiny yet potent seeds like chia and flaxseed. Consuming these fats has been linked to a plethora of health benefits, from reducing bad cholesterol levels to offering anti-inflammatory properties. They're not just nutrients; they're protective agents, guarding against heart diseases and supporting overall metabolic health.

The Mighty Omega-3s: Within the family of unsaturated fats, omega-3 fatty acids deserve a special mention. These essential fats, which our bodies cannot produce on their own, play a pivotal role in brain health, inflammation regulation, and even mood stabilization. Fatty fish, such as salmon, mackerel, and sardines, are treasure troves of these beneficial fats. Regular consumption of omega-3-rich foods can offer protection against a range of conditions, from cardiovascular diseases to certain mental health disorders.

The Cautionary Tale of Trans and Saturated Fats: On the other end of the spectrum lie trans fats and excessive saturated fats. While some amount of saturated fats, found in animal products and certain oils, can be part of a balanced diet, an overabundance can raise cholesterol levels, posing risks to heart health. Trans fats, often lurking in processed foods, baked goods, and some portions of margarine, are even more concerning. These artificially created fats not only elevate bad cholesterol but also lower the good cholesterol, doubling the risk to cardiovascular health.

Making Informed Choices: With fats, as with most things in life, balance and quality are key. Incorporating a variety of high-quality fat sources, while being wary of excessive saturated and trans fats, can pave the way for optimal health. It's not just about meeting daily caloric needs; it's about nourishing the body, supporting its functions, and safeguarding against potential ailments.

In conclusion, as we navigate the intricate world of fats, it's essential to remember that they're not mere numbers on a nutrition label. They're vital nutrients, each with its unique properties and effects on our health. We can also harness the true potential of fats, turning them into allies in our journey toward optimal health by prioritizing quality over mere quantity.

Harnessing the Power of Fats

In nutrition, fats emerge not as mere threads, but as vibrant patterns that shape the overall design. They are not just caloric contributors or taste enhancers; they are foundational pillars that support numerous physiological processes, from cellular functions to hormonal balances.

Understanding fats goes beyond merely knowing their types or sources. It's about recognizing their diverse roles in our health and well-being. They insulate our organs, facilitate the absorption of vital fat-soluble vitamins, and serve as a significant energy reserve. But beyond these functions, fats play a role in cognitive health, mood regulation, and even the texture and health of our skin.

However, like any powerful tool, the benefits of fats are best realized when used judiciously. It's not just about how much fat we consume, but where it comes from. The heart-healthy unsaturated fats from avocados, nuts, and olive oil differ vastly from the potentially harmful trans fats found in certain processed foods. Making informed choices, therefore, becomes paramount.

Physical activity, age, metabolic health, and even genetic factors can influence our fat requirements. While general guidelines provide a starting point, true dietary wisdom lies in adequate recommendations to one's unique needs and circumstances. It's a dance of balance, where listening to one's body and being aware of its signals is as crucial as understanding nutritional science.

In the end, fats are not mere dietary components to be measured, limited, or avoided. They are allies in our quest for optimal health, vitality, and performance. By embracing them with knowledge, respect, and discernment, we can harness their full potential, ensuring that they contribute positively to our health journey.

<u>**Calculating Caloric Needs: Metabolic Rate (BMR) and adjusting for your activity level.**</u>
Here's a step-by-step guide:
1. Calculate Basal Metabolic Rate (BMR): BMR represents the number of calories your body requires to maintain its current weight while at rest. There are several formulas to calculate BMR, but the Harris-Benedict equations are among the most popular:
For Men: BMR=88.362+(13.397×weight in kg)+(4.799×height in cm)−(5.677×age in years)
For Women: BMR=447.593+(9.247×weight in kg)+(3.098×height in cm)−(4.330×age in years)
2. Adjust for Activity Level: Once you have your BMR, you need to multiply it by an activity factor to get your daily caloric needs:
•**Sedentary (little or no exercise):** BMR x 1.2
•**Lightly active (light exercise/sports 1-3 days/week):** BMR x 1.375
•**Moderately active (moderate exercise/sports 3-5 days/week):** BMR x 1.55
•**Very active (hard exercise/sports 6-7 days a week):** BMR x 1.725
•**Extra active (very hard exercise/sports & a physical job):** BMR x 1.9
The result will give you the estimated number of calories you need to maintain your current weight based on your activity level.
3. Adjust for Goals: If you want to lose or gain weight, you'll need to adjust your caloric intake:
•**To lose weight:** Subtract 250-500 calories from your daily caloric needs (this will result in a 0.5 to 1 pound loss per week).
•**To gain weight:** Add 250-500 calories to your daily caloric needs (this will result in a 0.5 to 1 pound gain per week).
Note: These are general guidelines. Individual needs can vary. Consult with a healthcare professional when making changes to your diet.

Importance of Micronutrients and Hydration

Micronutrients

Micronutrients, comprising vitamins and minerals, might not provide energy or form the bulk of our tissues, but they are indispensable for the many physiological functions that sustain life. They are the conductors, ensuring that our body's processes play harmoniously, without missing a function.

Every enzyme that catalyzes a reaction, every hormone that sends a message, and every gene that expresses a trait relies on micronutrients, either directly or indirectly. They facilitate the extraction of energy from food, aid in the synthesis and repair of tissues, and ensure efficient communication between cells. In essence, while we might live on macronutrients, we function because of micronutrients.

For instance, consider the role of vitamin C. Beyond its famed association with immune function, it's crucial for the synthesis of collagen, a protein that lends structure to our skin, tendons, and blood vessels. Or take magnesium, a mineral involved in over 300 enzymatic reactions, including those that produce ATP, the cellular currency of energy.

However, the beauty and challenge of micronutrients lie in their balance. Too little, and we risk deficiencies that can derail normal physiological functions. Too much, especially of certain vitamins and minerals, can be toxic. Thus, ensuring an adequate and balanced intake is paramount.

In conclusion, while micronutrients might not grab headlines like their macro counterparts, their role in our health and well-being is monumental. They remind us that in nutrition, as in life, it's often the smallest things that make the most significant difference.

Key Vitamins and Minerals

Muscle growth and development is a multifaceted process, influenced by a myriad of factors ranging from training regimens to genetic predispositions. However, at the heart of this lies nutrition, and more specifically, certain vitamins and minerals that play pivotal roles in muscle physiology. Let's delve deeper into some of these essential micronutrients and their significance in muscle growth.

Vitamin D: The Sunshine Vitamin: Often associated with bone health due to its role in calcium absorption, Vitamin D also plays a crucial role in muscle function. It aids in the regulation of calcium and phosphate in the bloodstream, nutrients that are vital for muscle contraction. Moreover, there's emerging evidence suggesting that Vitamin D can influence protein synthesis and growth factor pathways within muscle cells, potentially enhancing muscle growth and repair. Given that many individuals, especially those in northern latitudes, are deficient in this vitamin, ensuring adequate intake or sun exposure is paramount for optimal muscle function.

Calcium: While the majority of the body's calcium is stored in bones, this mineral plays a vital role in muscle contraction. Calcium ions are released from storage sites in muscle cells during contraction, triggering a series of events that lead to the sliding of muscle filaments and subsequent muscle shortening. Without adequate calcium, this contraction process would be hampered, affecting muscle function and strength.

Iron: Iron's primary role in the body is to help red blood cells transport oxygen to tissues, including muscles. During exercise, muscles require a significant amount of oxygen to produce energy. An iron deficiency can lead to decreased oxygen delivery to muscles, reducing exercise capacity and affecting muscle recovery after exercise.

Magnesium: Magnesium is involved in over 300 enzymatic reactions in the body, many of which are related to energy production and muscle function. It plays a role in the process of muscle contraction and relaxation by acting as a cofactor for enzymes required in these processes. Moreover, magnesium aids in the synthesis of protein, a fundamental aspect of muscle growth and repair.

Zinc: Zinc is known for its role in immune function, but it's also vital for muscle growth. It plays a role in protein synthesis, hormone regulation (including testosterone, a key hormone for muscle growth), and cellular energy production. Zinc deficiency can hamper muscle growth, reduce appetite, and negatively affect exercise performance.

While macronutrients like proteins, carbohydrates, and fats often take center stage in discussions about muscle growth, it's essential not to overlook the role of these vital micronutrients. They work together, ensuring that our muscles have the resources they need to function, recover, and grow. Ensuring a diet rich in these vitamins and minerals, either through whole foods or supplementation, when necessary, can be a game-changer for those looking to optimize muscle health and performance.

Hydration

Water, the most basic of molecules, plays a profound role in our physiology. It's the medium in which all cellular processes occur, the transporter of nutrients, and the coolant that regulates our body temperature. When it comes to muscle function, performance, and overall health, hydration stands as a pillar, often overshadowed by discussions of macronutrients and training regimens, yet equally vital.

The Role of Hydration in Muscle Function and Overall Health: Muscles, being made up of approximately 75% water, rely heavily on adequate hydration. Water ensures that muscle cells can produce ATP, the energy currency, efficiently. It also plays a role in joint lubrication, ensuring smooth movement and reducing the risk of injuries. Beyond muscles, water supports digestion, nutrient absorption, and even cognitive function. Dehydration, even if mild, can impair concentration, coordination, and reaction time, all of which are crucial during physical activities.

The Crucial Role of Hydration During Exercise: As we exercise, our bodies generate heat. To prevent overheating, we sweat, releasing this heat in the form of water and electrolytes. This makes hydration during exercise not just beneficial but essential. Dehydration during physical activity can lead to reduced endurance, increased fatigue, reduced motivation, and increased perceived effort. For athletes and fitness enthusiasts, this can translate to reduced performance and increased risk of heat-related illnesses.

Monitoring Hydration Status: While thirst is a clear indicator that it's time to drink, relying solely on it, especially during intense physical activity, might not be sufficient. Some signs of dehydration include dark yellow urine, dry mouth, fatigue, and dizziness. A simple way to monitor hydration is the urine color test. A pale straw color indicates proper hydration, while a dark yellow or amber color suggests dehydration.

Electrolytes: The Silent Partners in Hydration: While water is vital, hydration isn't just about water. Electrolytes, including sodium, potassium, calcium, and magnesium, play crucial roles in muscle function and maintaining fluid balance. As we sweat, we lose these essential minerals. Replacing them, especially during prolonged physical activity, is crucial. Electrolytes support muscle contractions, and nerve function, and help maintain the body's pH level.

Sports drinks, often rich in electrolytes, can be beneficial during extended physical activities. However, for shorter workouts or general hydration, plain water, coupled with a balanced diet, should suffice.

In Conclusion

Hydration is a dynamic balance, influenced by factors like physical activity, environmental conditions, and individual physiology. By understanding the importance of hydration and being proactive in maintaining it, we can support muscle function, optimize performance, and promote overall health. Whether you're an athlete, a fitness enthusiast, or someone just trying to stay healthy, remember that every sip counts.

Pre-Workout Nutrition: Fueling the Body for Optimal Performance

In fitness and athletic performance, preparation is paramount. Just as an athlete stretches to prepare their muscles or a runner selects the right shoes for their feet, what one consumes before a workout can significantly influence the quality of the session. Pre-workout nutrition is not just about filling the stomach; it's about supplying the body with the right nutrients to optimize performance, endurance, and recovery.

Goals and Importance of Pre-Workout Nutrition: The primary goals of pre-workout nutrition are multifaceted:

1. **Energy Provision:** To provide the body with a ready source of energy to fuel the upcoming physical activity.

2. **Muscle Protection:** To reduce muscle glycogen depletion, decrease muscle protein breakdown, and reduce post-workout soreness.

3. **Performance Enhancement:** To improve exercise performance by increasing strength, endurance, and workout intensity.

4. **Hydration:** To ensure adequate hydration, which can enhance muscle function and delay fatigue.

5. **Mental Preparation:** A proper pre-workout meal can also boost mood and concentration, setting the stage for a focused and effective workout.

The importance of these goals cannot be overstated. Without the right energy, the body might get tired quickly, perform sub-optimally, or take longer to recover post-exercise. Moreover, inadequate nutrition can increase the risk of injuries.

Recommended Nutrient Intake Before a Workout

- **Carbohydrates:** They are the body's primary energy source during high-intensity workouts. Consuming carbohydrates before exercise can top up muscle and liver glycogen stores. Ideal sources include whole grains, fruits, and energy bars. The exact amount varies based on the individual and the nature of the workout, but a general guideline is 30-60 grams of carbohydrates 30 minutes to an hour before exercise.

- **Proteins:** While carbohydrates fuel the workout, proteins protect the muscles. Consuming protein before a workout can reduce muscle protein breakdown, promote muscle growth, and aid in recovery. Sources like whey protein, lean meats, or a combination of essential amino acids can be beneficial. Aim for 15-25 grams of protein in your pre-workout meal.

- **Fats:** For longer, lower-intensity workouts, fats can serve as a significant energy source. While they're not the primary focus of pre-workout nutrition (as they take longer to digest), including small amounts of healthy fats can be beneficial. Nuts, seeds, or avocados are essential supplements.

- **Hydration:** Begin every workout well-hydrated. Consume water in the hours leading up to your exercise, and consider including electrolytes if you're preparing for a prolonged or particularly sweaty session.

- **Timing:** While nutrient composition is crucial, so is timing. A larger meal can be consumed 2-3 hours before the workout, while a smaller, more carbohydrate-focused snack can be taken 30 minutes to an hour before the session.

Pre-workout nutrition is both an art and a science. While the science provides guidelines and recommendations, the art lies in tailoring these to individual preferences, workout goals, and how one's body responds. By giving pre-workout nutrition the attention it deserves, one can have a productive, effective, and enjoyable workout session.

Intra-Workout Nutrition: Sustaining the Body Through the Grind

Amidst the sweat, the pounding heart, and the high beat of a workout, the body is in a state of constant demand. While pre-workout nutrition sets the stage, intra-workout nutrition ensures that the performance curtain doesn't drop prematurely. It's about sustaining energy, delaying fatigue, and supporting the muscles as they work tirelessly.

Goals and Importance of Intra-Workout Nutrition

1. **Sustained Energy:** To provide a continuous source of fuel, ensuring that energy levels don't drop mid-workout.

2. **Hydration:** To replace fluids lost through sweat and support optimal muscle function.

3. **Electrolyte Balance:** To maintain the balance of essential minerals, aiding in muscle contractions and preventing cramps.

4. **Muscle Protection:** To reduce muscle protein breakdown and support ongoing muscle function.

5. **Endurance Enhancement:** To delay the onset of fatigue, especially during prolonged or high-intensity sessions.

The essence of intra-workout nutrition lies in its ability to bridge the gap between the initial energy from pre-workout meals and post-workout recovery. During longer sessions, especially the body can start to deplete its readily available energy sources, making intra-workout nutrition a crucial component for sustained performance.

Recommendations for Longer or High-Intensity Workouts

1. **Carbohydrates:** For workouts exceeding an hour, especially those of high intensity, a continuous supply of carbohydrates can be beneficial. Consider consuming 30-60 grams of carbohydrates every hour. Liquid solutions, gels, or simple carbohydrate snacks can be effective.

2. **Protein:** While not always necessary for shorter sessions, amino acid or small protein intakes can be beneficial for very long workouts to protect against muscle breakdown. Consider branched-chain amino acid (BCAA) supplements or small amounts of easily digestible proteins.

3. **Hydration:** Drink water throughout the workout. For longer sessions, especially in hot or humid conditions, consider isotonic drinks that replace both fluids and electrolytes.

4. **Electrolytes:** Sodium, potassium, and magnesium are essential for muscle function. Electrolyte tablets, powders, or specially formulated sports drinks can help maintain electrolyte balance during prolonged workouts.

5. **Adaptogens:** Some athletes swear by the benefits of adaptogens like Rhodiola Rosea or Ashwagandha during workouts. While not essential, they might help some individuals cope with physical stress.

6. **Caffeine:** For those who respond well to caffeine, it can be a powerful ally during workouts, enhancing focus, energy, and endurance. However, it's essential to be cautious with dosage and timing, especially if working out later in the day.

The Mid-Workout Boost

Intra-workout nutrition is like a pit stop in a race. It's a chance to refuel, rehydrate, and ensure that the body has everything it needs to perform optimally. By understanding the body's demands and channeling intra-workout nutrition to meet these needs, one can optimize performance, enhance endurance, and ensure that every workout is a step toward their fitness goals.

Post-Workout Nutrition: The Recovery Catalyst

The moments and hours following a workout are a golden window of opportunity, a time when the body is primed to receive nutrients and kickstart the recovery process. This phase, powered by post-workout nutrition, is where the groundwork for muscle repair, growth, and overall recovery is laid.

Goals and Importance of Post-Workout Nutrition

1. **Muscle Repair and Growth:** The stress of exercise causes microscopic tears in muscle fibers. Post-workout nutrition provides the essential building blocks, primarily proteins, to repair these tears, leading to muscle growth and increased strength over time.

2. **Replenishing Energy Stores:** Intense workouts deplete the body's primary energy store, glycogen. Consuming carbohydrates post-exercise helps refill these stores, ensuring the muscles have the energy they need for the next workout.

3. **Reducing Muscle Protein Breakdown:** While exercise increases muscle protein breakdown, consuming protein after a workout can help increase muscle protein synthesis, tipping the balance in favor of muscle growth.

4. **Enhancing Overall Recovery:** Beyond muscles, the body as a whole benefits from post-workout nutrition. Proper nutrient intake can reduce inflammation, decrease muscle soreness, and improve overall recovery rates.

Recommended Nutrient Intake

1. **Carbohydrates:** The body's primary energy source, essential for replenishing depleted glycogen stores. Depending on the workout's intensity and duration, aim for 0.5 to 1.2 grams of carbohydrates per kilogram of body weight within 30 minutes post-exercise.

- *Examples:* Whole grain bread, quinoa, fruits like bananas and berries, and starchy vegetables like sweet potatoes.

2. **Proteins:** The building blocks of muscles, vital for repair and growth. For optimal recovery, consume 15-25 grams of high-quality protein post-workout. This intake is best consumed within the 30-minute window post-exercise.

- *Examples:* Lean meats like chicken or turkey, tofu, legumes, dairy products like Greek yogurt, and protein shakes.

3. **Fats:** While not as immediate a concern as proteins and carbohydrates, including some healthy fats in your post-workout meal can support overall recovery and nutrient absorption.

- *Examples:* Avocado, nuts, seeds, and olive oil.

4. **Hydration:** Essential for replacing lost fluids and aiding in nutrient transport. The amount will vary based on the workout's intensity and duration and individual sweat rates.

- *Examples:* Water, electrolyte solutions, or sports drinks for particularly intense sessions.

Nourishing the Future

The choices made in the post-workout window set the stage for future workouts, dictating the speed and quality of recovery. By understanding the body's needs and tailoring nutrient intake to meet these demands, one can lay the foundation for consistent progress, ensuring each workout builds upon the last. In fitness, the journey doesn't end when the workout does; it's merely the beginning.

Bedtime Snack: The Silent Architect of Recovery

As the world outside dims and our bodies prepare for rest, there's a repair and rejuvenation that begins within us. The night, often overlooked in the context of nutrition, is a crucial period for muscle recovery and growth. While we dream, our bodies work diligently, repairing the wear and tear of the day. And like any craftsman, the body requires the right tools for the job. This is where the bedtime snack, a simple yet potent tool, comes into play.

Benefits of Overnight Recovery

1. **Sustained Muscle Protein Synthesis:** Consuming protein before bed provides the body with a steady supply of amino acids, supporting muscle protein synthesis throughout the night. This can be particularly beneficial for those engaged in regular resistance training or intense physical activity.

2. **Glycogen Restoration:** While the primary focus post-workout is to replenish glycogen stores, a bedtime snack containing carbohydrates can further assist in this restoration, ensuring muscles are energy-ready for the next day.

3. **Hormonal Advantages:** Sleep is associated with a surge in growth hormone, a key player in muscle repair and growth. Providing the body with the right nutrients can complement this natural hormonal advantage, optimizing the repair process.

4. **Prevention of Muscle Breakdown:** A prolonged fasting state, like the overnight period, can lead to muscle protein breakdown. A bedtime snack can help counteract this, preserving muscle mass.

Recommended Nutrient Sources

1. **Proteins:** Slow-digesting proteins are ideal for the night, providing a steady release of amino acids.

- *Examples:* Casein protein (found in dairy products like cottage cheese or as a supplement), Greek yogurt, and milk.

2. **Carbohydrates:** While not as critical as protein, a moderate amount of complex carbohydrates can support glycogen restoration.

- *Examples:* Oats, whole grain crackers, or a slice of whole grain bread.

3. **Fats:** Healthy fats can slow digestion, ensuring a sustained release of nutrients throughout the night.

- *Examples:* Nuts, seeds, avocados, or a spoonful of almond or peanut butter.

4. **Micronutrients:** Certain vitamins and minerals can support sleep quality and muscle function.

- *Examples:* Magnesium (found in nuts and seeds) and vitamin D (found in fortified dairy products).

The Night's Ally

In nutrition, the bedtime snack is the hero, quietly laying the groundwork for recovery while we rest. It's a testament to the idea that timing matters, and that understanding our body's needs can amplify the benefits of what we consume. As the day ends and we drift into sleep, the right snack ensures our bodies have what they need to build, repair, and emerge stronger with the dawn.

Supplements and Muscle Growth--Creatine

Creatine is one of the most researched and widely used supplements in the sports and fitness industry. Its popularity stems from its proven efficacy in enhancing muscle growth, strength, and athletic performance. Let's delve deeper into the role of creatine:

Role in Muscle Growth and Performance:

- **Energy Production**: Creatine plays a pivotal role in the production of adenosine triphosphate (ATP), the primary energy currency of the cell. During short, intense activity, like weightlifting or sprinting, creatine phosphate donates a phosphate group to produce ATP, providing immediate energy.
- **Enhanced Muscle Volume**: Creatine supplementation can increase the water content within muscle cells, leading to a more volumized or "full" appearance. This cellular hydration may also play a role in muscle growth by stimulating protein synthesis.
- **Improved Work Capacity**: Creatine also allows athletes to perform more work during high-intensity activities, leading to increased training adaptations over time by replenishing ATP stores more rapidly.

Mechanism of Action

- **Phosphocreatine System**: Creatine is stored in the muscles as phosphocreatine. During high-intensity activities, phosphocreatine donates its phosphate group to regenerate ATP from adenosine diphosphate (ADP). This rapid ATP production is crucial for activities that last between 5 to 10 seconds.
- **Cell Signaling**: Creatine may also enhance muscle growth by increasing the levels of certain growth-promoting hormones and amplifying the effects of resistance training on cell signaling pathways involved in muscle growth.

Recommended Supplementation Protocol:

- **Loading Phase**: To rapidly increase muscle creatine stores, a common approach is a loading phase of 20 grams per day (divided into 4 doses) for 5-7 days.
- **Maintenance Phase**: After the loading phase, a maintenance dose of 3-5 grams per day is sufficient to maintain elevated creatine stores.
- **No Loading**: Some individuals skip the loading phase and take 3-5 grams per day from the start. This approach will still increase muscle creatine stores, but it may take a few weeks longer.
- **Timing**: While the timing of creatine supplementation is not critical, some people prefer to take it post-workout, potentially benefiting from increased blood flow to the muscles.

- **Safety and Purity**: It's essential to choose a high-quality creatine monohydrate supplement without added fillers or contaminants. Most research supports the safety of creatine supplementation, but as with any supplement, it's advisable to consult with a healthcare professional before starting.

Creatine stands out as a supplement with robust scientific backing for its benefits in muscle growth and athletic performance. However, as with all supplements, individual responses can vary, and it's essential to use them as a complement to a balanced diet and structured training program.

Caffeine: The Stimulant for Enhanced Performance

Caffeine, a natural stimulant most commonly found in coffee, tea, and many energy drinks, has been a part of human diets for centuries. In the context of sports and exercise, caffeine has gained significant attention for its potential ergogenic (performance-enhancing) effects. Here's a closer look at its role, mechanism, and recommended supplementation:

Role in Muscle Growth and Performance:

- **Increased Alertness and Concentration**: Caffeine stimulates the central nervous system, leading to heightened alertness. This can be particularly beneficial for athletes or individuals who train early in the morning or those who need a boost in focus for their workouts.
- **Enhanced Endurance**: Several studies have shown that caffeine can increase endurance in aerobic activities, allowing athletes to train longer and at higher intensities.
- **Strength and Power**: Some research suggests that caffeine might enhance strength and power output, making it beneficial for weightlifters and sprinters.
- **Reduced Perception of Effort**: Caffeine can make a given workload feel less challenging, potentially allowing individuals to push harder during their workouts.

Mechanism of Action

- **Adenosine Receptor Blockade**: Caffeine primarily works by blocking adenosine receptors in the brain. Adenosine is a neurotransmitter that promotes relaxation and sleepiness. By blocking its effects, caffeine promotes alertness and wakefulness.

- **Release of Neurotransmitters**: Caffeine increases the release of certain neurotransmitters like dopamine and norepinephrine, which can enhance mood, focus, and concentration.
- **Mobilization of Calcium in Muscles**: Caffeine can increase the release of calcium stored in muscles, which might enhance muscle contraction and overall power output.
- **Increased Fat Oxidation**: Caffeine can increase the release of adrenaline, which in turn promotes the breakdown of fat. This means that during exercise, the body might use a higher proportion of fat for energy, preserving muscle glycogen.

Recommended Supplementation Protocol

- **Dosage**: For performance-enhancing benefits, research suggests a dose of 3-6 mg of caffeine per kilogram of body weight. For a 70 kg individual, this translates to 210-420 mg of caffeine.
- **Timing**: It's best to consume caffeine about 30-60 minutes before exercise to allow time for peak absorption and maximal effects.
- **Tolerance**: Regular caffeine consumers might develop a tolerance, meaning they might need higher doses to achieve the same effects. It's essential to monitor your body's response and adjust accordingly.
- **Side Effects**: High doses of caffeine can lead to jitters, insomnia, increased heart rate, and digestive issues. It's crucial to start with a lower dose and gauge tolerance.
- **Other Considerations:** While supplements can offer a range of benefits, especially for athletes and fitness enthusiasts, it's essential to approach them with a well-informed perspective. Here's a closer look at some crucial considerations when incorporating supplements into your regimen.

Caffeine, when used judiciously, can be a potent tool in an athlete's arsenal. It offers a range of benefits from increased focus to enhanced endurance. However, as with all supplements, it's essential to use caffeine in moderation and in conjunction with a balanced diet and training regimen.

Approach to Supplementation

- **Research and Evidence**: Before introducing any supplement into your routine, it's vital to research its efficacy, safety, and potential side effects. Look for supplements that have robust scientific evidence supporting their claims.
- **Quality Over Quantity**: It's easy to get lured into the idea that more supplements mean better results. However, it's more beneficial to focus on a few high-quality supplements that align with your goals rather than overwhelming your system with numerous products.

- **Natural Sources**: Whenever possible, prioritize getting nutrients from whole food sources. Supplements should complement your diet, not replace it.
- **Importance of Consulting Professionals**:
- **Personalized Recommendations**: Everyone's body and goals are unique. Consulting with a nutritionist, dietitian, or sports medicine professional can provide appropriate supplement recommendations that align with your specific needs and objectives.
- **Safety Concerns**: Some supplements can interact with medications or have contraindications for certain medical conditions. Professionals can guide you in making safe choices.
- **Dose Optimization**: While general guidelines exist for many supplements, professionals can help determine the optimal dose for your body weight, activity level, and goals.

Role of Supplements in a Comprehensive Approach to Nutrition and Training:

- **Holistic View**: Supplements are just one piece of the puzzle. A balanced diet, structured training regimen, adequate rest, and hydration are equally, if not more, important.
- **Performance versus Health**: While some supplements might enhance performance, it's essential to consider their long-term effects on health. Always prioritize your overall well-being over short-term gains.
- **Adapt and Evolve**: As you progress in your fitness journey, your body's needs might change. Regularly reassess your supplementation strategy in line with your evolving goals and physical demands.

While supplementation offers exciting possibilities for enhanced performance and health, it's crucial to navigate it with a discerning and informed approach. By doing so, you can harness the benefits of supplements while ensuring your overall well-being and long-term health.

The Triad of Nutrition, Training, and Supplementation

As we wrap up this exploration into supplementation, it's essential to reiterate a foundational principle: no supplement, no matter how potent or well-researched, can replace the foundational pillars of a nutrient-rich diet and structured training regimen. Supplements are precisely what their name suggests – a supplementary addition to an already solid foundation.

The Synergy of Diet, Training, and Supplementation

Nutrient-Rich Diet: At the heart of any fitness journey lies a balanced diet. Nutrients from whole foods provide the energy, building blocks, and sustenance our bodies need to function optimally. They lay the groundwork upon which all other efforts are built.

Structured Training: Supplements can support training, but they can't replace the sweat, effort, and consistency required in the gym or on the track. Training is where muscles are challenged, endurance is built, and character is forged.

Strategic Supplementation: With the foundation of diet and training in place, supplements can provide that extra edge, helping to optimize performance, recovery, and results. They fill the gaps, enhance processes, and can sometimes offer shortcuts to specific goals.

As we transition to the next chapter, we'll delve deeper into exercise and its impact on muscle growth. While supplements can play a supporting role, it's the act of training itself such as the repetitions, sets, challenges, and recoveries that truly drive muscle growth. We'll explore the science behind this process, offering insights and strategies to maximize every workout.

In essence, the journey to optimal fitness and health is a holistic one, where diet, training, and supplementation work in harmony. As we continue this exploration, always remember that the whole is greater than the sum of its parts, and every choice, from the foods you eat to the supplements you take, plays a role in making the final masterpiece that is your body.

CHAPTER 4

—◆—

UNDERSTANDING MUSCLE HYPERTROPHY AND ITS INFLUENCES

In human physiology, myriad processes, each with its unique role and significance exist. Yet, among these, muscle hypertrophy stands out, not just as a biological phenomenon, but as a symbol of human determination, discipline, and drive. It's more than just the bulging muscles of a bodybuilder or the toned figure of an athlete; it's a living, breathing testament to many hours of dedication, sweat, and sheer willpower. Every visible contour and definition tells a story of weights lifted, of boundaries pushed, and of difficulties faced head-on.

But to reduce muscle hypertrophy to its aesthetic appeal would be to do it a disservice. Beneath the skin, hidden from the naked eye, lies cellular machinery which functions in perfect harmony. Each repetition, each set, and each workout triggers biological events. Cells respond, proteins are synthesized, and fibers thicken and lengthen. This isn't just growth; it's a carefully planned biochemistry and biomechanics.

Furthermore, muscle hypertrophy is not an isolated event. It doesn't occur in a vacuum. Instead, it's the confluence of our genetic blueprint, the training regimens we adopt, and the nutrition we choose. The weights we lift provide the stimulus, and our genes set the stage, but it's the nutrients we consume that propel, and sustain this growth.

Therefore, muscle hypertrophy is a testament to the human body's adaptability and resilience. It reminds us that with the right stimulus, resources, and dedication, we can develop, mold, and transform ourselves. It's a celebration of what it means to challenge, overcome, and grow.

Definition and Significance of Muscle Hypertrophy

In fitness and physiology, muscle hypertrophy serves as a beacon of human adaptability and potential. But to truly grasp the role it plays, we must define it, and explore the profound implications it holds for our health, performance, and overall well-being.

Defining Muscle Hypertrophy

Muscle hypertrophy is a term that might sound complex, but its essence is relatively straightforward. It denotes the process wherein muscle fibers increase in diameter due to the accumulation of protein content. Contrary to a common misconception, hypertrophy doesn't involve the generation of new muscle cells, also known as hyperplasia. Instead, it focuses on maximizing the potential of existing muscle cells, making them larger and more robust.

The Multifaceted Significance of Muscle Growth

While the visual appeal of well-defined muscles is undeniable, the significance of muscle hypertrophy extends far beyond aesthetics:

Strength and Power Amplification: One of the most immediate benefits of muscle hypertrophy is the enhancement of strength and power. As muscle fibers grow in size, their capacity to generate force amplifies too. This not only translates to lifting heavier weights in the gym but also improves performance in various physical activities, from sprinting on a track to leaping in a basketball game.

A Boost to Metabolic Health: Muscles are metabolic powerhouses. The larger they are, the more energy they demand, even at rest. This increased energy expenditure can elevate the basal metabolic rate, aiding in calorie burning and weight management. Furthermore, with greater muscle mass comes enhanced glycogen storage capacity, a critical factor for endurance athletes. More so, muscles play an important role in glucose metabolism, and their growth can enhance insulin sensitivity, reducing the risk of type 2 diabetes.

Guardians of the Skeletal System: Muscles and bones share a symbiotic relationship. Strong muscles protect the joints, reducing the wear and tear that could lead to conditions like osteoarthritis. Moreover, the tension exerted on bones during resistance training promotes bone density, acting as a preventive measure against osteoporosis. Beyond protection, well-developed muscles also contribute to better posture, ensuring the skeletal system's alignment and functionality.

The Psychological Edge: The journey to muscle hypertrophy, marked by consistent effort and progress, can be incredibly empowering. Witnessing physical transformation often leads to enhanced self-confidence, body positivity, and a sense of accomplishment. Moreover, the discipline and dedication needed to achieve muscle growth can spill over into other areas of life, fostering a growth mindset.

In summary, muscle hypertrophy is not just a physiological process but a holistic experience. It embodies the human spirit's tenacity, the body's adaptability, and the profound interconnection between physical form and function. Whether one's goal is athletic prowess, health optimization, or personal fulfillment, understanding and harnessing the power of muscle hypertrophy can pave the way for a life of vitality and vigor.

The Relationship Between Resistance Training and Muscle Growth

Resistance training, or the act of challenging muscles by making them work against a weight or force, is the primary driver of muscle hypertrophy. When muscles face resistance, especially when it's more than they're used to, it results in microscopic damage or tears. While this might sound alarming, it's this damage that sets the stage for growth.

Post-workout, the body goes into repair mode. With adequate nutrition and rest, it doesn't just repair the damage – it overcompensates, building the muscle back stronger and larger in anticipation of future challenges. This cycle of stress, damage, repair, and growth, repeated over time, leads to muscle hypertrophy.

However, it's essential to understand that not all resistance training is created equal. Factors like load, volume, rest intervals, and training frequency can all influence the hypertrophic response. Again, individual factors like genetics, age, and nutrition determine the extent and rate of muscle growth.

The Growth Process

Muscle hypertrophy is more than just an aesthetic goal; it's a testament to the body's incredible adaptability and resilience. It's a cellular response, hormonal shift, and metabolic process, targeted at creating visible, and tangible growth. As we delve deeper into this topic, we'll explore the differences in training, the importance of nutrition, and the science that underpins every muscle fiber's growth.

Mechanisms of Muscle Hypertrophy

The Art and Science of Muscle Development

Muscle hypertrophy, while often associated with the sweat and grind of the gym, is as much an art as it is a science. It's where the raw determination of an athlete meets the intricate choreography of cellular events. Here, each repetition, each set, and each workout is a brushstroke on the canvas of our physiology, which gradually paints the masterpiece of muscle growth.

The Cellular Ballet Behind the Bulk

At the cellular level, muscle hypertrophy works with precision. Muscle cells, or myocytes, don't increase in number. Instead, they grow in size, as a result of increased protein synthesis and the addition of new contractile structures called myofibrils. This cellular enlargement is designed by a series of signaling pathways, activated in response to the mechanical stress of resistance training.

Biochemical Choreography: The Role of mTOR and Other Key Players

Central to this biochemical process is a protein called mTOR (Mammalian Target of Rapamycin). When muscles face tension such as lifting weights, mTOR is activated, serving as a master switch that accelerates protein synthesis. Alongside mTOR, other molecules like IGF-1 (Insulin-like Growth Factor-1) and hormones like testosterone and growth hormone play pivotal roles, each contributing a unique step to muscle growth.

Physiological Adaptations: Beyond the Muscle Fiber

While the muscle fiber is the star of the hypertrophy show, it doesn't work alone. Blood vessels expand and proliferate to supply more nutrients to the growing muscles. Connective tissues also strengthen to support the increased muscle mass. The nervous system, too, fine-tunes its control, improving the coordination and recruitment of muscle fibers. This holistic adaptation ensures that the muscle doesn't just grow in size but also in strength, functionality, and efficiency.

The Signals in Muscle Fiber: From Strain to Strength

Every time a weight is lifted, signals of various dimensions go through the body. The body swings into action through a coordinated response from the initial strain sensed by mechanoreceptors in the muscle to the biochemical events that amplify the signal. This response ensures that the muscle not only recovers from the immediate challenge but also prepares it for future ones, growing in size and capacity.

In Conclusion: The Elegance of Growth

Muscle hypertrophy, often seen as the rugged outcome of intense training, is, in essence, an elegant process. It's where biology's precision meets the athlete's passion. By understanding the intricacies of growth, we gain a deeper appreciation for every hour spent in the gym, every drop of sweat shed, and every ounce of muscle earned. It reminds us that behind the visible growth lies an intricate ballet of science, dedication, and the relentless spirit of adaptation.

Mechanical Tension and Microtrauma: The Catalysts of Growth

The Science of Strain: Understanding Mechanical Tension

Every time a muscle contracts against resistance, it experiences mechanical tension. This tension can be visualized as the tautness a rubber band experiences when stretched. In the context of our muscles, this tension is generated when muscle fibers actively slide and overlap, working against an external force. The greater the resistance, the higher the mechanical tension, pushing the muscle fibers to their limits.

Microtrauma: The Subtle Scars of Strength

As the muscle fights with this heightened tension, especially during resistance training exercises that push it beyond its usual capacity, the fibers undergo microscopic damage. This isn't the kind of damage one might associate with a significant injury. Instead, it's a series of minuscule tears within the muscle fibers, often at the points where the muscle fibers contract and generate force.

The Silver Lining of Stress

While the idea of causing deliberate damage to our muscles might seem counterintuitive, this microtrauma is a blessing in disguise. It acts as a potent stimulus, which signals to the body that the current muscle structure needs reinforcement. In response, the body initiates a series of adaptive processes, aimed not just to repair the damage but to fortify the muscle against future stressors.

The Repair and Reinforce Paradigm

Post-exercise, as the body recognizes the microtrauma, a flurry of repair processes is set into motion. Blood flow to the affected muscles increases, delivering essential nutrients and growth factors. These elements facilitate the repair of damaged muscle fibers. But the body, in its wisdom, doesn't stop at mere repair. It reinforces, and adds more protein to the muscle fibers, making them thicker and more robust. This adaptive response ensures that the next time the muscle encounters a similar challenge, it's better equipped to handle it.

The Cycle of Growth

This cycle of tension, microtrauma, repair, and reinforcement, when repeated consistently, leads to progressive muscle growth. Each resistance training nudges the muscle a step further on its growth journey, ensuring that over time, with consistent training and adequate recovery, the muscle not only recovers from the microtrauma but emerges larger and more potent than before.

In essence, mechanical tension and the resultant microtrauma are the foundational pillars of muscle hypertrophy. They serve as the initial triggers, setting off events that culminate in muscle growth. Recognizing their significance allows us to train smarter, optimize our workouts to maximize tension, and, by extension, improve muscle growth.

Satellite Cells: The Heroes of Muscle Growth

In muscle physiology, satellite cells stand out as pivotal players, often operating behind the scenes but holding immense significance in muscle growth. These cells, with their unique location and function, are central to the process of muscle repair and hypertrophy. Let's delve deeper into the satellite cells and uncover their role in developing our muscular physique.

Definition and Location: Satellite cells, aptly named for their peripheral location around muscle fibers, are a type of stem cell specifically associated with muscles. Residing just outside the muscle fiber, they lie sandwiched between the muscle cell membrane, known as the sarcolemma, and the surrounding protective sheath called the basal lamina. In their dormant state, they might seem inconspicuous, but their potential is immense. Often, sarcolemma which is referred to as 'muscle stem cells', holds the key to muscle regeneration and growth.

Activation and Significance

The journey of a satellite cell from dormancy to activity is triggered by muscle damage. When we engage in intense physical activity, especially resistance training, our muscle fibers experience microtrauma. This damage acts as a wake-up call for satellite cells. Springing into action, they begin to proliferate, multiplying in number, and then differentiate, preparing themselves to play their part in the repair process. But their role isn't just about numbers; it's about function. One of the most significant contributions of satellite cells is their ability to donate nuclei to muscle fibers. This addition of nuclei is very important because it enhances the muscle cell's capacity to produce proteins, and help in muscle growth and repair.

MUSCLE UNIVERSITY

Fusion Process and Its Impact on Muscle Growth

The story of satellite cells doesn't end with activation. Once they've proliferated and differentiated, they embark on a fusion mission. They merge with the damaged muscle fibers, integrating into their structure. This fusion is more than just a physical amalgamation; it's a functional enhancement. Satellite cells amplify the protein-synthesizing capacity of the muscle by donating their nuclei to muscle fibers. This not only aids in the immediate repair of the muscle but also fortifies it for future challenges. The muscle, now equipped with more nuclei, is better prepared to handle subsequent stress, ensuring continued growth and adaptation.

In Conclusion: The Silent Architects of Muscle Growth

Satellite cells might not be the most talked-about entities in fitness and bodybuilding, but their contribution is undeniable. They are the silent architects, that shape our muscles, ensuring their repair, and their growth. Every time we lift a weight, challenge our limits, and push our boundaries, these cells are at work, to ensure a complex repair and growth. Understanding their role gives us a profound appreciation of the intricate processes that transform our efforts in the gym into visible, tangible muscle growth.

Factors Influencing Muscle Hypertrophy

The process of muscle growth is an interplay of various elements, each contributing its unique essence to the grand tapestry of hypertrophy. While the sight of a well-defined muscle might seem straightforward, the path leading to its formation is anything but a path shaped by numerous factors, each as critical as the next. In fact, every decision plays a pivotal role in determining the trajectory of muscle development, from the weight you lift, the food you consume, the hours you rest to the exercises you choose. In this section, we will delve deep into these influential factors, unraveling the science and strategy behind each one, and illuminating the roadmap to optimal muscle growth.

Training Volume and Intensity: The Foundations of Growth

The Principle of Progressive Overload: At the heart of muscle development lies a simple yet powerful principle known as progressive overload. It explains that, for muscles to grow, they must be subjected to a stimulus that's beyond what they've previously experienced. This concept is likened to a blacksmith forging a blade, repeatedly subjecting it to heat and hammering, each time making it sharper and more resilient.

In the context of resistance training, progressive overload can be achieved in various ways:

Incremental Weight Increases: Incremental weight increases are the most straightforward method, which involves gradually adding more weight to your exercises. As your muscles adapt to a particular weight, they introduce a slightly heavier load which forces them to work harder, triggering growth.

Volume Manipulation: This refers to the total amount of work done in a training session, typically calculated as sets multiplied by repetitions. By increasing the number of sets or reps, you can enhance the muscle's time under tension, a crucial factor for hypertrophy.

Intensity Modulation: Intensity doesn't just refer to the weight lifted but also the effort expended in each set. Pushing a set to its limit, or near failure, can be a potent stimulus for muscle growth, even if the weight isn't maximal.

Altering Rest Periods: Shortening or occasionally lengthening rest intervals can change the muscle's metabolic response, potentially enhancing hypertrophic outcomes.

Exercise Tempo: The speed at which exercises are performed, especially the eccentric (or lowering) phase, can significantly influence muscle tension and, consequently, growth.

As one progresses in their training journey, the importance of listening to one's body becomes paramount. While the principle of progressive overload is foundational, it must be applied judiciously, to ensure that progression doesn't come at the expense of form or lead to injury. Balancing ambition with prudence, and challenge with recovery, is the art and science of effective resistance training.

Exercise Selection and Variation: The Art of Targeting

Importance of Targeting Different Muscle Groups: In the development of muscle, each muscle group plays a unique and vital role. Just as a maestro ensures every instrument contributes to the harmony, so must an individual ensure that every muscle group is given its due attention in the gym.

Holistic Development: Focusing on a comprehensive workout routine ensures that every muscle, from the major groups to the stabilizers, is developed. This not only enhances overall aesthetics but also ensures functional strength. For instance, while the quadriceps might be the star of the show during a squat, the stabilizing role of the core and the glutes cannot be overlooked.

Injury Prevention: Muscle imbalances, often a result of neglecting certain groups, can lead to postural issues and increase the risk of injuries. For example, overdeveloping the chest while neglecting the upper back can lead to a hunched posture.

Enhanced Performance: A well-rounded muscle development ensures better performance in physical activities, be it sports or daily tasks. Strong legs are important for running and jumping, but a robust core and upper body enhance balance and power.

Overcoming Plateaus: Introducing variations in exercises can shock the muscles, and push them out of their comfort zone. This can be particularly beneficial when one hits a challenge in their training progress.

Mental Engagement: A varied routine keeps things interesting. The excitement of trying a new exercise or challenging a different muscle group can reignite passion and motivation, essential for long-term adherence to a fitness regimen.

In essence, while every muscle might have its moment of glory, it's the collective effort of all muscle groups that leads to true physical prowess. By embracing variation and ensuring a holistic approach to exercise selection, one paves the way for balanced growth, peak performance, and a body that's not just pleasing but also functionally formidable.

Differences Between Sarcoplasmic and Myofibrillar Hypertrophy

The human muscle is wonderful, capable of adapting and growing in response to various stimuli. One of the primary ways this adaptability manifests is through changes in muscle size and composition, driven by different types of hypertrophy. Understanding the nuances between sarcoplasmic and myofibrillar hypertrophy can guide training decisions and help individuals direct their workouts to achieve specific goals.

Sarcoplasmic Hypertrophy: The Pursuit of Size

- **Nature of Growth:** Sarcoplasmic hypertrophy, as the name suggests, revolves around the sarcoplasm – the semi-fluid substance inside the muscle cell. When we talk about this kind of hypertrophy, we're referring to an expansion in the volume of this fluid, which contains elements like water, glycogen, and other substrates. What is then the result? It produces muscles that look fuller and more voluminous. However, it's crucial to note that the increase in muscle size, does not result in the density of muscle contractile proteins (actin and myosin). Hence, the strength gains might not be as pronounced as the size gains.
- **Training for Sarcoplasmic Growth:** Achieving sarcoplasmic hypertrophy isn't about lifting the heaviest weights in the gym. Instead, it's about volume and metabolic stress.

Therefore, exercises should be structured around higher repetitions, often in the range of 10-15 reps, sometimes, even going up to 20 reps for certain exercises. The idea is to engorge the muscle with blood, creating that 'pump' sensation. The chosen weights should be challenging enough that the final repetitions of each set are tough to complete, but not so heavy that form is compromised. Shorter rest intervals, typically ranging from 30 seconds to 90 seconds, further amplify the metabolic stress, pushing the muscle to its limits and promoting the expansion of the sarcoplasm.

- **Benefits:** For those looking to achieve that 'bodybuilder' look, sarcoplasmic hypertrophy is often the goal. The increased muscle volume gives a pronounced and aesthetic appearance, making muscles look fuller, especially under stage lights or in photographs. But it's not just about looks. The increased sarcoplasmic volume also means a greater storage capacity for energy substrates like glycogen, enhancing endurance. This can be particularly beneficial for athletes in sports that require sustained muscle contractions over long periods.

In Conclusion Sarcoplasmic hypertrophy offers a blend of aesthetic and functional benefits. While it might not provide the raw strength associated with myofibrillar hypertrophy, its contribution to muscle endurance and the coveted 'pumped' appearance makes it a vital component in the toolkit of many athletes and bodybuilders.

Myofibrillar Hypertrophy: The Quest for Strength

- **Nature of Growth:** Diving deep into the muscle fiber, we find the myofibrils – the contractile fibers in muscle cells responsible for muscle contraction. Myofibrillar hypertrophy is centered on these myofibrils. Unlike its sarcoplasmic counterpart, which focuses on volume, myofibrillar hypertrophy zeroes in on muscle density. It involves an increase in the size and number of these contractile proteins, specifically actin and myosin. The result is a muscle that's not just bigger, but denser and more capable of generating force.

- **Training for Myofibrillar Growth:** Building dense, powerful muscles requires a different approach to training. The emphasis here is on lifting heavy objects. Exercises should be structured around lower repetitions, usually in the range of 1-6 reps. This doesn't mean doing just one repetition and calling it a day. Instead, it's about performing multiple sets with weights that challenge the muscle to its maximum, where even six repetitions feel like a monumental task. Given the intensity of these sets, rest intervals are longer, often ranging from 2 to 5 minutes, ensuring the muscle and nervous system adequately recover before the next set.

- **Benefits:** Myofibrillar hypertrophy is beneficial to those who prioritize strength over size. Powerlifters, who aim to lift the heaviest weights possible in exercises like the squat, bench press, and deadlift, train specifically for this type of hypertrophy. Olympic weightlifters, who perform complex lifts like the snatch and clean and jerk, also benefit from the enhanced force production that comes with denser muscles. But it's not just limited to weightlifting; athletes in sports like sprinting, football, or any discipline where bursts of raw power are essential, often have training regimens to promote myofibrillar growth. The result is a physique that's not just about the show, but predominantly about go – muscles that deliver on the promise of strength and power.

In conclusion, myofibrillar hypertrophy underscores the principle that not all muscle growth is the same. While it might not offer the 'pumped' appearance associated with sarcoplasmic hypertrophy, its contributions to functional strength are unparalleled. For those on a quest for raw power, understanding and training for myofibrillar hypertrophy is a game-changer.

Striking a Balance: The Dual Path to Muscle Mastery

In muscle building, there's no one-size-fits-all approach. While the allure of bulging muscles might draw some to sarcoplasmic hypertrophy, and the raw power associated with myofibrillar hypertrophy might appeal to others, the truth is that the most well-rounded physiques and functional bodies often benefit from a blend of both.

Periodization: The Art of Muscle Cycling

Periodization is a structured approach to training that cycles through different phases, each with its own emphasis. By systematically varying the focus between muscle endurance (higher reps, lower weight) and muscle strength (lower reps, higher weight), one can tap into the benefits of both sarcoplasmic and myofibrillar hypertrophy.

For instance, an individual might spend a few weeks focusing on higher repetition workouts, emphasizing muscle endurance and promoting sarcoplasmic growth. This could be followed by a phase centered on lifting heavier weights with fewer repetitions, targeting myofibrillar hypertrophy. Such cyclical training not only ensures comprehensive muscle development but also keeps the training regimen fresh and challenging. It reduces the risk of overtraining specific muscle fibers and offers the body a chance to recover and adapt.

Benefits of a Balanced Approach: A dual focus on both types of hypertrophy offers several advantages:

1. **Comprehensive Muscle Development:** By targeting both the fluid and contractile components of the muscle, one can achieve a physique that's both pleasing and functionally powerful.

2. **Versatility:** Whether it's lifting heavy objects, engaging in endurance activities, or participating in sports that require a mix of strength and stamina, a balanced muscle development approach prepares the body for varied physical challenges.

3. **Prevention of Plateaus:** Different training stimuli keep the muscles guessing, thereby reducing the likelihood of hitting growth risks. It ensures that the body doesn't adapt too comfortably to one type of stimulus, which can stagnate progress.

Engaging Training for Desired Outcomes: Understanding the differences between these two types of hypertrophy allows individuals to direct their training regimens to their specific goals. For instance, someone who aims to build body competition might focus more on sarcoplasmic hypertrophy in the months leading up to the event. In contrast, an athlete preparing for powerlifting would prioritize myofibrillar hypertrophy.

Muscle growth is a process, influenced by training parameters, nutrition, genetics, and more. By understanding the underlying mechanisms of sarcoplasmic and myofibrillar hypertrophy, individuals can make informed decisions about their training, ensuring they're moving closer to their goals with each rep and set.

Rest and Recovery: The Pillars of Progress

Talking about fitness, much emphasis is placed on the intensity, duration, and type of workouts. However, what happens outside the gym is equally, if not more important. Rest and recovery are the heroes of muscle development, often overshadowed by the allure of relentless training. Yet, without them, the journey to muscle hypertrophy would be fraught with setbacks and stagnation.

The Recovery Phase: More Than Just Downtime

Nature of Recovery

The recovery phase isn't merely a period where the body is inactive. It's a dynamic process where the body gets to work repairing and rebuilding. Let's think of it as the body's response team arriving at the scene after a rigorous workout, patching up the damage, and fortifying the structure.

Microtears: The Precursors of Progress

Contrary to initial impressions, microtears are not the enemy. They are, in fact, the harbingers of growth. Each resistance training session, with its myriad lifts, pulls, and pushes, inflicts these tiny tears on our muscle fibers. But it's this very damage that signals the body to initiate repair mechanisms, leading to stronger, more robust muscle tissue.

Energy Restoration

In muscle recovery, while the repair of muscle fibers often takes center stage, another equally crucial process unfolds in the wings known as the restoration of energy. This process is paramount, ensuring that the body is not just repaired, but also recharged and ready to tackle the next physical challenge.

The Body's Adaptive Response

The human body is molded to adapt to changes. When subjected to the stresses of resistance training, it doesn't merely restore the muscle to its previous state. Instead, it fortifies it, and prepares it for future challenges. This adaptive response ensures that with consistent training, the muscle becomes increasingly resilient, allowing for progressive overload and continuous growth.

The Importance of Adequate Recovery

Systemic Recovery

While the spotlight often shines on muscle recovery after exercise, there's a broader, more encompassing process at play. Systemic recovery delves into the holistic rejuvenation of the whole body system, and ensures that every component, from the cardiovascular system to the nervous system, is restored and rebalanced after strenuous activity. It's this all-encompassing approach that guarantees sustained optimal performance and overall well-being.

- **Optimizing Muscle Growth:** Muscle doesn't grow during the workout; it grows afterward. By ensuring adequate recovery, one maximizes the potential for muscle hypertrophy.

- **Beyond Muscles:** Recovery isn't just about muscles. Intense training also impacts the nervous system, joints, and connective tissues. Adequate rest ensures that these systems have time to recuperate, maintaining optimal function and reducing injury risk.

- **Mental Refreshment:** Mental fatigue can be as infirmous as physical exhaustion. Rest days provide a mental break from the rigors of training, allowing for psychological rejuvenation.

Avoiding Overtraining:

- **Symptoms and Setbacks:** Overtraining, or the state of training beyond the body's ability to recover, can manifest in various ways such as persistent fatigue, decreased performance, increased susceptibility to injuries, sleep disturbances, and even mood swings.

- **The Importance of Listening to the Body:** While structured recovery days are essential, it's also crucial to listen to the body's signals. If muscles are sore beyond the usual post-workout ache or if there's a general feeling of tiredness, it might be wise to take an additional rest day.

Active Recovery:

During fitness and training, there's a common misconception that recovery equates to complete inactivity. However, the concept of active recovery challenges this notion, emphasizing the benefits of purposeful, gentle movement even during "rest" days. Active recovery bridges the gap between intense training sessions, ensuring that the body and mind remain on good terms. It's a reminder that sometimes, the gentlest activities can offer the most profound benefits.

- **Purposeful Movement:** Recovery doesn't always mean complete rest. Engaging in low-intensity activities like walking, stretching, or yoga can promote adequate blood flow, alleviate muscle stiffness, and speed up the healing process without tasking the body.

In conclusion, the path to muscle growth is a delicate balance of stress and rest. While training provides the stimulus for growth, it's during recovery that the body capitalizes on this stimulus. Embracing the dual importance of training and recovery ensures a journey marked by consistent progress, minimal setbacks, and a deep respect for the body's innate wisdom.

Role of Diet in Muscle Repair and Growth

Muscles aren't just built in the gym; they're also forged in the kitchen. Nutrition plays a vital role in muscle repair, recovery, and growth. A caloric surplus, where one consumes more calories than one burns is often essential for significant muscle growth. Moreover, the quality of these calories matters. A balanced intake of proteins, carbohydrates, and fats ensures that the muscles receive all the necessary nutrients for optimal growth. While the gym provides the stimulus for muscle growth, the kitchen determines the magnitude of that growth. A strategic approach to nutrition, understanding the roles of macronutrients and micronutrients, and recognizing the importance of a caloric surplus, can make the difference between modest gains and transformative growth.

Muscle growth is a journey that intertwines the realms of physiology, nutrition, and dedication. It's not just about the weights lifted or the repetitions completed; it's about the cellular responses, the harmony of metabolic processes, and the recovery cycles. Every meal consumed, every night's rest, and even the moments of intentional rest contribute to growth. The intensity of a workout, the quality of nutrients ingested, the adequacy of sleep, and the mindfulness of recovery all converge to influence the outcome. It's a delicate balance of strain and rest, challenge and recovery, discipline and patience. By delving deep into each influencing factor and harmonizing them, individuals can craft a journey of muscle development that's not just about size, but also about strength, health, and overall well-being.

The Role of Protein Synthesis and Breakdown in Muscle Growth

Muscle growth is a captivating process, a harmonious blend of creation and destruction, building and breaking. At the heart of this process lie two primary actors: protein synthesis and protein breakdown. Like two dancers on a stage, they move in tandem, their actions and reactions setting the pace for muscle development, repair, and overall health. This process is not just about the physical act of building muscle; it's a reflection of the body's ability to adapt, recover, and evolve. Understanding these processes, the science that underpins them, and the factors that can either enhance or hinder their optimal performance are important.

The Protein Creation Synthesis

Protein synthesis is akin to a master craftsman at work, carefully constructing new proteins to replace old ones or to accommodate increased demands. Every time we engage in activities that stress our muscles, like resistance training, we create a demand. Protein synthesis responds, by building new muscle proteins to repair the damage and, ideally, making the muscle stronger in anticipation of future stressors. This process is the essence of muscle growth and adaptation.

The Necessary Balance of Protein Breakdown

On the other side is protein breakdown, and the process responsible for degrading and recycling old or damaged proteins. Protein breakdown refines and reshapes our muscles, ensuring they function optimally. While it might seem counterintuitive, this process of breaking down is just as crucial as building up. It ensures that our muscles are not bogged down by damaged or non-functional proteins.

The Delicacy of Balancing Synthesis and Breakdown

The relationship between protein synthesis and breakdown is a delicate balance, a seesaw that determines the fate of our muscles. When synthesis exceeds breakdown, we experience muscle growth. When breakdown overshadows synthesis, we face muscle loss. The goal for many, especially those aiming for muscle growth, is to tip this balance in favor of synthesis, ensuring consistent muscle growth.

In our body, protein synthesis and breakdown are not mere background players; they play very crucial roles. Their performance, influenced by factors like nutrition, training, and recovery, dictates muscle health and growth. As we examine muscle physiology deeper, understanding the relationship between these two processes offers a foundation to make informed decisions, optimize training outcomes, and truly appreciate the mystery that is muscle growth.

Protein Synthesis: The Architect of Muscle Growth

- **Definition:** Protein synthesis is the cellular process of constructing new proteins. It can be likened to a construction site where raw materials (amino acids) are assembled, following the blueprint (mRNA) to build structures (proteins).
- **Importance:** In muscle health, protein synthesis is akin to the architect of growth. Every time we engage in activities that stress our muscles, microtears occur. Protein synthesis steps in, to repair these tears, add a bit extra, and fortify the muscle against future stress. This continuous cycle of damage and repair, underpinned by protein synthesis, is the essence of muscle adaptation and growth.
- **Activation:** The spark that ignites the protein synthesis machinery can come from various sources. Resistance training, for instance, sends a powerful signal to the muscles, emphasizing the need for repair and growth. Nutritionally, consuming essential amino acids, especially leucine, acts as a key that unlocks the protein

synthesis process. Additionally, hormones like insulin and growth hormone play pivotal roles in modulating and enhancing protein synthesis.

Muscle Protein Breakdown: The Sculptor of Muscle Health

- **Definition:** Muscle protein breakdown is the systematic process where old, damaged, or surplus proteins are broken down into their constituent amino acids. These amino acids can then be recycled within the muscle or transported to the liver.
- **Importance:** At first glance, breaking down muscle protein might seem like a step backward. However, this process is more of a molder than a demolisher. By removing damaged or non-functional proteins, muscle protein breakdown ensures the muscle's integrity and functionality. It's a refining process, removing the unnecessary ones, and ensuring that the muscle remains a masterpiece of efficiency and strength.
- **Triggers:** Several factors can accelerate muscle protein breakdown such as prolonged periods of inactivity, like bed rest, which can signal the body to degrade muscle protein, leading to muscle atrophy. Also, nutritional deficits, especially a lack of essential amino acids, can ramp up protein breakdown. Certain conditions or illnesses, like chronic infections, severe burns, or specific hormonal imbalances, can contribute to muscle protein breakdown rates.

In muscle health, protein synthesis, and breakdown are two sides of the same coin: one builds, the other refines. Together, they ensure that our muscles remain robust, functional, and ever-adapting to the challenges we throw their way.

Factors Influencing Protein Synthesis and Breakdown

Adequate Protein Intake: The Cornerstone of Muscle Growth

- **Definition:** Protein intake refers to the amount of protein an individual consumes through dietary sources.

- **Significance:** Protein is more than just a macronutrient; it's the primary raw material for muscle repair and growth. By taking protein adequately, we provide our muscles with a steady supply of amino acids, which are the building blocks necessary for protein synthesis.

- **Optimal Sources:** High-quality protein is obtained from lean meats, dairy, eggs, legumes, and plant-based proteins like quinoa and tofu.

Essential Amino Acids

- **Definition:** These are essential molecules that the body cannot produce on its own and must be obtained through the diet.

- **Significance:** Essential amino acids, especially leucine, play a crucial role in initiating the protein production machinery. Without them, the process can be interrupted, regardless of other favorable conditions.

- **Sources:** Foods rich in essential amino acids include meats, dairy, eggs, and certain plant-based foods like soy.

Nutrient Timing: The Strategic Consumption

- **Definition:** Nutrient timing involves consuming specific nutrients, like protein, at strategic times to boost physiological responses.

- **Significance:** After exercise, there's a heightened sensitivity to protein intake, often termed the 'anabolic window'. Consuming protein during this period can amplify the muscle protein synthesis response, optimizing recovery and growth.

- **Recommendation:** Aim to consume a protein-rich meal or shake within 1-2 hours post-exercise.

Resistance Training

- **Definition:** Resistance training is an exercise that makes muscles work against a weight or force.

- **Significance:** Resistance training acts as a potent stimulus for muscle protein synthesis. By inducing microtrauma in muscle fibers, it signals the need for repair, setting the stage for growth.

- **Recommendation:** Incorporate compound movements like squats, deadlifts, and bench presses, which engage multiple muscle groups, for optimal muscle stimulation.

Sleep/Recovery

- **Definition:** Sleep is the restorative period where the body undergoes repair, recovery, and growth.

- **Significance:** During deep sleep, the body enters a heightened state of recovery. Also, growth hormone releases peaks, further accelerating protein synthesis and muscle repair.

- **Recommendation:** Aim for 7-9 hours of quality sleep nightly. Consider practices like meditation, reading, or a nighttime routine to improve sleep quality.

In essence, the journey of muscle growth is a harmonious interplay of various factors. From the food on our plate to the weights we lift and the sleep we cherish, each element plays a pivotal role in muscle protein synthesis and breakdown. By understanding and optimizing these factors, we can develop a physique that's not just pleasing but also a testament to our health and vitality.

The relationship between protein synthesis and breakdown is at the heart of muscle growth and health. By understanding and optimizing the factors that influence these processes, one can create an environment conducive to muscle development and longevity.

Hormonal Influences on Muscle Growth

In muscle growth, if the muscles themselves are the instruments, hormones are the conductors. These biochemical messengers play a pivotal role in orchestrating the myriad processes that culminate in muscle hypertrophy. This section delves into the key hormones that influence muscle growth, shedding light on their roles, production mechanisms, and the factors that can optimize their levels.

Testosterone: The Anabolic Maestro of Muscle Development

During muscle growth, testosterone stands tall as a key player, often hailed as the 'king' of anabolic hormones. Its influence on muscle development, strength, and overall physical performance is profound, making it a focal point of interest for athletes, bodybuilders, and anyone keen on building their muscles.

Role in Muscle Development and Beyond

Testosterone, commonly associated with male virility and vitality, is more than just a hormone that defines masculinity. Its anabolic properties make it a cornerstone for muscle development. Here's how:

- **Protein Synthesis:** Testosterone enhances the body's ability to build proteins, the primary building blocks of muscle. This means that with adequate testosterone levels, the muscle repair and rebuilding process post-exercise is more efficient.

- **Inhibition of Protein Breakdown:** While promoting protein synthesis, testosterone also acts to reduce protein degradation. This dual action ensures that the balance is directed in favor of muscle growth.

- **Satellite Cell Activation:** Satellite cells are often termed the 'reserve cells' of muscles. Testosterone can activate these cells, which then contribute additional nuclei to muscle fibers, aiding in repair and growth.

The Production Centers: While testosterone is synonymous with males, it's essential to understand that it's present in both genders, albeit in different concentrations.

- **In Males:** The testes are the primary production centers, responsible for the bulk of testosterone production.

- **In Females:** The ovaries produce testosterone, but in much smaller quantities compared to males. This is why females naturally have a lower muscle mass compared to their male counterparts.

- **Adrenal Glands:** Both genders also produce small amounts of testosterone in their adrenal glands, which sit atop the kidneys.

Factors Modulating Testosterone Levels

Testosterone levels aren't static; they can fluctuate based on various internal and external factors such as:

- **Age:** Testosterone levels peak during adolescence and early adulthood; at post adulthood, there's a gradual decline, especially after the age of 30.

- **Diet:** Certain nutrients, like zinc and vitamin D, can influence and boost testosterone production. A well-balanced diet rich in these nutrients can support optimal levels.

- **Sleep:** Quality sleep is crucial for testosterone production. Chronic sleep deprivation can lead to reduced levels of testosterone.

- **Stress:** Chronic stress, and the consequent elevated cortisol levels, can negatively impact testosterone production.

- **Exercise:** Resistance training, especially compound movements like squats and deadlifts, can lead to short-term spikes in testosterone levels. However, overtraining without adequate recovery can have the opposite effect.

Generally, testosterone is a pivotal hormone in the muscle growth equation. By understanding its role, production, and the factors that influence its levels, individuals can make informed choices, be it in training, nutrition, or lifestyle, to boost their muscle growth potential.

Growth Hormone (GH): The Repair and Regrowth Maestro

Growth hormone, often shrouded in mystery and intrigue, is a pivotal player in the body's growth and repair mechanisms. While its name might suggest a singular focus on growth, its roles are diverse, touching various facets of metabolism, repair, and overall health. In the context of muscle development, growth hormone emerges as a key player, ensuring that muscles not only grow but also repair efficiently.

Role in Muscle Development and Beyond

Growth hormone's influence on muscle development is both direct and indirect, making it a central figure in the anabolic processes.

- **Protein Synthesis:** Growth hormone directly stimulates the production of proteins in muscle, ensuring that the building blocks of muscle are laid down efficiently after exercise.

- **Fat Metabolism:** One of growth hormone's standout roles is its ability to mobilize and burn fat stores. This not only aids in achieving a lean physique but also ensures that muscles are well-defined.

- **Stimulation of IGF-1 Production:** IGF-1, or Insulin-like Growth Factor-1, is a hormone that works in tandem with growth hormone. As a potent anabolic agent, it is produced in the liver in response to GH, and IGF-1, and further amplifies the muscle-building effects of growth hormone.

The Production Epicenter: The body's endocrine system works wonders with various glands producing a plethora of hormones. For growth hormone, the production center is the anterior pituitary gland, a pea-sized gland located at the base of the brain. This gland releases growth hormone in pulses, with the most significant pulse typically occurring shortly after the onset of deep sleep.

Factors Modulating GH Release: The release of growth hormone isn't constant; it's influenced by many factors, some within our control and others not.

- **Sleep:** The relationship between sleep and growth hormone is profound. The deep stages of sleep, particularly the first deep sleep cycle of the night, witness the most significant growth hormone release. This underscores the importance of quality sleep for muscle repair and growth.

- **Exercise:** Physical activity, especially high-intensity workouts or resistance training, can lead to acute spikes in growth hormone levels. This is one of the reasons exercise is so beneficial for overall health and muscle development.

- **Nutrition:** Certain amino acids, like arginine and lysine, when consumed, can stimulate growth hormone release. This has led to interest in amino acid supplementation among athletes and bodybuilders.

- **Fasting and Nutrient Deprivation:** Short-term fasting or periods of low blood sugar can stimulate growth hormone release. This is the body's adaptive response, ensuring that muscle tissue is preserved even in the absence of adequate nutrition.

In conclusion, growth hormone is a cornerstone in the process of muscle development. Its roles are diverse, touching upon growth, repair, and metabolism. By understanding its functions, production, and the factors that modulate its release, individuals can make informed decisions in their training, nutrition, and recovery strategies to harness the full potential of growth hormone.

Insulin-like Growth Factor-1 (IGF-1): The Anabolic Maestro of Muscle Development

In the hormones that influence muscle growth, Insulin-like Growth Factor-1 (IGF-1) stands out as a skilled performer. Its role in muscle development is profound; it acts as a bridge between the initial stimulus of growth (like resistance training) and the actual process of muscle protein synthesis. Let's delve deeper into the multifaceted world of IGF-1 and its significance in muscle growth.

The Anabolic Role of IGF-1: IGF-1's influence on muscle is both direct and indirect, which makes it a central figure in the muscle-building process.

- **Muscle Protein Synthesis:** IGF-1 directly stimulates the synthesis of proteins in muscle cells, ensuring that the building blocks of muscle are laid down efficiently after a workout.

- **Cell Proliferation and Differentiation:** IGF-1 promotes the proliferation of satellite cells, which are essential for muscle repair and growth. These cells, once activated, can differentiate and fuse with muscle fibers, aiding in muscle hypertrophy.

- **Anti-Catabolic Effects:** Apart from its muscle-building properties, IGF-1 also has anti-catabolic effects. It helps in reducing protein breakdown, ensuring that the hard-earned muscle is preserved.

The Production Hub: While many hormones have a direct link to the tissues they influence, IGF-1's production is a bit more indirect. It's primarily produced in the liver in response to growth hormone (GH) stimulation. This makes IGF-1 a secondary responder, coming into play after the growth hormone has set the stage.

Factors Modulating IGF-1 Release: The release and production of IGF-1 are influenced by many factors, some of which are within our control.

- **Growth Hormone (GH):** Since growth hormone stimulates IGF-1 production, anything that boosts growth hormone levels, like deep sleep or resistance training, will indirectly enhance IGF-1 levels.

- **Nutrition:** Amino acids, especially essential ones, play a role in modulating IGF-1 levels. Leucine, in particular, has been shown to stimulate IGF-1 production.

- **Age:** IGF-1 levels are highest during the growth spurts of puberty and gradually decrease with age.

- **Other Hormones:** Insulin, another anabolic hormone, can influence IGF-1 levels. Proper carbohydrate intake after a workout can lead to insulin release, which might synergize with IGF-1's anabolic effects.

In conclusion, IGF-1 is a linchpin in the muscle development process. Its roles are diverse, touching upon growth, repair, and even preservation of muscle tissue. By understanding its functions, production, and the factors that modulate its release, individuals can make informed decisions in their training and nutrition strategies to harness the full potential of IGF-1.

Estrogen: The Underappreciated Architect of Muscle

Often overshadowed by its more talked-about counterparts like testosterone and growth hormone, estrogen plays a subtle yet significant role in muscle health and development. While it's primarily recognized for its role in female reproductive health, estrogen's influence extends to various physiological processes, including those related to muscle growth and repair.

Role in Muscle Health and Development

- **Muscle Repair and Recovery:** Estrogen has anti-inflammatory properties, which can aid in muscle recovery post-exercise. By modulating the inflammatory response, estrogen can potentially reduce muscle soreness and expedite the repair process.

- **Protection Against Muscle Damage:** Some studies suggest that estrogen can reduce muscle damage caused by intense exercise. This protective effect might be one reason why females often experience less muscle soreness than males after similar workouts.

- **Muscle Metabolism:** Estrogen influences how muscles use energy substrates. It can enhance the use of fats as an energy source during exercise, potentially preserving muscle glycogen stores.

- **Bone Health:** While not directly related to muscle, it's worth noting that estrogen plays a crucial role in maintaining bone density. Strong bones provide a robust framework for muscles, and any compromise in bone health can indirectly affect muscular strength and function.

Production and Sources

- **Ovaries:** In females, the primary source of estrogen is the ovaries. Levels fluctuate throughout the menstrual cycle, with a peak around ovulation.

- **Adipose Tissue:** Both males and females produce estrogen in adipose (fat) tissues. This production becomes especially significant in postmenopausal women, where the ovaries significantly reduce estrogen output.

- **Testes:** In males, the testes produce small amounts of estrogen, which is essential for modulating libido, erectile function, and spermatogenesis.

Factors Influencing Estrogen Levels

- **Age:** Estrogen levels peak during the reproductive years and decline during menopause.

- **Body Fat:** Since adipose tissue can produce estrogen, individuals with higher body fat percentages might have elevated estrogen levels.

- **Diet and Lifestyle:** Certain foods, like soy products, contain phytoestrogens, which can influence estrogen activity. Additionally, lifestyle factors like stress, exercise, and alcohol consumption can modulate estrogen levels.

In conclusion, its role in muscle health and development is multifaceted. Estrogen proves itself as a key player in the muscle growth narrative by supporting muscle recovery, protecting against damage, and influencing muscle metabolism. Recognizing and appreciating its role can lead to more holistic training and recovery strategies, especially for female athletes.

Multifactorial Effects of Hormones on Muscle Hypertrophy

The human body is an interconnected system, and when it comes to muscle growth, the hormonal system stands at the forefront. Each hormone, while having its distinct role, doesn't work in isolation. Instead, they weave complex interactions that collectively influence muscle growth.

Synergistic Interactions

- **Testosterone and IGF-1:** While testosterone sets the stage for an anabolic environment, IGF-1 takes it a step further by directly stimulating protein synthesis and activating satellite cells. The combined action of these two hormones can lead to more pronounced muscle growth than either would achieve individually.

- **Growth Hormone and Fat Metabolism:** The growth hormone's ability to promote fat metabolism means that as muscles grow, they do so with a leaner composition. This lean muscle growth is not just pleasing but also functionally beneficial, as it can lead to improved muscle definition and strength without unnecessary bulk.

- **Estrogen and Muscle Recovery:** The anti-inflammatory properties of estrogen can enhance the muscle recovery process, ensuring that the muscle is primed for growth after each training session. When combined with the anabolic effects of other hormones, this can lead to more efficient muscle development cycles.

- **Hormonal Feedback Loops:** It's also worth noting that the body's hormonal system operates on feedback loops. For instance, elevated levels of one hormone might suppress the production of another. This delicate balance ensures that muscle growth is regulated and sustainable.

Optimizing the Hormonal Environment: Diet, exercise, sleep, and stress management are all pivotal in modulating the body's hormonal environment. For instance, resistance training can boost testosterone and growth hormone levels, while adequate sleep can optimize the release of most growth-related hormones. Consuming a protein-rich diet can support the anabolic actions of hormones, ensuring that the muscle has the necessary building blocks for growth.

Muscle growth is not just about lifting weights; it's about understanding and harnessing the body's internal hormonal elements. Each hormone plays its part, and their collective performance dictates the pace and quality of muscle growth. By recognizing the multifactorial effects of hormones and channeling lifestyle and training choices accordingly, one can truly master the art and science of muscle development.

The Impact of Genetic Factors on Muscle Growth

Muscle growth is a fascinating interplay between the genes we inherit and the environment we create for our bodies. While the dedication we pour into our workouts, the nutrition we prioritize, and the recovery we ensure are pivotal, our genetic code lays the foundational framework. This section takes a deeper look into the genetic determinants of muscle growth, shedding light on how our DNA can influence our muscle-building journey and how we can harness this knowledge for optimal results.

Muscle Fiber Type Composition: The Genetic Spectrum of Strength and Stamina

- **Overview:** Every muscle in our body is a mosaic of type I (slow-twitch) and type II (fast-twitch) fibers. While type I fibers excel in endurance and are fatigue-resistant, type II fibers are powerhouses designed for short bursts of strength and speed.

- **Genetic Influence:** Our genes largely dictate the ratio of these fiber types. Thanks to their genetic endowment, some individuals might naturally possess a higher percentage of type I fibers, predisposing them to excel in endurance sports like marathon running. Conversely, those with a genetic tilt towards type II fibers might find themselves naturally adept at powerlifting or sprinting.

Hormone Receptor Density

- **Role:** Let's think of hormone receptors as molecular docking stations on muscle cells. They allow hormones, the body's chemical messengers, to bind and relay signals that stimulate muscle growth.

- **Genetic Influence:** The number and sensitivity of these receptors can vary among individuals due to genetic variations. Given the enhanced hormonal signaling, those blessed with a higher density or more sensitive receptors might experience more pronounced muscle growth in response to training.

Metabolic Factors: Genetic Tuning of the Muscle's Metabolism

- **Overview:** Our muscles' metabolic machinery, comprising enzymes, energy pathways, and nutrient transport systems, fuels every contraction and supports growth.

- **Genetic Influence:** Genetic variations can influence the efficiency of these metabolic processes. For instance, an individual might genetically have a more efficient ATP production pathway, allowing for better performance during high-intensity workouts.

Harnessing Genetic Potential

Understanding one's genetic predispositions can be empowering. It offers a roadmap, guiding training, and nutritional strategies. For instance, someone with a genetic inclination towards type I fibers might benefit from periodized training, incorporating both endurance and strength phases. Similarly, understanding one's metabolic genetic makeup can guide nutritional choices, ensuring that the muscle gets the right ingredient at the right time.

Our genes set the stage, but our actions determine the play. While genetics can provide insights and set certain boundaries, the potential within these boundaries is vast. We can navigate our genetic landscape, maximizing muscle growth and achieving our top fitness with informed choices, consistent effort, and a dash of patience.

Conclusion: Navigating the Path to Peak Muscle Potential

In muscle growth, understanding the many factors that influence muscle growth is akin to possessing a map. This map, detailed with the nuances of genetics, hormonal influences, and evidence-based practices, provides a clearer path toward our muscle-building goals.

Optimizing Genetic Predispositions

Every individual is bestowed with a unique genetic blueprint. While these genes set certain parameters, they are by no means a definitive fate. Instead, they offer a starting point, a baseline. With the right knowledge and strategies, we can optimize these predispositions, pushing the boundaries and tapping into the vast potential that lies within these genetic confines.

Evidence-Based Practices

In a world engulfed with myths and misconceptions about muscle building, turning to evidence-based practices is our watchword. Scientific research, empirical evidence, and time-tested strategies have provided us with reliable guidance. So, by aligning our training, nutrition, and recovery with these practices, we ensure that every drop of sweat, every meal, and every moment of rest propels us closer to our goals.

A Holistic Approach: Seeing the Forest for the Trees

Muscle growth is not just about lifting weights or consuming protein. It's a holistic process, interwoven with our biology, lifestyle, mindset, and even our emotions. Recognizing this interconnectedness allows us to adopt a comprehensive approach. It's about nurturing the body, challenging it, feeding it, resting it, and understanding it.

In essence, muscle growth is a testament to the body's remarkable adaptability and resilience. While the journey is complex, armed with knowledge, dedication, and a holistic perspective, we can go through the path to peak muscle potential, crafting physiques that are not only good but also formidable in function.

CHAPTER 5

EXERCISE AND MUSCLE GROWTH

In fitness and physical development, resistance training emerges as a strong pillar, supporting the aspirations of those seeking muscular growth and strength. It's more than just lifting weights or doing push-ups; it's a deliberate challenge posed to our muscles: a challenge that demands response, adaptation, and growth.

When we engage in resistance training, we're essentially having a dialogue with our muscles. We challenge them, and they respond. We push them to their limits, and they rebuild stronger, preparing for the next challenge. This cycle of stress, adaptation, and growth is the essence of enlargement. The microtears that occur during intense workouts might seem like setbacks, but they're the opposite. They're opportunities for muscles to rebuild, reinforce, and rise to greater heights.

But resistance training isn't a monolithic entity. It's a spectrum, a diverse range of exercises and modalities, each with its nuances, benefits, and considerations. From the raw power of weightlifting to the functional strength of bodyweight exercises, and the versatility of resistance bands, each form of resistance training contributes uniquely to muscle growth.

As we delve deeper into this chapter, we'll explore these varied forms, and understand their roles, benefits, and how they fit into the grand scheme of muscle development. Whether you're a seasoned athlete or a starter on your fitness journey, understanding the intricacies of resistance training is important in sculpting a physique that's not just aesthetically pleasing but also functionally formidable.

Definition and Importance of Resistance Training for Muscle Growth

Resistance training, at its essence, is a systematic approach to challenging the muscles, compelling them to adapt, strengthen, and grow. It's not just about moving weights or performing repetitions; it's about creating an environment where muscles are pushed beyond their comfort zones, prompting them to respond.

Defining Resistance Training: Resistance training is a form of exercise where muscles contract against an external force to enhance strength, tone, muscle mass, or endurance. The "resistance" part of the equation can be provided by various means – from the gravitational pull acting on dumbbells, barbells, or kettlebells, to the tension in resistance bands, or even the weight of one's own body when doing push-ups, squats, or pull-ups.

The Pivotal Role in Muscle Growth: The human body is remarkably adaptable. When subjected to challenges, it seeks to overcome them, to be better prepared for the next encounter. This is the foundational principle behind resistance training. When muscles face resistance, they experience microscopic tears. While this might sound dangerous, it's a natural and beneficial process. These micro tears signal the body to repair and reinforce the muscle fibers, making them thicker and stronger – a process we recognize as muscle growth or enlargement.

Moreover, resistance training doesn't just impact the muscles in isolation. It boosts bone density, enhances metabolic rate, improves insulin sensitivity, and fosters better physical functionality. It's a holistic approach to health, going beyond aesthetics.

The Symbiotic Relationship with Muscle Growth: Muscle growth isn't just about size; it's about strength, functionality, and resilience. Resistance training nurtures this growth, providing the stimulus muscles need to develop. Every rep, every set, and every session is a step towards a stronger version of oneself. Whether the goal is to lift heavier objects, run faster, jump higher, or simply lead a healthier life, resistance training is the bridge that connects ambition to reality.

In conclusion, resistance training is more than a component of a workout regimen; it's a catalyst for physical change. It's the challenge that muscles need, the stimulus that drives growth, and the foundation upon which physical strength and endurance are built.

The Evolution of Weightlifting: From the ancient Greeks lifting heavy stones to prove their physical prowess, to modern-day athletes hoisting barbells in state-of-the-art gyms, weightlifting has been a testament to human strength and determination. This age-long discipline has not only evolved in technique but also in its tools, transitioning from rudimentary objects to meticulously designed equipment.

Diving into the Types of Weightlifting--Free Weights: The Essence of Raw Strength

The Legacy: Tracing back to ancient civilizations, free weights have been an integral part of human strength training. From warriors preparing for battle to athletes competing in early Olympic games, the allure of lifting raw, unguided weight has been a timeless pursuit. Even today, amidst a sea of advanced gym machinery, the simplicity and effectiveness of free weights continue to captivate fitness enthusiasts worldwide.

Versatility in Motion: The world of free weights is vast and varied. Dumbbells, suitable for isolated and compound movements; barbells, perfect for heavy lifting and foundational exercises; kettlebells, offering a blend of strength and cardio with their unique design. The exercises one can perform with these tools are nearly limitless. Deadlifts, bench presses, kettlebell swings, and goblet squats - the list goes on, each exercise sculpting a different facet of our musculature.

Pros: One of the standout advantages of free weights is their unparalleled ability to simulate real-world movements. When you lift a dumbbell or a barbell, you're not just working on the target muscle. You're engaging a network of stabilizing muscles, enhancing balance, coordination, and overall functional fitness. This kind of training ensures that the strength gained in the gym translates seamlessly to daily activities, be it lifting a heavy box or playing a sport.

Cons: But this raw, unbridled strength training comes with its set of challenges. The very aspect that makes free weights so effective - their unguided nature also introduces an element of risk. Without proper form, the chances of strains, sprains, or more severe injuries rise significantly, especially when venturing into heavier weights, the margin for error narrows. It's a matter of strength and technique, where both must be in harmony for optimal results.

Machine Weights: Precision-Engineered Strength

The Evolution: In the ever-evolving world of fitness, machine weights represent the intersection of science, engineering, and biomechanics. These machines have become staples in gyms worldwide, offering precision-targeted workouts tailored to individual needs.

Purpose-Driven Design: Each machine is a testament to human ingenuity, meticulously designed to target specific muscle groups. The chest fly machine, for instance, isolates the pectoral muscles, ensuring they bear the brunt of the resistance. The hamstring curl machine, on the other hand, zeroes in on the back of the thighs. This specificity ensures that each workout is laser-focused, maximizing gains in the targeted area.

Pros: Machine weights democratize strength training. For those new to the world of lifting, the guided motion of machines offers a safe entry point, reducing the intimidation factor. The controlled movement path minimizes the risk of injury, allowing users to focus solely on muscle engagement. Additionally, for those recovering from injuries or with specific physical limitations, machines can offer a safer alternative to free weights.

Cons: Every coin has two sides. The very guidance that makes machine weights so beginner-friendly can also be their Achilles' heel. The fixed motion can sometimes bypass the engagement of stabilizing muscles, which are crucial for functional strength and injury prevention. Furthermore, since everyone's body is unique, the one-size-fits-all design of some machines might not accommodate every individual's biomechanics, potentially leading to discomfort or suboptimal muscle engagement.

In conclusion, the world of weightlifting is vast and varied, with each tool offering its unique set of advantages and challenges. Machine weights, with their precision engineering, have carved a niche for themselves, catering to both novices and seasoned lifters. As with any tool, the key lies in understanding its strengths and limitations, ensuring that every workout is not just effective but also safe.

Cable Machines: Dynamic Resistance and Versatility

Bridging the Gap: Cable machines represent a harmonious blend of the structured resistance of machine weights and the adaptable nature of free weights. Through a sophisticated system of pulleys, weights, and cables, they offer a unique resistance experience that's both controlled and versatile.

Endless Possibilities: One of the standout features of cable machines is their adaptability. With a simple adjustment of the pulley height or attachment, one can transition from a high-intensity cable crossover to a focused triceps extension. This adaptability ensures a comprehensive workout, targeting muscles from various angles and intensities.

Pros: The continuous tension provided by the cables is a game-changer. Unlike free weights, where tension can sometimes be lost at certain points in a lift, cables ensure that muscles remain engaged throughout the entire range of motion. This constant tension can lead to enhanced muscle activation and growth. Additionally, the semi-guided nature of cables offers a balance between structure and freedom, making them suitable for both beginners and seasoned lifters.

Cons: However, the versatility that makes cable machines so appealing can also be a double-edged sword. It's crucial to ensure that each movement is executed with proper form with so many possible exercises and adjustments. Incorrect usage cannot only diminish the effectiveness of the exercise but also pose a risk of strain or injury.

The realm of weightlifting is rich and diverse, with each piece of equipment adding its unique flavor to the mix. Cable machines, with their blend of structure and adaptability, have secured their place as a favorite among many. They remind us that the development of strength and growth is not just about the destination but also the diverse paths we can take to get there.

Bodyweight Exercises: Mastery Through Simplicity

Harnessing Inherent Strength: Bodyweight exercises are a testament to the power and potential of the human body. Without the need for external equipment, they challenge individuals to push, pull, and lift using nothing but their own mass, making every movement a direct dialogue between the individual and gravity.

The Essence of Functional Fitness: At the core of bodyweight exercises lies the principle of functional fitness. Movements like squats, push-ups, and lunges aren't just exercises; they're fundamental human motions. Training with bodyweight hones these natural movements, enhancing everyday performance and agility.

Pros: One of the most compelling attributes of bodyweight exercises is their unparalleled accessibility. Regardless of location, whether it's a hotel room, a park, or a living room, the opportunity for a robust workout is always at hand. This accessibility is complemented by the holistic engagement these exercises offer. Many of them are compound movements, meaning they engage multiple muscle groups simultaneously, ensuring a balanced workout and fostering harmonious muscle development. Furthermore, the inherent safety and scalability of bodyweight exercises cannot be overlooked. Without the addition of external weights, the risk of certain injuries is naturally reduced. Each exercise can also be tailored to match individual fitness levels, ensuring that both novices and seasoned practitioners find challenge and growth.

Cons: However, as with all things, bodyweight exercises come with their set of challenges. As one's strength and proficiency grow, the resistance offered by standard bodyweight exercises might plateau. To continue experiencing growth, one might need to delve into advanced variations or even consider integrating additional resistance. In addition, while bodyweight exercises can be comprehensive, they might not equally challenge all muscle groups. For instance, sculpting a robust back might require specific setups or additional tools, which can be a limitation for some.

Bodyweight exercises stand as a testament to the body's innate strength and capability. They serve as a reminder that viable workouts are always within reach, even without a gym or equipment. Individuals can leverage their weight to sculpt a physique that's both pleasing and functionally formidable through dedication, creativity, and a deep understanding of one's body.

Resistance Bands: Elasticity Meets Strength

Stretching the Limits: Resistance bands, with their simple yet effective design, have revolutionized the way we perceive resistance in workouts. These stretchable bands, ranging from light to heavy tension, offer a unique resistance experience, challenging muscles in ways traditional weights often can't.

Adaptable and Accessible: The beauty of resistance bands lies in their adaptability. Whether you're performing a bicep curl, a squat, or even a chest press, these bands can seamlessly integrate into the movement, adding that extra layer of challenge. Their lightweight and portable nature means that they can be a travel partner, ensuring that your workouts aren't confined to the four walls of a gym.

Pros: The versatility of resistance bands is truly commendable. They can amplify a bodyweight workout, assist in pull-ups, or even serve as the primary resistance in exercises. This adaptability is supported by the different resistances they offer; as the band stretches, the resistance increases, ensuring that muscles are engaged throughout the entire motion. This dynamic resistance can lead to enhanced muscle activation and growth. Furthermore, resistance bands are a boon for rehabilitation. Their gentle yet effective resistance is perfect for slowly building strength post-injury. For beginners or those intimidated by traditional gym equipment, resistance bands offer a welcoming entry point into the world of strength training.

Cons: While resistance bands are a valuable tool, they come with a set of considerations. Over time, they can wear out and potentially snap, so regular inspection is always required. Additionally, while they offer variable resistance, gauging the exact resistance can be challenging, especially when compared to the definitive weights of dumbbells or barbells. This ambiguity might make progression tracking a tad more complex.

Resistance bands, in their simplicity, encapsulate the essence of innovation in fitness. They remind us that strength training isn't just about heavy weights and machines but about challenging muscles in diverse ways. With a resistance band in hand, one is equipped with a tool that's as versatile as it is effective, paving the way for strength, flexibility, and resilience.

Conclusion for Resistance Training: The Symphony of Strength

Harmonizing Modalities: In resistance training, each modality - be it weightlifting, bodyweight exercises, or resistance bands - plays its distinct tune. But when harmonized, they create a rhythm of strength and growth that resonates with the body's innate potential.

The Power of Diversity: Just as a musician wouldn't rely on a single note to compose a masterpiece, fitness enthusiasts shouldn't confine themselves to one mode of resistance training. Weightlifting offers the raw power of lifting heavy, pushing one's limits in strength and endurance. Bodyweight exercises, on the other hand, bring in the element of functional fitness, enhancing agility, balance, and core strength. Resistance bands, with their unique elastic resistance, add a layer of dynamic tension, challenging muscles in ways traditional weights might not.

Crafting the Perfect Regimen: The key lies in understanding one's goals, strengths, and limitations. For someone aiming for sheer muscle size, weightlifting might take precedence, but integrating bodyweight exercises can ensure functional strength. Similarly, resistance bands can be a perfect tool for rehabilitation, muscle activation, or adding variety to routine workouts. By weaving these modalities into a cohesive training plan, one ensures that every muscle fiber, and every sinew is engaged, challenged, and nurtured.

Resistance training, in its varied forms, is a testament to the human body's adaptability and resilience. It's not about choosing one over the other but about integrating each, crafting a regimen that's as diverse as it is effective. In this holistic approach lies the promise of not just muscle growth but a journey of self-discovery, discipline, and unparalleled strength.

High-Intensity Interval Training (HIIT): The Powerhouse of Modern Fitness

In the ever-evolving world of fitness, HIIT has emerged as a shining star. It has captured the attention of fitness enthusiasts, athletes, and casual gym-goers alike with promises of rapid results in less time. But what lies beneath the hype? Let's dive deep into the world of HIIT.

Definition and Popularity of HIIT

High-Intensity Interval Training, or HIIT as it's widely recognized, is a distinctive approach to cardiovascular conditioning. It's structured around alternating cycles: intense, all-out bursts of activity are followed by shorter, more relaxed recovery phases or complete rest. This rhythm of pushing the body to its limits, only to let it catch its breath momentarily, is the essence of HIIT.

But what's behind its soaring popularity? For one, in our fast-paced world, time is a luxury. HIIT offers a solution to the time-crunched individual, delivering a potent workout in a fraction of the time traditional workouts might demand. Imagine achieving comparable, if not superior, results from a grueling hour-long session in just 20 minutes; that's the allure of HIIT. Furthermore, the claims of accelerated calorie burn, even post-workout, have drawn many to its fold, especially those on a weight loss journey. The blend of efficiency, effectiveness, and the sheer challenge it presents has positioned HIIT not just as a workout, but as a movement in the fitness realm

Principles of HIIT

Intensity: The Heartbeat of HIIT: Intensity is the lifeblood of High-Intensity Interval Training. It's not just about working hard; it's about pushing oneself to the brink. This isn't a leisurely jog in the park; it's a sprint with the metaphorical bear chasing you. The objective during these intense intervals is to reach an effort level that's close to your maximum capacity. This could be anywhere from 80% to 95% of your maximal heart rate, depending on the specific protocol. This level of exertion rapidly accelerates heart rate, taxes the muscles, and challenges one's aerobic and anaerobic systems, leading to physiological adaptations that can improve both strength and endurance.

Short Duration: Efficiency at its Best: In today's fast-paced world, time is a luxury. HIIT, with its condensed format, respects that too. Despite its shorter duration, the benefits reaped can be comparable to, if not greater than, traditional longer workouts. But it's essential to note that it's the quality, not just the quantity, of the workout that matters. Those brief minutes are packed with effort, sweat, and, often, a good deal of heavy breathing. The idea is to achieve more in less time, anchoring on the body's ability to work at peak levels in short bursts.

Interval Structure: An Exertion and Recovery: HIIT is likened to a well-composed piece of music, with crescendos of intense activity followed by decrescendos of rest. This structured alternation is carefully designed to provide the body with moments of extreme challenge, followed by brief respites to recover. But these recovery periods aren't just about catching one's breath. They're strategic, ensuring that the body can maintain its performance throughout the workout. By oscillating between high-intensity work and rest, HIIT leverages the body's energy systems efficiently, tapping into both aerobic and anaerobic reserves, which leads to a comprehensive cardiovascular workout.

Effects on Muscle Growth

Muscle Fiber Recruitment: The Dual Engagement: Every muscle in our body is made up of a mix of slow-twitch (Type I) and fast-twitch (Type II) fibers. Slow-twitch fibers are endurance-oriented, while fast-twitch fibers are all about power and strength. Traditional steady-state cardio primarily engages slow-twitch fibers. HIIT, with its bursts of intense effort, calls upon those fast-twitch fibers, pushing them to their limits. This dual engagement ensures a more comprehensive muscle workout. Over time, as these fibers are repeatedly activated and stressed, they adapt and grow, leading to gains in both muscle strength and endurance.

EPOC: The Caloric Afterglow: One of the standout advantages of HIIT is the metabolic boost it provides even after the workout. This phenomenon, known as Excess Post-exercise Oxygen Consumption or EPOC, is a period where the body's metabolism remains elevated, burning more calories than it would at rest. This is caused due to the body working overtime to restore itself to a pre-exercise state, repairing muscle tissue, replenishing energy stores, and balancing hormones. This increased caloric expenditure can aid in fat loss, revealing more defined muscles and contributing to the overall appearance of muscle growth.

Hormonal Response: Nature's Muscle Boosters: The body's hormonal response to HIIT is highly impressive. The intense nature of the workout can stimulate the release of anabolic hormones like growth hormone and testosterone. Growth hormone, often dubbed the 'fountain of youth', plays a pivotal role in tissue repair, muscle growth, and fat metabolism. Testosterone, on the other hand, is a primary player in muscle synthesis. Both these hormones work together, repairing the microtears caused by intense exercise and facilitating muscle growth. This hormonal surge not only helps in muscle development but ensures faster recovery, preparing the body for the next bout of intense activity.

Considerations for HIIT

Fitness Level: Starting on the Right Foot: High-intensity interval Training, by its very nature, demands a lot from the body. For those new to exercise or returning after a long hiatus, jumping straight into a HIIT routine might be overwhelming and potentially risky. It's essential to have a foundational level of cardiovascular and muscular endurance before incorporating HIIT into one's regimen. Starting with more moderate forms of exercise and gradually increasing intensity can prepare the body for the rigors of HIIT.

Recovery: The Silent Component of Growth: The intensity of HIIT places significant stress on the muscles, cardiovascular system, and central nervous system. This stress, while beneficial in promoting adaptation and growth, also necessitates a period of recovery. Without adequate rest between sessions, the risk of overtraining, injuries, and burnout increases. It's crucial to listen to one's body and allow sufficient time for muscles to repair and energy stores to replenish.

Proper Technique: The Guardian of Safety and Efficacy: The fast-paced nature of HIIT can sometimes lead to a compromise in form, especially when fatigue sets in. However, maintaining proper technique is non-negotiable. Not only does it ensure that the targeted muscles are effectively engaged, but it also minimizes the risk of strains, sprains, and other injuries. In essence, every movement should be executed with precision and control whether it's a sprint, a burpee, or a kettlebell swing.

Individualization: Crafting a Personal Blueprint: The world of HIIT is vast, with countless routines, exercises, and interval structures. While this variety is one of HIIT's strengths, it also means that what works for one person might not work for another. Factors like age, fitness level, goals, and even personal preferences play a role in determining the ideal HIIT routine. Tailoring the workout to one's unique needs ensures not only better results but also a more enjoyable and sustainable exercise experience.

Conclusion for HIIT

A Symphony of Modalities: High-intensity Interval Training, with its pulsating rhythms of exertion and rest, has undeniably carved a niche for itself in the fitness world. Its allure lies in its promise of maximum results in minimal time. However, like any powerful instrument, it's most effective when harmonized with other forms of exercise. Just as a symphony is incomplete with only one instrument, a fitness regimen thrives on diversity.

Strength, Flexibility, and Endurance: While HIIT excels in boosting cardiovascular health and metabolic rate, other training modalities address different facets of fitness. Strength training lays the foundation of muscle mass and bone density. Flexibility exercises, like yoga or pilates, ensure that our bodies remain agile, limber, and less prone to injuries. Traditional, steady-state cardio, on the other hand, offers a different kind of endurance training, building a robust cardiovascular system over longer durations.

Beyond the Trend: In an age of fleeting fads and transient trends, it might be tempting to dismiss HIIT as just another blip on the fitness radar. But its enduring popularity and the plethora of scientific studies vouching for its efficacy suggest otherwise. HIIT is more than just a workout; it's a celebration of the body's ability to push boundaries, adapt, and evolve.

The Transformative Journey: Embarking on a fitness journey with HIIT at the helm can be transformative. But it's essential to remember that the journey is as crucial as the destination. By integrating HIIT with a balanced, holistic approach to health and fitness, one cannot only achieve their goals but also discover the joy, empowerment, and fulfillment that comes with every heartbeat, every drop of sweat, and every challenge overcome.

Cardiovascular Exercise and Muscle Growth

The world of fitness is a vast tapestry, woven with various threads, each representing a different form of exercise. Among these, resistance training, with its promise of bulging biceps and chiseled abs, often stands out, capturing the limelight. However, in the shadows, working diligently and consistently is cardiovascular exercise. It might not promise the immediate allure of pumped muscles, but its role is just as vital, if not more so. Cardiovascular exercise is the conductor behind the scenes, ensuring that every part of the body, especially the muscles, receives the life-giving oxygen and nutrients it deserves. It's the steady beat, the consistent rhythm that underpins the explosive crescendos of weightlifting, ensuring that the body plays harmoniously, without missing a note. As we delve deeper into this topic, we'll uncover the intricate dance between cardiovascular exercise and muscle growth, revealing how they complement each other in the pursuit of holistic fitness.

MUSCLE UNIVERSITY

Importance of Cardiovascular Exercise in a Fitness Program

Cardiovascular exercise, also known as 'cardio,' is more than just a routine to elevate one's heart rate or shed a few extra calories. It's the silent partner in the dance of fitness, gracefully complementing the robust and dynamic moves of resistance training. While the allure of muscle growth and strength often draws individuals to the weights section of the gym, the treadmills, ellipticals, and open tracks hold their own unique charm and set of benefits.

At its core, cardiovascular exercise is about endurance, stamina, and the heart's health. But its influence extends far beyond just the circulatory system. It acts as a support system for resistance training, enhancing the body's ability to recover, improving circulation to deliver essential nutrients to the muscles, and aiding in the removal of waste products that accumulate during intense workouts. Furthermore, it ensures that the body's respiratory and circulatory systems are optimized, providing a solid foundation upon which muscles can grow and thrive.

In essence, while resistance training builds the structure – the muscles, the strength, the power; cardiovascular exercise ensures that this structure has a robust and efficient supply chain, delivering oxygen and nutrients and removing waste products. It's a harmonious partnership, where one without the other would be akin to building a magnificent structure without the necessary infrastructure to support it. In the theater of fitness, if resistance training is the lead actor, cardiovascular exercise is the director, ensuring that every scene plays out actively.

Benefits of Cardiovascular Exercise for Muscle Growth

In fitness, cardiovascular exercise plays a melody that resonates with the rhythm of muscle growth. While it might not be the first thing that comes to mind when one thinks of hypertrophy, its role is undeniably significant. Let's delve into the relationship between cardiovascular exercise and muscle development.

Improved Blood Circulation: At the heart of cardiovascular exercise is, well, the heart. As one engages in activities that elevate the heart rate, the heart pumps blood more vigorously, ensuring that every nook and cranny of the body receives a rich supply of oxygenated blood. For muscles, this is similar to receiving a fresh supply of building materials and workers continuously. The enhanced blood flow ensures that muscles are well-fed with the nutrients they need to repair and grow. After a grueling resistance training session, as microtears form in the muscle fibers, this improved circulation plays a pivotal role in transporting the necessary resources for repair. It's like having a dedicated highway for muscle recovery, ensuring minimal traffic jams and maximum efficiency.

Enhanced Endurance: Let's create this scene for clarity: you're in the middle of a weightlifting session, and just as you're about to hit that last rep, your muscles scream in fatigue. Now, infuse this scenario with the stamina built from regular cardiovascular exercise. The result is that you push through, not just completing that rep but maybe even adding a few more. Cardiovascular training conditions the body to endure, and to persevere. It trains the heart, lungs, and muscles to work in unison, to withstand fatigue. This endurance is a boon for resistance training, allowing one to push boundaries, challenge limits, and in the process, stimulate greater muscle growth.

Fat Utilization: The aesthetics of muscle growth aren't just about size and strength; definition plays a crucial role. Cardiovascular exercise is a master sculptor in this regard. As one engages in sustained cardio, the body taps into its fat reserves for energy. This process of fat utilization ensures that as muscles grow, they aren't hidden under a layer of fat. Instead, they emerge defined, pronounced, and sculpted. It's the difference between a rough block of marble and a finely chiseled statue. Cardio ensures that the beauty of muscle growth isn't just felt but also seen.

In essence, cardiovascular exercise isn't just the backdrop against which the drama of muscle growth unfolds; it's an active player, setting the stage, supporting the actors, and ensuring that the performance is nothing short of spectacular.

Considerations for Cardiovascular Exercise

Cardiovascular exercise offers a plethora of pathways to improved health and fitness. However, as with any journey, it's essential to navigate with a map and compass, ensuring that the chosen path aligns with one's destination. Let's delve into the considerations that can guide this journey, ensuring it complements and enhances the quest for muscle growth.

Balance with Resistance Training: Imagine a seesaw. On one side, you have resistance training, with its weights, reps, and sets. On the other, you have cardiovascular exercise, with its rhythms, beats, and breaths. For optimal muscle growth, this seesaw needs to be in balance. Overindulging can tip the balance, potentially eating into the muscle gains achieved through resistance training while the rhythmic pulse of cardio is still crucial, especially when not supported by adequate caloric intake, excessive cardio can lead the body to utilize muscle protein for energy, hindering organ enlargement. Thus, it's a dance of balance, ensuring that while the heart races, the muscles also flex, lift, and grow.

Intensity and Duration: Cardiovascular exercise is not a monolith; it's a spectrum. On one end, you have the short, explosive bursts of high-intensity interval training (HIIT). On the other, the long, steady strides of a marathon runner. Both have their merits. Shorter, high-intensity sessions can be incredibly effective, offering the benefits of cardio in a condensed timeframe and even stimulating muscle growth pathways similar to resistance training. On the other hand, longer sessions can enhance endurance, stamina, and fat utilization. The key is to listen to one's body, understand its needs, and adjust the intensity and duration accordingly.

Individualization: The world of fitness is rich with stories. Each individual brings to it their unique narrative of goals, challenges, preferences, and experiences. Cardiovascular exercise, in all its forms, should align with this narrative. A sprinter's regimen will differ vastly from that of a long-distance cyclist. Someone aiming for muscle definition might approach cardio differently from someone training for a triathlon. It's essential to tailor cardiovascular exercise to one's unique goals, fitness levels, and even joys. After all, the most effective workout is the one that's sustainable, enjoyable, and aligned with one's aspirations.

In conclusion, while cardiovascular exercise offers great benefits, it's essential to approach it with mindfulness, understanding, and strategy. It's not just about moving; it's about moving with purpose, direction, and balance, ensuring that every heartbeat, every step, and every breath aligns with the overarching goal of holistic health, fitness, and muscle growth.

Variety in Cardiovascular Exercises

The tapestry of cardiovascular exercises is rich and varied, each thread offering its unique hue and texture to the overall picture. Let's explore the myriad ways one can elevate their heart rate, enhance endurance, and contribute to overall fitness.

Running: Running has been an integral part of our existence. From hunting to escaping predators to today's marathons and sprints, running is deeply ingrained in our DNA. It's the epitome of simplicity; all you need is a pair of shoes and the open road. Whether you're pushing the limits with a high-intensity sprint or finding your rhythm in a long-distance jog, running offers a spectrum of intensities, each catering to different fitness goals and preferences.

Cycling: There's a certain freedom that comes with cycling. The wind in your hair, the world rushing by, and the rhythmic pedaling create a meditative experience. Beyond the joy of movement, cycling offers a potent cardiovascular workout. Its low-impact nature makes it especially beneficial for those with joint concerns. Whether you're tackling challenging terrains outdoors or pushing your limits on a stationary bike, cycling is a versatile addition to any fitness regimen.

Swimming: Swimming is the art of immersing oneself in water. It is not just a cardiovascular exercise; it's a rhythm of strength, endurance, and technique. The water's resistance ensures that muscles are engaged throughout, offering a comprehensive workout. From the butterfly to the freestyle, each stroke brings its challenges and rewards.

Group Fitness Classes: There are infectious energy in group fitness classes. The beat of the music, the guidance of the instructor, and the collective spirit of participants create a motivating environment. Whether you're grooving to the beats of Zumba, pushing through a high-intensity interval class, or finding your balance in aerobics, group classes offer structure, variety, and a sense of community.

Sports: Beyond the structured workouts and exercises lies the playful world of sports. Sports offer a unique skill, strategy, and fitness through the strategic game of tennis, the teamwork of basketball, or the endurance test of soccer. They remind us that at the heart of every fitness journey lies the joy of movement, competition, and camaraderie.

During cardiovascular exercises, one thing becomes clear: variety is not just the spice of life; it's the essence of a holistic fitness journey. Each modality offers its unique benefits, challenges, and joys, ensuring that the heart, remains ever-engaged, ever-challenged, and ever-joyful.

Conclusion for Cardiovascular Exercise:

The element of fitness is composed of various instruments, each playing its unique tune. Among them, cardiovascular exercise plays seamlessly the powerful beats of resistance training. It's not merely an accompaniment but a vital component that elevates the entire composition.

In fact, cardiovascular exercise is the bridge that connects strength and endurance. Importantly, it's the rhythmic pulse of cardiovascular activity that ensures these muscles are nourished, oxygenated, and primed for growth. It also reminds us of the importance of stamina, the joy of movement, and the balance between pushing limits and flowing with grace.

Moreover, the versatility of cardiovascular exercise means that it can be tailored to individual needs, preferences, and goals. There's a form of cardio that speaks to every soul no matter the session or challenge of the team.

In fitness, cardiovascular exercise reminds us that in the journey of physical betterment, it's not just about the peaks of strength but also the valleys of recovery, the plateaus of consistency, and the ever-evolving path of holistic health. As we step back in admiration, the message is clear: to truly thrive, to truly grow, and to truly shine, one must embrace the dance of strength and endurance, of power and grace.

The Principle of Progressive Overload

In fitness and strength training, certain principles stand as pillars, guiding and shaping the journey of muscle development. Among these, the principle of progressive overload reigns supreme. It's the golden rule, the secret sauce, the key to unlocking consistent and sustainable gains.

Definition and Importance of Progressive Overload

In fitness, progressive overload is a beacon, responsible for muscle growth and strength development. Equally, progressive overload is the intentional and systematic increase of stress the body carries during exercise. It's a multifaceted concept other than seen as adding more weight to the barbell. Progressive overload encapsulates not just resistance, but also the volume, intensity, and frequency of workouts.

Why Does It Matter?

The human body likes to adapt to emerging situations. When subjected to stress, it seeks equilibrium by fortifying itself against future similar stresses. In the context of muscle training, this means that when we consistently push our muscles beyond their current limits, they respond. They grow, they strengthen, and they prepare. Our muscles would have no reason to change, and our workouts would yield diminishing returns without progressive overload.

Delving Deeper into Progressive Overload

Resistance is a broader concept. It's the challenge that our muscles face, and the hurdle they must overcome. For some, resistance is the weight of their own body, as seen in push-ups or squats. For others, it might be the elastic tug of resistance bands or the gentle yet persistent pushback from water in aquatic exercises. But regardless of its form, the principle remains the same: as our muscles adapt and grow stronger, the resistance must grow as well. This ensures that the muscles are challenged, fostering continuous growth and development.

Volume is the collective effort expended in a workout. It's a numeric representation of how much work the muscles have done. Consider doing 3 sets of 10 repetitions of a particular exercise; that's a story of 30 efforts. But the history of progressive overload demands evolution. So, to continue the story, one might add another chapter, perhaps increasing the narrative to 4 sets of 10, or adding a twist with 3 sets of 12. The story grows, and so do the muscles.

Intensity is less about numbers and more about feeling. It's the fiery challenge that courses through the muscles during a particularly grueling set. It's the breathlessness after a sprint, the trembling of muscles pushed to their limit. Intensity is malleable. It can be heightened by adding more weight, reducing the pause between sets, or even changing the tempo of each repetition. It's a reminder that sometimes, it's not about how long you train, but how fervently you engage with each moment of the workout.

Frequency is the cadence of one's training regimen. It's the recurring workouts in the week. Training a muscle group once a week sets a particular rhythm. Training the same muscle group twice a week changes the dance. But with this increased training, one must also be attuned to the silent beats - the rests, the recovery periods

Therefore, progressive overload is these elements - resistance, volume, intensity, and frequency - put together to create growth, challenge, and triumph.

General Workout/Recovery Cycle

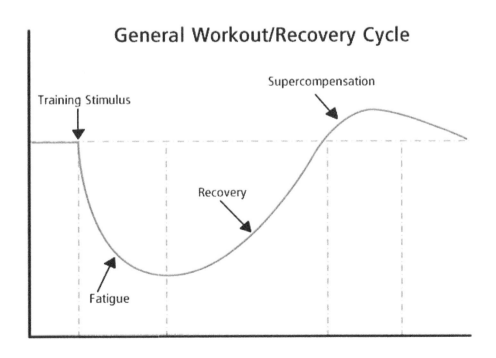

The Role of Progressive Overload in Muscle Growth

Increased Muscle Strength

Every time we challenge our muscles with greater resistance or intensity, we're essentially sending them a message: "You need to be stronger." And our muscles, being the adaptive powerhouses they are, respond. They rebuild themselves stronger than before, preparing for the next challenge. It's a continuous cycle of stress, recovery, and adaptation, leading to a steady increase in muscle strength.

Hypertrophy

At the heart of muscle growth lies the principle of enlargement. When we engage in resistance training, especially under the guidance of progressive overload, we induce microscopic tears in our muscle fibers. While this might sound alarming, it's a natural and essential process. During recovery, these tiny tears repair and regrow thicker and stronger, leading to muscle growth. Progressive overload ensures that this process continues unabated, driving consistent hypertrophy.

Improved Definition

Improved definition gives the finishing touches to the muscular masterpiece. Progressive overload, by continually challenging the muscles, ensures that they not only grow in size but also achieve that sought-after toned and chiseled look. It's the difference between a rough sculpture and a finely detailed statue.

Enhanced Performance

While the aesthetic benefits of progressive overload are evident, its impact goes beyond skin deep. By consistently pushing our boundaries, we're not just building muscle; we're enhancing our overall physical performance. This improvement translates to various facets of life, including effortlessly carrying groceries to excelling in sports. It's about building a body that's not just good to look at, but also highly functional and efficient.

Essentially, progressive overload isn't just a training principle; it's a philosophy. It's about understanding that growth, whether physical or personal, comes from consistently pushing our boundaries and embracing challenges. It's the thread of muscle growth, which gives it strength, form, and function.

The Art and Science of Applying Progressive Overload

Gradual Progression

Imagine climbing a mountain. If you try to scale it too quickly, you risk exhaustion or even injury. But with steady, measured steps, you can reach the mountaintop safely and enjoy the view. Similarly, in fitness, it's crucial to approach progressive overload with patience. By gradually increasing the demands on our body, we allow it to adapt at a natural pace, ensuring that growth is not only effective but also sustainable.

Tracking

In the quest for muscle growth, knowledge is power. By carefully tracking our workouts, we create a roadmap of progress. This record serves multiple purposes. It's a motivator, showing us how far we've come. It's a planner that helps us determine the next steps. And it's a safety net, ensuring we don't push too hard, or too fast. Tracking is the compass that guides our progressive overload journey be it a traditional workout log, a mobile app, or even mental notes.

Variation

While the core principle of progressive overload revolves around consistent progression, monotony can be a growth killer. Our muscles are adaptive, and over time, they can become accustomed to the same exercises and routines. This is where variation steps in. By introducing new exercises, tweaking angles, or even changing the order of workouts, we can keep our muscles guessing. This element of surprise can reinvigorate our training, stimulating muscles in novel ways and paving the path for continued growth.

Listening to Your Body

Our bodies are incredibly communicative, and constantly sending us signals. These signals include the burn of a good workout, the ache of growing muscles, or the sharp pain warning us of potential injury. In the pursuit of progressive overload, it's paramount to tune into these signals. While pushing boundaries is the essence of progression, it should never come at the cost of our well-being. Recognizing when to push harder and when to pull back is important, one that's honed over time and experience.

Applying progressive overload revolves around ambition and caution. It's about dreaming big but taking measured steps. It's about challenging limits but respecting boundaries. Essentially, it's about understanding that true strength isn't just physical; it's also the wisdom to know when to push and when to rest.

Navigating the Path of Progressive Overload:

In fitness, progressive overload stands out as a golden strand. It's the guiding principle that ensures continuous growth and evolution. It ensures that our bodies are always moving, always adapting, and always growing.

The beauty of this principle lies in its simplicity. It doesn't demand difficult feats of strength overnight. Instead, it asks for consistency, patience, and ambition.

As a matter of fact, progressive overload comes with a responsibility. It's not about reckless progression but thoughtful, measured steps forward. It's about following the intricacies of our muscles, and understanding the fine line between pushing limits and overstepping boundaries.

In fitness history, progressive overload is a timeless chapter. It reminds us that growth isn't just about the destination but the journey. It's about celebrating every extra rep, every added pound, and every small victory along the way. As things continue to evolve, the principle of progressive overload lights the way, promising a journey that's as rewarding as the destination.

Exercise and Aging

Time is a constant, with each tick of the clock marking our journey through life. As we journey through the years, our bodies remind us of time, showcasing changes that are both visible and invisible. Among these changes, our muscles narrate a particularly poignant story. They've supported us through our youthful time, and carried us through challenges, and now, as we grow older, they too transform. Obviously, aging brings about shifts in our muscle structure and function. Fortunately, our actions, especially our commitment to exercise, can shape the narrative, ensuring that our muscles remain robust and resilient, even as the years go by.

Effects of Aging on Muscle

- **Sarcopenia:** As human beings age, there's the gradual loss of muscle mass associated with aging. It's a silent process, initiating as early as our third decade of life. If not checked, sarcopenia can strip away our independence, making tasks we once took for granted, like lifting groceries or climbing stairs, increasingly challenging.
- **Muscle Atrophy:** Beyond just the loss of muscle mass, aging muscles can undergo atrophy, where they diminish in size. Muscle atrophy translates to a decline in strength and can affect our endurance, making prolonged activities more taxing.

- **Decreased Strength:** Time, which is a reminder of our experiences, can be tough on our muscles too. The combination of natural cellular changes, hormonal fluctuations, and years of wear and tear culminate in a decline in muscle strength. This reduction can subtly creep into our daily lives, making activities that once seemed effortless require a bit more exertion.

Benefits of Exercise for Older Adults

The golden years, often characterized by retirement, relaxation, and reflection, also present an opportunity—a chance to invest in one's health and well-being. Exercise, which functions as a panacea for numerous ailments, holds particular significance for older adults. Its benefits, both tangible and intangible, are improved quality of life, resilience, and vitality.

- **Improved Muscle Mass:** The natural ebb of muscle mass due to aging might seem like an unchangeable fate. However, exercise is a strong hope for aging muscles. Regular physical activity, especially strength training, acts as a bulwark against sarcopenia. It ensures they remain dense, robust, and functional. The adage "use it or lose it" rings particularly true here. By actively engaging muscles through exercise, older adults can not only halt the decline but even witness a resurgence in muscle mass.
- **Strength:** The strength of our muscles is foundational, underpinning every movement, and every gesture. As we grow older, this strength can decline. Yet, resistance training is a panacea. Muscles adapt, and grow stronger and more resilient by challenging them and making them work against resistance. This renewed strength translates to many benefits – from the ease of lifting a grandchild to the confidence of climbing stairs without hesitation.
- **Balance:** Balance during older age is often underappreciated until it's compromised. For older adults, maintaining balance is key to enjoying a healthy lifestyle. A misstep or a wobble can lead to falls, which can have negative health implications. Thankfully, exercises tailored to enhance balance, from tai chi to specific balance-focused routines, can fortify this skill. By improving proprioception and strengthening and stabilizing muscles, these exercises ensure that older adults move with assurance and poise.
- **Overall Health:** Exercise extends far beyond muscles. It courses through the arteries, ensuring heart health. It fortifies the bones, reducing the risk of osteoporosis. And perhaps most importantly, it nurtures the mind. The endorphins released during exercise act as a balm for the soul, warding off feelings of loneliness, anxiety, and

depression. In essence, exercise for older adults is not just a regimen; it promotes holistic well-being.

Types of Exercises for Older Adults

As the body matures, it craves movement, keeping it vibrant and agile. For older adults, exercise isn't just a recommendation; it's a bridge to a life of vitality, independence, and joy. Let's explore the diverse exercises for this phase of life.

- **Resistance Training:** For older adults, resistance training is a cornerstone. Resistance training is akin to a conversation with one's muscles. It's a dialogue where challenges are posed, and the body responds by growing stronger. Over time, this consistent engagement not only builds muscle mass but also fortifies bones, making them more resilient against fractures.
- **Cardiovascular Exercise:** The heart, that tireless engine, benefits immensely from cardiovascular exercises. For older adults, the beauty of cardio lies in its adaptability. A brisk morning walk, a leisurely cycle around the park, or even gentle laps in the community pool can invigorate the heart, ensuring it pumps with vigor and efficiency. Also, cardiovascular exercises enhance lung capacity, stamina, and even mood.
- **Flexibility:** As the seasons of life change, maintaining flexibility becomes paramount. It's the grace that allows one to bend down and play with a grandchild or reach up to pluck a book from a high shelf. Stretching exercises, whether they're part of a structured routine or interspersed throughout the day, ensure that the muscles remain supple. This suppleness translates to a better range of motion, reduced muscle tension, and a lower risk of injuries. It's the silent guardian that ensures fluidity in movement, no matter the age.
- **Balance Exercises:** Balance is crucial in the later stages of life. Physically, exercises like Tai Chi, with its flowing movements, or yoga, with its emphasis on groundedness offer stability. These exercises, not only strengthen the stabilizing muscles but also enhance proprioception, the body's ability to sense its position in space. The result is that it gives a confident stride, a steady stance, and a reduced risk of falls.

Considerations for Exercise in Older Adults

The older phase of life is marked by wisdom, experience, and often, introspection. As older adults embark on the journey of fitness, it's not just about movement but moving right. Embarking on exercises in this phase is intricate, demanding, and a delicate balance of enthusiasm and caution. Let's delve into the considerations for exercise in older adults.

- **Safety:** The adage, "Safety first", holds profound significance in the context of older adults and exercise. As the body matures, it might not bounce back from injuries as swiftly as it once did. Hence, the emphasis on safety becomes paramount. Therefore, older people while using supportive equipment like belts or braces, must be cautious to avoid slippery workout surfaces, or even seek professional guidance from fitness coaches. Moreover, regular health check-ups and consultations with physicians can provide valuable insights, ensuring that the exercise regimen aligns with one's health status.

- **Individualization:** Individual differences mark out the uniqueness of every man. This individuality extends to fitness as well. An exercise regimen that works for one might not suit another. Factors like pre-existing health conditions, past injuries, and even personal preferences play a pivotal role. Appropriate exercises for one's body and spirit ensure not just effectiveness but also longevity in the fitness journey.

- **Consistency:** Exercise, especially in the later stages of life, lies in consistency. It's not about the occasional intense workout but the gentle, consistent training of muscles and joints, day in and day out. This consistency aids in maintaining muscle mass, ensuring joint flexibility, and even fostering mental well-being.

- **Progression:** Age is but a number, and even in the golden years, the body's potential to grow and adapt is remarkable. Embracing the principle of progressive overload, older adults can gradually increase the intensity, duration, or complexity of exercises. However, this progression is a gentle slope, marked by patience and keen awareness. It's about recognizing achievements, no matter how small, and building upon them, to ensure that the body is consistently, yet safely, challenged.

Overcoming Barriers to Exercise in Aging

The golden years can sometimes be accompanied by challenges, especially when it comes to maintaining an active lifestyle. As time passes, barriers, both physical and psychological, might emerge on the path to fitness. Yet, with determination and the right strategies, these barriers can be surmounted, paving the way for a vibrant and active life. Let's explore the ways to navigate these challenges.

- **Motivation:** As the days meld into a routine, finding motivation can sometimes be difficult. Nevertheless, setting clear, tangible goals can guide, and inspire. Whether it's walking a certain distance, lifting a specific weight, or even mastering a yoga pose, these goals become milestones in the journey. Tracking progress, celebrating small victories, and even visual reminders can inspire motivation. Additionally, joining group classes can introduce an element of camaraderie and fun, making exercise less of a chore and more of an interesting venture.

- **Accessibility:** Sometimes, the most effective workouts can be found in the corners of one's home or the halls of community centers. The key is adaptability. Exercises can be modified to suit one's environment, ensuring they're always within reach just with the application of online resources. Be it chair exercises, resistance band workouts, or even simple stretches, exercises are vast and varied.
- **Health Concerns:** Life is often marked by various health challenges. These concerns, while valid, shouldn't become insurmountable walls but rather checkpoints that guide the fitness journey. Regular consultations with healthcare professionals can provide invaluable insights, tailoring exercises to align with one's unique health profile. This personalized approach ensures safety, effectiveness, and peace of mind.
- **Social Support:** Humans, by nature, are social beings. The presence of a supportive community, a friend, or even a family member can transform the fitness journey. Engaging in group activities, be it a dance class, a walking group, or a Tai Chi session in the park, can infuse workouts with laughter, encouragement, and a sense of belonging. For those who prefer a more intimate setting, enlisting a workout buddy can provide the necessary nudge on days when motivation wanes, ensuring consistency and accountability.

Conclusion for Exercise and Aging

The older age, often perceived as a period of slowing down, can instead be filled with vigor, vitality, and renewed purpose. Central to this rejuvenated narrative is the role of exercise.

Aging, with its intricate experiences, brings with it certain physiological changes. Muscles might not be as robust, joints not as flexible, and energy levels might see some ebb and flow. Yet, within this very point lies the potential for growth, strength, and rejuvenation. Exercise, in its forms, becomes the thread that propels these potentials into reality.

Whether it's a morning walk, yoga, or resistance training, each movement becomes a testament to the body's enduring spirit. It's a declaration that older age does not translate into inactivity but rather an opportunity to embrace movement in new, adaptive, and enriching ways.

Beyond the physical, exercise in older ages also nurtures the mind and soul. It becomes a bridge to social connections, a balm for mental well-being, and a catalyst for self-confidence. Each step taken, each rep completed, and each breath during meditation becomes a celebration of life's journey and the potential that still lies ahead.

In life, the later chapters can be as vibrant, if not more so, than the preceding ones. With exercise as a steadfast companion, the golden years can truly become blissful, reflecting a life of movement, purpose, and boundless possibilities. It's a gentle reminder that age is but a number, and the spirit of vitality knows no bounds.

Conclusion--Exercise and Muscle Growth

Throughout this chapter, we've embarked on a comprehensive exploration of the multifaceted relationship between exercise and muscle growth. From the foundational principles of resistance training to the pulsating rhythms of HIIT, the intricate dance of cardiovascular workouts, the steadfast progression of overload, and the graceful adaptations of exercise in aging, we've delved deep into the mechanics, benefits, and considerations of each.

Resistance training, with its myriad forms, stands as a testament to the body's raw power and potential for growth. HIIT, on the other hand, challenges the conventional norms of exercise, proving that intensity can sometimes outweigh duration. Cardiovascular exercises, often seen as the antithesis of muscle building, have shown their worth in sculpting, defining, and supporting muscular growth. The principle of progressive overload serves as a reminder that growth is a continuous journey, which requires consistent challenge and adaptation. Lastly, the segment on exercise and aging encapsulates the timeless nature of fitness, proving that the pursuit of muscle health and vitality knows no age.

In essence, muscle growth is not just a product of lifting weights or performing specific exercises. It has various training modalities, each contributing its unique notes to its growth. As we conclude this chapter, let's remember that the journey to muscle growth is as diverse as it is rewarding. It's a blend of science, dedication, adaptability, and passion. And as with any journey, it's not just the destination that matters, but the experiences, learnings, and transformations along the way.

CHAPTER 6

THE SCIENCE OF
PERIODIZATION PROGRAMMING

Periodization, a term often echoed in the corridors of elite training facilities and among seasoned coaches, stands as a testament to the evolution of training methodologies. But what exactly is periodization, and why has it become such a pivotal concept in sports and fitness?

Definition of Periodization

Periodization is the art and science of organizing training. It's not about random workouts or sporadic efforts; it's about a calculated approach to training that is designed with a clear end goal in mind.

- **Systematic Planning:** Periodization isn't a haphazard approach. It's a meticulous plan where every workout, every set, and every repetition has a purpose. This planning isn't just for the short term; it spans weeks, months, and even years, ensuring that an athlete or individual progresses steadily toward their optimal performance.

- **Aim:** The ultimate goal of periodization is to ensure that an athlete or fitness enthusiast is at their absolute best when it matters the most. This could be an Olympic event, a local marathon, a bodybuilding competition, or even a personal fitness milestone. The training is structured in such a way that the individual peaks at this crucial juncture, having the best possible physical and mental condition.

- **Progressive Cycling:** One of the unique aspects of periodization is the idea of cycling through various training aspects. This could mean focusing on endurance in one phase, strength in another, and power in yet another. This cycling ensures that the body is constantly challenged in new ways, preventing risks and fostering multifaceted development.

Importance of Periodization in Exercise Physiology

Exercise physiology delves into the intricate workings of the human body during physical activity. It seeks to understand how our muscles, cardiovascular system, and metabolism respond to exercise stimuli. Periodization, in this context, becomes immensely significant for several reasons:

- **Maximizing Adaptive Responses:** The human body is a marvel of adaptation. When subjected to stress, like exercise, it adapts by becoming stronger, faster, or more enduring. Periodization ensures that these adaptive responses are maximized. By varying the training stimulus and ensuring that the body doesn't get too accustomed to a particular type of stress, periodization fosters continuous growth and improvement.

- **Minimizing Overtraining Risks:** Overtraining is a real and prevalent risk among athletes and fitness enthusiasts. It's the result of pushing the body too hard without adequate recovery, leading to fatigue, injuries, and even regression in performance. Periodization, with its structured approach and built-in recovery phases, ensures that individuals train hard but also smart, giving their bodies the necessary time to recover and rejuvenate.

- **Optimal Performance Timing:** Imagine training hard for months, only to find that you're fatigued and underperforming on the day of your main event. Periodization prevents such scenarios. By structuring training in a way that aligns with competition or performance dates, it ensures that individuals are not just ready, but are at their absolute best when the spotlight is on them.

Ideally, periodization is more than just a training schedule; it's a philosophy that believes in the power of structured effort. It respects the body's need for varied stimuli, recognizes the importance of recovery, and always keeps the end goal in sight. Whether you're an elite athlete or someone just starting their fitness journey, periodization offers a roadmap to success, ensuring that every drop of sweat is a step towards greatness.

Role in Optimizing Training Programs and Achieving Fitness Outcomes

The world of fitness and athletic training is vast, with goals and objectives that individuals might pursue. From the casual gym-goer looking to shed a few pounds to the elite athlete training for the Olympics, everyone has a unique endpoint in mind. Periodization, in this vast landscape, serves as a compass, guiding individuals toward their goals with precision and efficiency.

Optimizing Training Programs

Training without a plan is similar to embarking on a journey without a map. You might make some progress, but there's a high chance you'll end up lost or, worse, injured. Periodization provides this much-needed map for training.

Structured Approach: Periodization isn't about random workouts; it's a meticulously crafted plan. It ensures that the body is always presented with a challenge, but one that it can handle by increasing or decreasing the training load in a structured manner. This balance is crucial to prevent burnout and injuries.

Preventing Stagnation: One of the biggest challenges in any fitness journey is the dreaded risk– a phase where, despite consistent efforts, progress seems to halt. Periodization, with its varied phases and focus, ensures that the body never gets too accustomed to a particular type of training stimulus. This variation keeps the body guessing, promoting continuous improvement and preventing stagnation.

Achieving Fitness Outcomes

Every individual's fitness journey is driven by specific outcomes they wish to achieve. These outcomes can be as varied as the individuals themselves.

Alignment with Objectives: Periodization is not a one-size-fits-all approach. It's expected to align with specific objectives. Whether someone's goal is muscle growth, strength gains, endurance enhancement, or peaking for a competition, periodization structures the training to cater to these specific needs.

Making Success Attainable: By aligning training with objectives, periodization makes success more tangible. It breaks down the journey into manageable chunks, each with its own set of goals and milestones. This step-by-step approach not only makes the journey more manageable but also provides regular feedback, ensuring that individuals remain motivated and on track.

Division of Training into Distinct Phases for Specific Focuses

One of the hallmarks of periodization is its division of training into distinct phases. This division is not arbitrary; it's designed to ensure that training remains varied, comprehensive, and aligned with goals.

Purpose of Phases: Each phase in a periodized program serves a specific purpose. It's designed to target certain physiological adaptations, ensuring holistic development. For instance, while one phase might focus on building a cardiovascular base, another might zero in on muscle strength.

Examples of Phases

1. **Foundational Phase:** Often, this phase as the starting point is about building general fitness. It lays the groundwork, focusing on overall conditioning, flexibility, and basic strength.
2. **Hypertrophy Phase:** As the name suggests, this phase is all about muscle growth. The training focuses on exercises and rep ranges that promote muscle growth.
3. **Strength Phase:** Building on the muscle mass gained in the hypertrophy phase, this phase aims to increase overall strength. The weights lifted become heavier, with a focus on compound movements.
4. **Power Phase:** This phase is about converting the strength gained into explosive power. It's especially crucial for athletes who need short intense effort in their sport.
5. **Peaking or Tapering Phase:** The culmination of all the previous phases, this is where individuals prepare for a competition or performance. The training becomes very specific, aiming to ensure peak performance at the desired time.

So, periodization is a dynamic approach to training. It respects the body's need for varied stimuli and recovery, understands the importance of aligned goals, and provides a structured path to success. Whether you're just starting out or are a seasoned athlete, periodization offers a roadmap to ensure that every effort is a step in the right direction.

Primary Objectives of Periodization

The concept of periodization is not just a random division of training into phases. It's a strategic approach, rooted in scientific principles and real-world results. The primary objectives of periodization underscore its importance and effectiveness in training programs. Let's critically look into these objectives:

Overcoming Training Risks

- **The Challenge of Adaptation:** The human body is an incredible machine, capable of adapting to various stimuli. While this adaptability is a testament to our resilience, it can also pose challenges in a training context. When exposed to the same type of training stimulus over extended periods, the body adapts, leading to diminished returns from the same effort – a phenomenon known as a training plateau.
- **The Role of Variation:** Periodization introduces variation in training, ensuring that the body is constantly exposed to different types of stimuli. This continuous change prevents the body from getting too accustomed to any single type of training,

thereby averting plateaus. It's like giving the body a new puzzle to solve just as it's getting comfortable with the current one, ensuring continuous progress.

Emphasizing Progressive Overload

- **The Backbone of Progress:** Progressive overload is a foundational principle in strength and conditioning. It's the idea that, for muscles to grow and strength to increase, the body must be subjected to demands that surpass its current capabilities.

- **Structured Progression with Periodization:** While the idea of progressive overload is simple, its implementation requires careful planning. Periodization provides this structure. It ensures that the body is continuously challenged but within its recovery capacity by systematically increasing the training load over specific periods. This balance is crucial to prevent burnout and injuries.

Strategies for Injury Prevention

- **The Risk of Overtraining:** In the quest for progress, there's a temptation to push harder continuously. However, without adequate recovery, this can lead to overuse injuries. These injuries not only hamper individuals but can also lead to long-term complications.

- **Balancing Work and Recovery:** Periodization acknowledges the importance of recovery. Varying training intensity and volume and incorporating rest or deload phases can ensure that the body gets the necessary time to heal and recover. This proactive approach reduces the risk of injuries and ensures that individuals remain fit and ready to tackle the next challenge.

Timing for Optimal Performance Peaks

- **The Art of Peaking:** For athletes, merely being in good shape isn't enough. They need to be in their best possible shape at the right time, especially for major competitions or events. This requires precise timing in training.

- **Strategic Planning with Periodization:** Periodization can be geared toward ensuring that athletes reach their peak performance when it matters most. By adjusting the duration and focus of each phase, coaches can ensure that athletes are in top form right in time for major competitions. This strategic approach can make the difference between a good performance and a gold medal.

Therefore, the primary objectives of periodization highlight its comprehensive approach to training. It's not just about working hard but working smart, ensuring that every effort brings individuals one step closer to their goals. Whether it's breaking through plateaus, preventing injuries, or peaking at the right time, periodization offers a structured path to success.

Different Models of Periodization – An Overview

Periodization, as a concept, has evolved over the years, leading to the development of various models. Each model offers a unique approach to structuring training, catering to different needs, goals, and training experiences. Let's delve deeper into these models to understand their nuances and applications:

Linear Periodization:

The Basics: Linear periodization, as the name suggests, follows a linear approach to training progression. It starts with high volume and low intensity and gradually moves to low volume and high intensity over a specified period.

Phased Approach: This model typically divides training into distinct phases, such as endurance, growth, strength, and power. Each phase has a clear focus and lasts for several weeks to months.

Advantages

- **Predictability:** The structured and phased approach makes it easy to plan and follow.

- **Foundation Building:** The initial phases, focusing on endurance and growth, lay a strong foundation for subsequent phases.

- **Considerations:** While effective, especially for those new to structured training, linear periodization can become predictable over time, potentially leading to plateaus for more advanced trainees.

Undulating Periodization (Nonlinear)

The Basics: Undulating periodization introduces more frequent changes in training volume and intensity. Instead of progressing linearly over extended periods, changes can occur daily or weekly.

Microcycles: Training is divided into short cycles, known as microcycles, each lasting a week or so. Within each microcycle, there's a mix of high, medium, and low-intensity sessions.

Advantages

- **Variability:** The constant changes keep the body guessing, reducing the chances of adaptation and plateaus.
- **Flexibility:** It allows for adjustments based on how one feels on a particular day or week, making it adaptable to real-life scenarios.
- **Considerations:** This model requires a deeper understanding of one's body and more meticulous planning. It might be overwhelming for beginners but can be highly effective for intermediate to advanced trainees.

Block Periodization

The Basics: In block periodization, training is segmented into blocks, with each block lasting several weeks. Each block has a specific focus, allowing for a concentrated development of particular fitness aspects.

Types of Blocks

- **Accumulation Block:** Focuses on building volume, endurance, and general physical preparedness.
- **Transmutation Block:** Transforms the gains from the accumulation phase into specific performance attributes, like strength or power.
- **Realization Block:** Also known as the peaking phase, fine-tunes the athlete for peak performance.

Advantages

- **Focused Training:** Concentrating on specific attributes in each block, allows for targeted and efficient training.
- **Versatility:** It can be channeled for various sports and goals, making it a favorite among elite athletes.

152

- **Considerations:** Block periodization requires careful planning and a clear understanding of the end goal. It's best suited for advanced athletes or those with specific performance targets.

In conclusion, the choice of periodization model should align with an individual or team's goals, training experience, and preferences. While all models are rooted in the same foundational principles, their application can vary, offering trainers and athletes a range of tools to optimize training outcomes.

Implementation Considerations for Periodization

Successfully implementing periodization in training requires more than just understanding its principles. It involves a series of considerations that ensure the training program is not only effective but also sustainable and aligned with the individual's or team's goals. These considerations include:

Planning

- **The Blueprint:** Think of planning as creating a blueprint for the training journey. It provides a roadmap, detailing each step and phase, ensuring there's a clear direction.

- **Duration Decisions:** Determining the overall duration of the training cycle is crucial. Whether it's a 12-week program, a 6-month plan, or a year-long journey, this decision will influence the length and focus of each phase.

- **Phase Goals:** Each phase within the periodization model should have a clear objective. For instance, in a hypertrophy phase, the goal might be muscle growth, while in a strength phase, it could be lifting heavier weights. Setting these goals ensures each phase has purpose and direction.

Individual Needs and Goals

- **Personalization:** A one-size-fits-all approach rarely works in training. Each individual has unique strengths, weaknesses, aspirations, and limitations. Creating the periodization model to these factors ensures better outcomes and reduces the risk of injuries or burnout.

Factors to Consider

- **Age:** Younger individuals might recover faster and adapt differently than older adults.

- **Training Experience:** Beginners might benefit from longer foundational phases, while advanced trainees might need more specialized blocks.

- **Fitness Level:** Someone already in shape might have different needs than someone just starting their fitness journey.

- **Specific Goals:** Training for a marathon requires a different approach than preparing for a bodybuilding competition.

Monitoring

- **The Feedback Loop:** Monitoring is the feedback loop in the training process. It provides insights into how effective the program is and whether the individual is moving closer to their goals.

- **Methods:** This can involve various methods, from performance tests (like time trials or strength tests) to physiological measures (like heart rate or muscle soreness). Subjective feedback, such as how the individual feels, is equally valuable.

- **Frequency:** While continuous monitoring is ideal, having structured check-ins, say every week or at the end of a phase, can provide a clearer picture of progress.

Adjustments

- **Staying Dynamic:** Training is not static. As individuals progress, face challenges, or even as their goals evolve, the training program should adapt.

- **Triggers for Change:** If monitoring reveals a plateau, increased fatigue, or if an individual feels they're not being challenged enough, it's time to adjust.

Types of Adjustments: This could involve:

- **Duration Changes:** Extending or shortening a phase based on progress.

- **Exercise Modifications:** Introducing new exercises or changing the sequence.

- **Intensity and Volume Tweaks:** Increasing weights, altering rep counts, or adjusting rest periods.

In essence, while periodization provides a structured approach to training, its implementation changes. It's a blend of science, where you follow proven principles, and art, where intuition, experience, and individual nuances play a significant role. Proper consideration and continuous engagement ensure that the training journey is not only effective but also enjoyable and fulfilling. Periodization stands harmoniously between science and art, evidence-based principles, and individual understanding. Let's delve deeper into these principles:

The Scientific Foundation

- **Evidence-Based Principles:** Periodization is built on decades of research and empirical evidence. Scientists and sports researchers have studied how the human body responds to different training stimuli, leading to the development of periodization models.

- **Physiological Adaptations:** The body's ability to adapt to training, whether it's building muscle, improving endurance, or enhancing power, is a complex physiological process. Periodization leverages this understanding, ensuring training aligns with the body's natural rhythms and recovery capacities.

The Artistic Touch

- **Individual Understanding:** No two individuals are the same. While science provides a framework, art ensures that this framework achieves the unique needs, goals, and circumstances of each person.

- **Intuition:** Often, the best coaches or athletes have a keen sense of intuition. They can sense when to push harder, when to pull back, and when to introduce variation. This intuition, honed over years of experience, adds an artistic touch to the structured world of periodization.

- **Flexibility:** Just as an artist might change a brush stroke in response to the evolving canvas, periodization requires the flexibility to adjust based on feedback. Whether it's an unexpected injury, a sudden change in goals, or simply a gut feeling, the ability to adapt the plan is where the art truly shines.

The Power of the Blend

- **Synergy:** When science and art come together in periodization, there's a synergy that amplifies the benefits of both. The structured approach ensures systematic progress, while the artistic touch ensures the journey is personalized and adaptable.

- **A Tool for All:** Periodization isn't just for elite athletes. The beauty of this combination is that it can be applied to anyone, from a beginner taking their first steps in fitness to a seasoned athlete aiming for Olympic gold. It's about maximizing potential, no matter where one starts.

In conclusion, periodization is more than just a training methodology; it's a philosophy. It respects the science of the human body, values the art of individual understanding, and, when done right, transforms training from a mundane routine into a dynamic journey of growth and discovery. Whether you're an athlete, coach, or someone passionate about fitness, embracing both the science and art of periodization can be a game-changer in your pursuit of excellence.

Types of Periodization

The realm of athletic training and physical fitness is vast and varied. From marathon runners to powerlifters, from ballet dancers to rugby players, the spectrum of physical activities and their demands is wide. Given this diversity, it's only logical that a single training approach wouldn't solve everyone's needs. This is where the brilliance of periodization comes in.

Training Approaches

Periodization is similar to a vast toolbox, brimming with various tools designed for specific tasks. Just as a carpenter wouldn't use a hammer for every job, an athlete or coach wouldn't employ the same training regimen for every goal or sport. Periodization acknowledges the unique demands of different activities and offers special strategies to meet them.

Adaptable to Individual Journeys

Every athlete has a unique journey. Some might be beginners, taking their first steps into the world of fitness. Others might be seasoned professionals, looking to fine-tune their performance for the next big competition. Then there are those recovering from injuries, aiming to regain their former prowess. Periodization, with its adaptable models, caters to all these scenarios. By allowing for structured variations in intensity, volume, and focus, it ensures that training remains relevant, challenging, and effective, regardless of where one is on their fitness journey.

A Dynamic Response to Changing Needs

The body's response to training isn't static. As one progresses, the challenges they face evolve too. Early plateaus, the need for skill refinement, or the desire to peak at the right moment for competition are all part and parcel of the athletic journey. Periodization, in its versatility, offers solutions to these challenges. It ensures that the body is always adapting, growing, and improving by cycling through different training focuses.

Incorporating Feedback and Real-world Results

One of the standout features of periodization is its feedback-driven approach. Segmenting training into distinct phases allows for regular assessment points. Athletes and coaches can evaluate performance, gauge progress, and make necessary adjustments. This iterative approach ensures that training remains aligned with goals and responsive to the athlete's evolving needs.

In athletic training, periodization stands out as a beacon of adaptability and precision. Its versatility is not just about offering different models but about understanding the demands of diverse physical activities and individual journeys. It's a testament to the marriage of science and art in the realm of physical training, ensuring that every athlete, regardless of their goals or experience, has a roadmap to success.

Linear Periodization

The Essence of Linearity in Training

Linear periodization, as the name suggests, follows a linear or sequential approach to training. Imagine climbing a mountain; you start at the base, gradually ascend, and eventually reach the peak. Similarly, in linear periodization, athletes start with foundational training and progressively move toward peak performance. This methodical progression ensures that each phase builds upon the previous one, paving a clear path towards the ultimate goal.

A Closer Look at the Phases--General Preparation Phase

Building the Base

- **The Foundation of Athletic Success:** Just as architects prioritize a sturdy foundation for skyscrapers, trainers, and athletes emphasize a solid base of fitness. Without this foundational strength and endurance, advanced training can lead to injuries and hinder performance.
- **Starting Slow:** The initial stages of the general preparation phase might seem basic, especially for seasoned athletes. However, these foundational exercises and routines are crucial. They set the stage for more advanced training down the line and ensure that the body is prepared for the increasing demands.

- **Mental and Physical Preparedness:** Beyond physical readiness, this phase also cultivates mental resilience. Athletes learn discipline, consistency, and patience, understanding that success is a gradual process built upon persistent effort.

Holistic Development

- **Beyond Muscle:** While muscle development is a significant component, holistic development encompasses cardiovascular endurance, flexibility, balance, and coordination. This comprehensive approach ensures that athletes are well-rounded and prepared for a variety of challenges.
- **The Power of Compound Exercises:** Compound exercises, like squats, deadlifts, and bench presses, are multi-joint movements that engage several muscle groups simultaneously. They not only promote muscle synergy but also mimic real-world or sports-specific movements, making them invaluable in training.
- **Functional Fitness:** The focus on compound exercises also leans into the realm of functional fitness. This means training the body for activities performed in daily life or sports, ensuring that the strength and endurance gained are not just for show but have practical applications.

Volume versus Intensity

The interplay between volume and intensity is a foundational concept in the realm of athletic training. These two parameters, while distinct, are deeply interconnected and play pivotal roles in shaping an athlete's training regimen and outcomes. Let's go deeper into their relationship and significance:

The Role of Repetitions in Skill Acquisition: The general preparation phase of an athlete's training is often characterized by a focus on volume, specifically in terms of repetitions and sets. This emphasis on high volume serves multiple purposes:

- **Technique Refinement:** By repeatedly performing a movement or exercise, athletes can hone their technique, ensuring that every aspect of the movement is executed correctly. This meticulous attention to detail can lead to more efficient and effective performance in the long run.

- **Muscle Memory Development:** Repetition is the mother of skill. The more an athlete repeats a particular movement, the more ingrained it becomes in their muscle memory. Over time, this can make complex movements feel almost automatic, allowing athletes to execute them with minimal conscious effort.

- **Endurance Building:** High-volume training, especially with resistance exercises, can also contribute to muscular endurance. Muscles are conditioned to sustain effort over extended periods, which can be beneficial in various sports and activities by performing more repetitions.

The Importance of Controlled Intensity: While volume is emphasized during the general preparation phase, it's crucial to balance it with appropriate intensity levels.

- **Injury Prevention:** Pushing too hard, especially when focusing on high volume, can strain muscles, tendons, and ligaments. By moderating the intensity, athletes can reduce the risk of injuries, ensuring a smoother and more sustainable training progression.

- **Sustainable Progress:** A moderated intensity ensures that athletes can maintain consistency in their training. They can steadily progress, building strength, endurance, and skill over time instead of facing extreme fatigue or burnout from overly intense sessions.

Striking the Right Balance for Optimal Adaptation: The synergy between volume and intensity is what drives effective training adaptations.

- **Physiological Adaptations:** The body responds to the specific demands placed upon it. A balance between volume and intensity ensures that muscles, cardiovascular systems, and neural pathways adapt optimally, leading to improvements in strength, endurance, and coordination.

- **Recovery Considerations:** Training is only one part of the equation. Recovery is equally vital. Therefore, athletes can optimize their recovery periods, allowing muscles to repair and grow, and energy systems to replenish by ensuring that intensity doesn't overshadow volume.

- **Psychological Benefits:** A balanced approach also has psychological advantages. Athletes can experience the satisfaction of completing high-volume sessions without the demotivation that can come from excessive fatigue or the risk of injury.

  Here, volume and intensity are two sides of the same coin. While they serve different purposes in training, their coordinated application is what leads to holistic athletic development. Athletes can pave the way for success both in training and performance.

Specific Preparation Phase

Transitioning to Specificity

The specific preparation phase is a pivotal point in an athlete's training journey. It's the bridge between foundational conditioning and the pinnacle of performance.

The preparation phase and its significance:

Embracing Sport-Specific Training: The overall theme of the specific preparation phase is specialization. As athletes transition from the broader strokes of general conditioning, this phase narrows the focus, honing in on the unique demands of their respective sports or events.

- **Purpose-Driven Approach:** Every exercise, drill, and training session in this phase serves a clear purpose. It's not about merely staying fit or building strength; it's about preparing the athlete for the specific challenges they'll face in competition. A sprinter, for instance, might shift their focus to explosive starts and speed drills, while a wrestler might emphasize grip strength and mat techniques.

- **Simulating Competitive Conditions:** One of the hallmarks of the specific preparation phase is its emphasis on replicating competition scenarios. This is more than just practicing the sport; it's about creating training environments that closely mimic the conditions of actual competitions. A tennis player might practice serves and volleys under varying wind conditions, or a triathlete might train transitions between swimming, cycling, and running to optimize their race-day performance.

- **Individualized Training Regimens:** The specific preparation phase recognizes the uniqueness of each athlete. While two athletes might compete in the same sport, their training needs can differ based on their roles, physical attributes, and personal goals. A goalkeeper in soccer will have a different training focus compared to a forward. This phase is characterized by its adaptability, ensuring that each athlete's regimen is crafted to their specific needs and objectives.

The Science Behind Specificity: The principle of specificity is rooted in the understanding of how our bodies adapt to training stimuli. When our bodies are exposed to specific demands consistently, they undergo physiological changes to better handle those demands in the future.

- **Neuromuscular Adaptations:** Repeatedly practicing specific movements or skills can lead to enhanced neuromuscular coordination. This means that the brain and muscles communicate more efficiently, allowing for smoother and more precise execution of those movements.

- **Energy System Optimization:** Different sports and events rely on different energy systems. A 100-meter sprinter taps into their anaerobic system, while a marathoner predominantly uses their aerobic system. The specific preparation phase ensures that training targets the relevant energy system, optimizing its efficiency for competition.

- **Tactical and Strategic Development:** Beyond physical preparation, this phase also emphasizes the tactical and strategic aspects of the sport. Athletes engage in scenario-based training, game plan discussions, and strategy sessions to ensure they're mentally prepared for the many situations they might encounter in competition.

So, the specific preparation phase is where the general conditioning is overlaid with the intricate details of sport-specific training. It's a period of refinement, where athletes sharpen their skills, strategies, and bodies to meet the exacting demands of their sport or event. Through a combination of purpose-driven training, real-world simulations, and individualized regimens, athletes are primed to perform at their best when it matters most.

Balancing Act

In the athlete's journey, this phase is characterized by a heightened focus on pushing boundaries while maintaining a delicate balance to ensure optimal performance and safety. Let's delve deeper into this intricate balancing act:

Intensity and Volume: The specific preparation phase is marked by a shift in the training dynamics, where intensity and volume play pivotal roles, each complementing the other.

- **The Rise of Intensity:** As athletes transition into this phase, there's a noticeable uptick in the intensity of their training sessions. Whether it's lifting heavier weights in the gym, sprinting at faster speeds on the track, or executing more complex drills on the field, the emphasis is on pushing the envelope. This surge in intensity is vital for simulating competition conditions and preparing the athlete for the rigors of their sport or event.

- **Volume's Strategic Retreat:** While intensity climbs, volume—measured in terms of repetitions, sets, or duration takes a deliberate step back. This isn't a sign of reduced effort but a strategic move. So, athletes can focus on the quality of each repetition or drill by reducing volume, ensuring precision and effectiveness. Moreover, this reduction safeguards against overtraining, which can be a risk when intensity levels soar.

The Imperative of Recovery: With the heightened demands of the specific preparation phase, recovery emerges as a cornerstone of the training regimen.

- **Physiological Necessity:** As athletes push their bodies to new limits, the physiological stress increases. Muscles undergo micro-tears, energy stores deplete, and the nervous system gets tasked. Recovery periods, whether in the form of rest days, light training sessions, or specific recovery techniques like foam rolling or massage, allow the body to heal and rebuild. This process of repair and rejuvenation is what leads to strength gains and performance improvements.
- **Setting the Stage for Adaptation:** Recovery isn't just about resting; it's about adaptation. The body's response to training stimuli, especially at high intensities, is to adapt and become more resilient. Adequate recovery ensures that these adaptations occur optimally, preparing the athlete for subsequent training sessions and, ultimately, peak performance.
- **Mental Refreshment:** Beyond the physical aspect, recovery also plays a role in mental well-being. Intense training sessions can be mentally tasking. Periods of rest and lighter training can help refresh the mind, ensuring that athletes remain focused, motivated, and ready for the challenges ahead.

In summary, the specific preparation phase is a masterclass in balance and precision. It's where athletes refine their skills, push their boundaries, and prepare for the pinnacle of their sport or event. Through a judicious mix of intensity, volume, and recovery, they ensure that they're not just working hard but working smart, setting the stage for success when it counts the most.

Competition Phase: The Apex of Athletic Preparation

The Competition Phase stands as the pinnacle of the athletes' journey. This isn't just another chapter in their story; it's the climax, the moment when every drop of sweat, every hour of training, and every sacrifice converges.

Let's picture Lucas, a dedicated swimmer. For him, water isn't just a medium; it's a place where he finds his true self. He's been training for the most significant championship of his life. Every stroke, every lap, has led him to this moment: The Competition Phase, or as he calls it, "The Final Push".

The pool, which once felt vast and intimidating, now seems like home. But Lucas knows that this phase is different. It's not about building; it's about refining. Every dive, every turn, is scrutinized, analyzed, and perfected. This is the phase of "Strategic Intensification". His coach, a seasoned veteran, leaves no stone unturned. They dissect every movement, ensuring that Lucas isn't just prepared but is in the prime shape of his life.

But Lucas's preparation isn't just physical. The Competition Phase brings with it a weight, a pressure that can be crushing. The bright lights, the roaring crowd, and the weight of expectations constitute a mental battlefield. Lucas undergoes rigorous mental conditioning sessions, learning to harness his nerves, and channeling them into focus, calmness, and unwavering confidence.

The essence of the Competition Phase is "Peak Performance". It's where every element of Lucas's training must come together in perfect agreement. His coach often speaks of "Synchronized Excellence". It's not just about training hard but training smart, ensuring that Lucas peaks at the exact moment he dives into the pool during the championship.

To mimic the pressures of the big day, Lucas engages in "Tactical Rehearsals". He competes in mock races, simulating the championship environment. The tension, the competition, and the unpredictability are a mirror to the main event, ensuring Lucas is ready for any scenario.

As the championship draws near, Lucas's diet consciously changes. Every meal, every drink, is chosen with precision. "Nutrition and Hydration" become his mantras. Specialized diets, rich in proteins, essential fats, and hydrating fluids, ensure his body is a well-oiled machine, ready to deliver a performance that's nothing short of spectacular.

In the grand tapestry of athletic training, the Competition Phase is the crowning jewel. For Lucas, it's more than just a phase; it's a testament to his dedication, his passion, and his unwavering spirit. As he stands at the edge of the pool, ready to dive into destiny, he knows he's prepared, not just in body, but in soul. The Competition Phase has forged him into a champion, ready to conquer the waves and etch his name in history.

Active Rest Phase

In linear periodization, there's a phase often overlooked by many but cherished by seasoned athletes: the Active Rest Phase. Imagine an athlete, let's call him Alex, who has just completed an intense training cycle. His muscles are sore, his joints slightly achy, and mentally, he's exhausted. He knows that pushing further without a break might lead to burnout or, worse, an injury.

He enters the Active Rest Phase. Instead of completely sidelining himself, Alex decides to engage in this phase, a period designed not for pushing boundaries but for healing and rejuvenation. It's not about sitting on the couch all day; it's about staying active, but at a much gentler pace.

Each morning, Alex swaps his heavy weights and sprinting sessions for light jogs in the park. Some days, he dives into the pool, letting cool his tired muscles with water as he swims at a leisurely pace. On others, he rolls out his yoga mat, stretching and breathing, focusing on flexibility and mindfulness.

This phase, which might last a week or even a month, offers Alex numerous benefits. His muscles are grateful for the respite, repair, and grow stronger. The light activities keep the blood flowing, aiding in recovery. Mentally, the change of pace is refreshing. The intense focus and determination required during his training cycles give way to a sense of calm and enjoyment.

But it's not just about physical and mental recovery. This phase prepares Alex for the challenges ahead. As the days go by, he feels his energy returning, his enthusiasm for his sport reigniting. He knows that when this phase ends, he'll be ready to move back into his training, stronger and more focused than before.

The main aspect of the Active Rest Phase is to halve the amount of intensity or volume of the other phases. In essence, the Active Rest Phase is like the calm after a storm, a period of tranquility and healing that ensures Alex is not just recovering, but also evolving, setting the stage for greater achievements in the future.

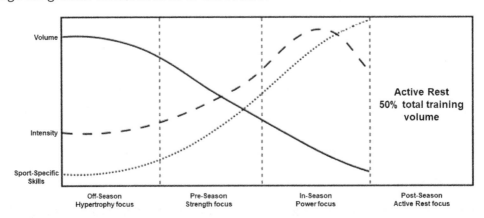

Who Stands to Benefit?

Linear periodization is particularly beneficial for those with clear, long-term objectives. Whether it's an athlete preparing for a championship several months away or an individual training for a marathon, this model offers a structured roadmap. The predictable nature of linear periodization, with its clear progression from one phase to the next, makes it ideal for those who have set competition dates or milestones.

In Conclusion

The primary principle of Linear Periodization is that the program starts with high volume, lower intensity at the beginning of the off-season, and progressively inverts while moving towards the year's main event. Additionally, throughout the year, sport-specific drills continuously increase from the off-season to the main event.

Linear Periodization is a tried-and-true method, rooted in the principles of progressive overload and specificity. It offers athletes a systematic and structured approach to achieving their peak potential by segmenting training into distinct phases, each with its unique focus and intensity. Whether you're a novice looking to embark on a fitness journey or a seasoned athlete aiming for gold, linear periodization provides a clear and effective path to success.

Undulating Periodization

Undulating periodization is a methodology that defies the conventional, challenges the predictable, and embraces the dynamic in athletic training. Let's embark on a journey to understand this concept more deeply.

The Essence of Fluidity: Imagine a vast ocean, its waves rising and falling, never static, always in motion. This is the spirit captured by undulating periodization. It's a methodology that refuses to be boxed into a set pattern, choosing instead to flow and adapt, much like water. The essence of this approach is its fluidity, ensuring that training remains dynamic and ever-evolving.

The Intensity and Volume: In undulating periodization, intensity, and volume are like partners, moving in tandem but always varying their steps. On some days, intensity takes the lead, pushing the athlete to their limits, while volume might take a step back. On others, volume takes the lead, demanding more repetitions or longer durations, while intensity might be dialed down. This symbiotic relationship ensures that the body is continuously challenged in diverse ways.

Breaking the Monotony: Routine can be both a friend and a foe. While it brings a sense of familiarity, it can also lead to monotony. Undulating periodization breaks this cycle. By constantly shifting the training parameters, it ensures that every session brings with it a new challenge, a new adventure. For an athlete, this means that every day is a fresh start, and a new puzzle to solve.

Adapting to the Unpredictable: Life is unpredictable, and so is training under undulating periodization. This unpredictability is its strength. The body, when exposed to varied stimuli, is forced to adapt, grow, and evolve. It can't settle or become complacent because the next challenge is always just around the corner.

The Philosophy of Change: Undulating periodization is rooted in the philosophy of change. It acknowledges that for growth to occur, change is essential. It ensures that athletes are not just going through the motions but are actively engaged, mentally and physically, in their training journey by introducing this change in a structured yet varied manner.

In conclusion, the core concept of undulating periodization is not just about varying workouts; it's about embracing change, challenging the status quo, and pushing boundaries. It's a testament to the idea that growth occurs not in comfort but in adaptation, ensuring that athletes are always on a path of discovery, evolution, and peak performance.

Dynamic Nature

Training: Training is the essence of the dynamic nature of undulating periodization. Each training session, with its unique intensity and volume, contributes to a larger, harmonious training plan, ensuring that no two days are ever truly the same.

The Roller Coaster of Effort: For an athlete, let's revisit our friend, Jake, whose training under undulating periodization is akin to riding a roller coaster. There are highs, where he pushes his limits to the maximum, feeling every muscle burn with effort. Then there are the lows, where he allows his body to recover, preparing for the next ascent. This continuous ebb and flow ensures that Jake's body and mind are always engaged, and always anticipating the next challenge.

Breaking Predictability: In many training regimens, predictability is the norm. Monday might always be leg day, and Tuesday might always focus on cardio. But undulating periodization shatters this predictability. Jake might find himself lifting heavy weights one day and focusing on endurance the next. This unpredictability keeps him on his toes, ensuring that every training session is a new adventure.

The Balance of Challenge and Recovery: The dynamic nature of undulating periodization isn't just about introducing variability; it's about striking a balance. While it's essential to challenge the body, recovery is equally crucial. By varying the intensity and volume, this approach ensures that while the body is pushed to its limits on some days, it's also given time to recover and rejuvenate on others.

Embracing the Unknown: One of the most exciting aspects of the dynamic nature of undulating periodization is the element of surprise. Jake never truly knows what to expect from his next training session. This sense of the unknown keeps him motivated, curious, and eager to train, ensuring that his passion and enthusiasm never waned.

In essence, the dynamic nature of undulating periodization is its most defining feature. It's a matter of effort and recovery, challenge and rest, known and unknown. For athletes like Jake, it ensures that training is not just a routine but a journey of discovery, growth, and continuous evolution.

Contrast with Linear Model

The Straightforward Path versus The Winding Trail: Imagine two roads: one is a straight highway, stretching endlessly, its path clear and direct. This represents the linear model, where progression is steady and predictable. The other road is a winding road, with unexpected turns, ascents, and descents. This embodies undulating periodization, where the journey is filled with varied challenges and surprises.

The Predictability of Linear Progression: In the linear model, there's a sense of comfort in its predictability. An athlete, let's name her Sophie, knows that each week she'll push a little harder, run a little further, or lift a little heavier. It's a gradual climb, where the end goal is clear, and the path to it is methodically charted.

The Dynamic Shifts of Undulating Periodization: Contrast this with Jake, our athlete earlier mentioned, who follows undulating periodization. His training is a mosaic of intensities and volumes. One week might see him pushing his boundaries with high-intensity sessions, while the next could focus on volume, with longer but less intense workouts. The unpredictability ensures that Jake's body is always adapting, always evolving.

The Evolution of Adaptation: While both models aim for progress, their approach to adaptation differs. In the linear model, the body adapts to increasing demands over extended periods. Sophie's body gets used to the steady increments, preparing for the next predictable increase. In undulating periodization, the body is kept guessing. Jake's muscles and cardiovascular system are continuously challenged in new ways, ensuring that adaptation is multifaceted and comprehensive.

The Flexibility of Undulating Periodization: One of the standout features of undulating periodization is its inherent flexibility. While the linear model follows a set trajectory, undulating periodization can be channeled to an athlete's needs, goals, and even external factors like competitions or recovery from minor injuries. This adaptability ensures that training remains relevant, effective, and aligned with the athlete's objectives.

In athletic training, both linear and undulating periodization have their merits. While the linear model offers clarity and a straightforward path, undulating periodization thrives on variability and adaptability. For athletes, the choice between the two often boils down to their goals, preferences, and the challenges they wish to embrace. Both roads lead to progress, but the journey on each is distinct and unique.

The Role of Variability

The Spice of Training: Just as variety is said to be the spice of life, variability is the spice of training. It introduces an element of unpredictability, ensuring that workouts remain fresh, engaging, and challenging. Without variability, training can become monotonous, leading to decreased motivation and potential risks.

The Science Behind Variability: From a physiological perspective, variability plays a crucial role in preventing the body from adapting too quickly to a specific stimulus. When the body is exposed to the same type of training repeatedly, it becomes more efficient, leading to decreased energy expenditure and, eventually, diminished results. By introducing variability, undulating periodization ensures that the body is always facing new challenges, prompting continuous adaptation and growth.

Tailored Challenges: Variability isn't about random changes; it's about tailored challenges. Depending on the athlete's goals, strengths, and weaknesses, the variability in their training can be designed to target specific areas. For instance, if an athlete struggles with endurance, certain phases might focus more on volume, while others might emphasize strength or speed.

Mental Engagement and Motivation: Beyond the physical benefits, variability plays a pivotal role in keeping athletes mentally engaged. Knowing that each training session brings something different can be a significant motivator. It adds an element of curiosity and excitement, ensuring that athletes remain eager and committed to their training regimen.

Adapting to External Factors: Life is unpredictable. Athletes might face unexpected challenges, from minor injuries to changes in their competition schedules. The inherent variability in undulating periodization allows for flexibility, ensuring that training can be adapted based on external factors, and keeping athletes on track even when faced with unforeseen circumstances.

In summary, variability is the heartbeat of undulating periodization. It's what sets it apart, ensuring that training remains a dynamic journey of continuous growth and adaptation. Sticking to variability helps athletes not just go through the motions but also on a path of discovery, challenge, and peak performance.

Continuous Adaptation

The Ever-Changing Landscape of Training: In athletics, staying static is akin to moving backward. The beauty of undulating periodization lies in its ever-changing landscape, ensuring that athletes are always on a path of evolution. Each session, with its varied intensity and volume, presents a new challenge, prompting the body to adapt and grow.

The Body's Remarkable Resilience: Our bodies are not just vessels; they're dynamic entities, constantly learning and adapting. When we face a new challenge, we recalibrate, finding ways to become more efficient and resilient. While this adaptability is a testament to our body's incredible capabilities, it can be a double-edged sword in training. If the challenges become too predictable, the body's adaptive responses can lead to plateaus.

The Catalyst of Change: Undulating periodization acts as a catalyst, constantly introducing new variables into the training equation. Just as the body starts to adapt to a particular regimen, the parameters shift, reigniting the adaptive response. This ensures that the body is always in a state of flux, continuously growing and improving.

Mental and Physical Symbiosis: Adaptation isn't just a physical phenomenon; it's a mental one as well. The varied nature of undulating periodization ensures that athletes remain mentally engaged, always anticipating the next challenge. This mental engagement, combined with the physical challenges, creates a symbiotic relationship where the mind and body work together, driving continuous progress.

The Long-Term Perspective: While the immediate benefits of continuous adaptation are evident in short-term progress, the real magic lies in the long-term perspective. Athletes training under undulating periodization are better equipped to handle the rigors of their sport over extended periods. The constant adaptation prepares them for varied challenges, ensuring they remain at the top of their game, season after season.

In conclusion, continuous adaptation is the heartbeat of undulating periodization. It ensures that training is not just a series of exercises but a dynamic journey of growth, challenge, and evolution. For athletes, it offers the promise of never-ending progress, ensuring that every session, every challenge, brings them closer to their peak potential.

Prevention of Stagnation

The Invisible Wall: Every athlete, at some point in their journey, encounters what feels like an invisible wall: the dreaded plateau. It's a phase where, despite pouring in consistent effort, progress seems unattainable. The routines that once yielded results now seem ineffective. Stagnation is not just a physical challenge but a mental one, often leading to frustration and dwindling motivation.

The Adaptive Nature of the Human Body: Our bodies are marvels of adaptation. When subjected to consistent stimuli, they learn, adapt, and become more efficient. While this adaptability is a testament to our evolutionary prowess, it poses challenges in a training context. The routines that once pushed our boundaries become the new norm, leading to diminished returns.

The Magic of Variability: Undulating periodization, with its inherent variability, acts as a powerful antidote to stagnation. It ensures that the body never truly settles into a routine by continuously changing the training parameters. Just as it begins to adapt to a particular stimulus, a new challenge is introduced, reigniting the cycle of growth and adaptation.

Mental Rejuvenation: Beyond the physical benefits, the variability in undulating periodization offers a mental respite. The ever-changing nature of the workouts brings a sense of novelty and excitement. For athletes, this means that every session presents a new challenge, a new puzzle to solve, ensuring that their mental engagement remains high and burnout is kept at bay.

Long-Term Consistency: One of the most significant advantages of preventing stagnation is the promotion of long-term consistency. When athletes see continuous progress, their motivation remains high, leading to sustained effort over extended periods. Undulating periodization, by preventing plateaus, ensures that athletes remain committed to their training journey, always eager to discover what the next session holds.

In essence, the prevention of stagnation is one of the most compelling arguments in favor of undulating periodization. It ensures that the journey of training remains dynamic, rewarding, and progressive. For athletes, it offers the promise of continuous growth, ensuring that every drop of sweat, every hour of effort, brings them one step closer to their goals.

Key Characteristics

Variability:

- **Essence of the Model:** Variability is not just a feature of undulating periodization; it's its very essence. It's what sets this training approach apart from others. Instead of a predictable, steady increase or consistent pattern, undulating periodization thrives on change, ensuring that no two training sessions or cycles are exactly alike.
- **Fluctuations in Intensity and Volume:** The two primary parameters that see a constant change in this model are intensity and volume. Intensity refers to how hard a workout or exercise session is, often gauged by the amount of weight lifted, the speed of a run, or the resistance in a cycling session. Volume, on the other hand, pertains to the quantity of work done, such as the number of repetitions, sets, or the distance covered. In undulating periodization, both these parameters are in a state of flux, ensuring a multifaceted training experience.
- **Daily versus Weekly Variations:** The frequency of these changes can differ based on the specific program or the goals of the individual. Some might experience these shifts, where every day of training within a week has a distinct focus. For instance, Monday could be high-intensity but low-volume, while Tuesday might be moderate on both counts, and Wednesday could be low-intensity but high-volume. On the other hand, some programs might introduce these changes every week, where the focus of one week differs significantly from the next.
- **Benefits of Variability:** This constant change has multiple benefits. Firstly, it ensures that the body is always being challenged in new ways, promoting continuous adaptation and growth. Secondly, it reduces the risk of overuse injuries, as no single muscle group or joint is being subjected to the same kind of stress repeatedly. Lastly, it keeps the training regimen fresh and engaging, reducing the likelihood of boredom or burnout.
- **Adaptable to Individual Needs:** Another noteworthy characteristic of the variability in undulating periodization is its adaptability. Depending on an individual's goals, fitness

level, and other factors, the degree and frequency of changes can be adjusted. This makes it a versatile tool that can be channeled to meet diverse training needs.

In summary, the variability inherent in undulating periodization is both its defining feature and its greatest strength. By constantly changing the training stimuli, it offers a holistic, adaptable, and engaging approach to fitness that caters to a wide range of goals and needs.

The Architectural Blueprint: The Structure of Undulating Periodization

Microcycles - The Building Blocks: Imagine constructing a building. Before the skyscraper stands tall, it starts with the laying of individual bricks. In undulating periodization, these bricks are microcycles. Spanning typically between one to four weeks, microcycles are the foundational units of this training approach. Each microcycle is meticulously designed, with days earmarked for specific intensities and volumes. Picture an athlete, let's call him Leo. His week might kick off with a session that pushes him to his limits, a high-intensity day. As the week progresses, he might find himself in a moderate-intensity session, allowing for a bit of recovery while still challenging his body. By the week's end, a low-intensity day ensures he's recuperating, gearing up for the challenges of the next microcycle.

The Art of Variation - Weekly Fluctuations: If microcycles are the bricks, then weekly fluctuations are the patterns and designs that give the building its unique character. Undulating periodization thrives on variability, and this is most evident in its weekly fluctuations. Each week presents a new challenge, a new combination of intensity and volume. For Leo, this means that no two weeks are the same. One week might focus heavily on building strength, while the next could emphasize endurance. This constant shift ensures that Leo's body never settles into a routine. It's always adapting, always evolving, ensuring that plateaus are kept at bay.

The Training Stimuli: The beauty of undulating periodization lies in its training stimuli. This approach ensures that every aspect of an athlete's training is harmoniously integrated. The highs and lows, the intense days, and the recovery days, all come together to create a training regimen that's both challenging and sustainable.

The Long-Term Vision: While the immediate focus might be on the microcycles and weekly fluctuations, undulating periodization is designed with a long-term vision in mind. Each microcycle builds on the previous one, and each week's fluctuations are designed to complement the next. For Leo, this means that while each day and week presents its unique challenges, they all contribute to his overarching training goals, be it a marathon, a weightlifting competition, or simply achieving overall physical fitness.

In this regard, the structure of undulating periodization is both an art and a science. It's meticulously designed to ensure continuous growth, prevent stagnation, and keep athletes engaged and motivated. It's a journey of peaks and valleys, challenges, and recoveries, all leading to the ultimate goal of optimal performance.

Ideal Candidates

Athletes

In competitive sports, athletes are always in pursuit of methods and techniques that can enhance their performance. Achieving peak performance often requires a multifaceted approach, targeting various aspects of an athlete's physical capabilities.

For instance, a sprinter, while primarily focused on explosive power, also needs a degree of endurance to maintain speed throughout a race. Similarly, a marathon runner, although predominantly concerned with endurance, can benefit from strength training to improve running economy and reduce the risk of injuries. A soccer player, on the other hand, requires a combination of agility, strength, speed, and endurance to go through the demands of a 90-minute game effectively.

Undulating periodization caters to these diverse needs by providing a structured training regimen that emphasizes different physical attributes at different times. Scientific studies have shown that varying training stimuli can lead to better overall athletic adaptation. For example, a research study might reveal that athletes who incorporated both strength and endurance training in varied cycles achieved better overall performance metrics than those who focused on just one aspect.

Athletes can also ensure that they're not only developing one aspect of their fitness but are achieving a comprehensive, well-rounded athletic profile by employing undulating periodization. This approach allows for targeted training phases. An athlete might focus on strength and power during one phase, utilizing exercises like squats, deadlifts, and plyometrics. In another phase, the emphasis might shift to cardiovascular endurance, with longer, aerobic sessions or interval training.

Furthermore, the varied nature of undulating periodization can help in injury prevention. Overtraining or excessively focusing on one type of training can lead to overuse injuries.

By diversifying the training stimuli, athletes can reduce the risk of such injuries, ensuring they remain in optimal shape throughout their competitive season.

In summary, undulating periodization provides athletes with a scientifically-backed approach to achieve holistic development, ensuring they are prepared for the multifaceted demands of their respective sports.

Fitness Enthusiasts

Fitness enthusiasts, whether they're regulars at the local gym, participants in park boot camps, or dedicated home workout practitioners, often seek continuous improvement and personal growth. Their goals might range from achieving a specific body composition, increasing their cardiovascular fitness, or simply enhancing overall well-being. For such individuals, undulating periodization offers a structured and scientifically-backed approach to achieving these objectives.

Research has shown that the body responds best to varied training stimuli. By continuously changing the intensity and volume of workouts, undulating periodization prevents the body from adapting too quickly to a specific routine. For instance, a fitness enthusiast might incorporate heavy resistance training exercises in one week to target muscle growth. The following week, they might shift to high-intensity interval training (HIIT) sessions, which are known to boost cardiovascular fitness and enhance metabolic rate.

Such variation has multiple benefits. From a physiological viewpoint, it ensures that different energy systems and muscle groups are targeted, leading to comprehensive fitness improvements. For example, alternating between strength training and aerobic exercises can optimize both anaerobic and aerobic energy pathways, ensuring balanced development.

Furthermore, the varied nature of undulating periodization can combat the plateau effect. When the body is subjected to the same type of training stimulus over extended periods, it becomes efficient, leading to diminished returns. Fitness enthusiasts can ensure that they're consistently making progress, be it in terms of muscle gain, fat loss, or endurance enhancement just by introducing regular changes in the workout regimen.

Lastly, from a psychological perspective, the varied nature of workouts can help maintain high levels of motivation and commitment. Repeating the same exercises and routines can become tedious over time. However, with undulating periodization, every week presents a new set of challenges and goals, ensuring that the training journey remains engaging and goal-oriented.

Benefits of Undulating Periodization

Prevention of Plateaus: One of the most common challenges faced by individuals in a consistent training regimen is the dreaded plateau. This occurs when the body becomes too efficient at a specific type of exercise, leading to diminished returns. With undulating periodization, the frequent shifts in intensity and volume ensure that the body is always exposed to varied stimuli. Scientifically, this constant variation challenges the body's homeostasis, forcing it to adapt and grow continuously. As a result, individuals experience consistent progress in their fitness journey.

Keeps Training Engaging: Repetitiveness can lead to decreased motivation and enthusiasm for workouts. Undulating periodization, with its ever-changing focus, ensures that every session is different from the last. This not only provides a physical challenge but also keeps the training sessions mentally stimulating. The anticipation of what each session holds can be a significant motivator, ensuring that individuals remain committed to their training regimen.

Psychological Benefits: Training isn't just a physical endeavor; it's a mental one as well. The varied nature of undulating periodization ensures that individuals are always mentally engaged, anticipating the challenges of each session. This continuous engagement can lead to a heightened sense of accomplishment as individuals conquer diverse challenges. Furthermore, achieving small milestones in varied domains (strength, endurance, agility) can boost confidence and foster a positive mindset, essential for long-term commitment and success in any fitness journey.

Flexibility and Customization: Undulating periodization stands out for its adaptability. It's not a one-size-fits-all approach. Instead, it can be designed to meet individual needs. For instance, a sprinter might focus more on power and speed, with occasional endurance sessions, while a triathlete might have a more balanced approach, targeting strength, endurance, and agility in equal measures. This adaptability ensures that individuals can mold their training regimen based on their specific goals, strengths, and areas of improvement.

In Conclusion

The primary principle of Undulating periodization is the change of high intensity-low volume to low intensity-high volume. Unlike the progressive one-time change of linear periodization, this change constantly occurs throughout the year with Undulating periodization, creating a constant flux of intensity and volume.

Undulating periodization is more than just a training model; it's a holistic approach to fitness. It recognizes the multifaceted nature of athletic performance and personal fitness goals, offering a dynamic and adaptable path to achieve them. Undulating periodization emerges as a preferred choice for those serious about their fitness journey by ensuring physical and mental engagement, preventing plateaus, and allowing for customization. Whether you're aiming for the podium or personal milestones, this approach provides the tools and framework to achieve success.

Block Periodization: A Comprehensive Look

Introduction to Block Periodization:

Block periodization stands as a beacon in the realm of athletic training methodologies. It's a systematic and strategic approach that segments an athlete's training regimen into distinct periods or "blocks". Each of these blocks is meticulously designed to concentrate on specific athletic attributes, ensuring that every facet of an athlete's performance is addressed in a structured manner.

The beauty of block periodization lies in its clarity and focus. Instead of juggling multiple training objectives simultaneously, athletes can channel their energy and efforts into honing a particular skill or attribute during each block. This concentrated approach not only allows for deeper mastery but also ensures that the foundational elements are firmly in place before advancing to more specialized training.

For instance, before an athlete can work on their technique or strategy, they must first possess the requisite strength, endurance, and basic skills. Block periodization recognizes this hierarchy of needs and structures training accordingly.

Moreover, this method is rooted in the science of human physiology and adaptation. The body responds optimally when subjected to specific stimuli over a consistent period, allowing for targeted adaptations. By dedicating blocks of time to particular training focuses, athletes can achieve more profound and lasting physiological changes, be it in muscle growth, aerobic capacity, or neuromuscular efficiency.

Furthermore, block periodization also considers the psychological aspects of training. Achieving mastery or noticeable improvement in a specific area during a block can boost an athlete's confidence and motivation, setting a positive tone for subsequent blocks.

In essence, block periodization is not just a training schedule; it's a philosophy. It emphasizes depth over breadth, mastery over mere participation, and structured progression over random activity. For athletes serious about achieving their peak potential, block periodization offers a clear, focused, and scientifically-backed path forward.

Diving Deeper into the Concept of Block Periodization

Block periodization, as a training methodology, is more than just a division of training into separate blocks. It's a reflection of a deep understanding of how the human body adapts, grows, and evolves in response to specific training stimuli over time. This approach is rooted in both the science of sports physiology and the practical experiences of elite athletes and coaches.

Block periodization is mostly about optimizing the training process. It allows athletes to channel their efforts more effectively by segmenting training into distinct phases, each with a clear focus. This ensures that every training session is purposeful and contributes to a larger, overarching goal.

For instance, consider the process of building a house. Before one can decorate the interiors or paint the walls, a solid foundation must be laid, and the basic structure must be erected. Similarly, in block periodization, the foundational skills and attributes are developed first, setting the stage for more specialized and advanced training later on.

The segmentation also allows for better monitoring and evaluation. Coaches and athletes can assess progress at the end of each block, making necessary adjustments for subsequent phases. This iterative process ensures that training remains aligned with the athlete's goals and that any potential issues are addressed promptly.

From a physiological perspective, block periodization aligns with the body's natural adaptation mechanisms. The human body responds best when exposed to consistent, specific stimuli over a period. By dedicating blocks of time to particular training focuses, such as strength, endurance, or power, athletes can achieve more profound and lasting physiological adaptations. This targeted approach ensures that the body isn't overwhelmed with too many stimuli at once, leading to more effective and efficient training adaptations.

Moreover, the concept of block periodization acknowledges the interconnectedness of different athletic attributes. While each block has a primary focus, the training often incorporates elements from previous blocks, ensuring a holistic development. For example, even in a block dedicated to power development, elements of endurance or foundational strength might still be included to maintain and support the primary training focus.

In summary, the concept of block periodization is a testament to the intricacies of athletic training. It's a method that respects the complexity of human physiology, the psychology of motivation and progress, and the practicalities of athletic performance.

Types of Blocks Periodization

Block Periodization: A Structured Journey Towards Athletic Mastery

Block periodization is a systematic approach to training, where the athlete's journey is divided into distinct phases, each channeled to specific developmental needs. This methodical progression ensures that athletes evolve fully, addressing every facet of their athletic prowess. Let's explore each block in detail:

The Accumulation Phase: Building the Foundation

The accumulation phase is the initial step in the block periodization journey, setting the stage for all subsequent training phases. It's a time of foundational work, where athletes focus on building the essential components of their athletic profile. Let's delve deeper into the intricacies and objectives of this phase:

- **Muscle Development:** While muscle growth, is a primary goal during this phase, it's not just about increasing muscle size. It's about creating a muscular foundation that can support the more intense and specialized training that follows. Athletes engage in resistance training routines, often using moderate weights with higher repetitions, to stimulate muscle fibers and promote growth.

- **Strength:** Alongside muscle development, there's a significant emphasis on developing foundational strength. This isn't about lifting the heaviest weights but about building a base level of strength that's sustainable and can be built upon in later phases. Compound exercises, which engage multiple muscle groups simultaneously, are staples during this phase. These exercises, such as squats, deadlifts, and bench presses, ensure a holistic development of strength across the body.

- **Skill Development:** The accumulation phase is also a crucial period for skill acquisition and refinement. Athletes dedicate significant time to mastering the fundamental techniques and movements integral to their sport. This could involve a tennis player working on their serve mechanics, a swimmer focusing on their kick technique, or a gymnast perfecting their basic routines. The idea is to ingrain these movements so deeply that they become second nature, allowing the athlete to execute them flawlessly under the pressures of competition.

- **Endurance and Cardiovascular Fitness:** Beyond strength and skill, the accumulation phase often incorporates cardiovascular training. Whether it's through steady-state runs, interval training, or sport-specific cardio drills, the aim is to enhance the athlete's stamina and cardiovascular efficiency. This foundational cardiovascular fitness will support the increased intensities in the subsequent phases.

- **Flexibility and Mobility:** An often-overlooked aspect of the accumulation phase is the emphasis on flexibility and mobility. Athletes engage in stretching routines, mobility drills, and even practices like yoga to ensure their joints and muscles remain supple. This flexibility is crucial for preventing injuries and ensuring a full range of motion in sport-specific movements.

In essence, the accumulation phase is a multifaceted period of training, where athletes focus on building a robust and versatile athletic foundation. It's about creating a well-rounded profile, ensuring that athletes have the strength, skills, endurance, and flexibility to support the more specialized and intense training that lies ahead.

The Transmutation Phase:

The transmutation phase represents a pivotal transition in the block periodization model. As athletes move from the foundational work of the accumulation phase, they now begin to refine and specialize their training to closely align with their sport's specific demands. This phase is characterized by its emphasis on converting general athletic attributes into performance-enhancing skills and strengths. Let's explore the transmutation phase:

- **Elevating Intensity:** One of the defining features of the transmutation phase is the marked increase in training intensity. Athletes are now expected to push themselves harder, challenging their limits. In resistance training, this might mean lifting heavier weights or engaging in more complex and demanding exercise variations. For cardiovascular training, it could translate to faster-paced runs or more intense interval sessions.

- **Volume Moderation - Quality Over Quantity:** As intensity rises, there's a strategic reduction in training volume. This means that while individual sessions or exercises might be more challenging, athletes might perform fewer repetitions or shorter durations. This balance ensures that while athletes are pushing their boundaries, they aren't overextending themselves, which could lead to injuries or burnout.

- **Sport-Specific Focus:** The transmutation phase is characterized by its heightened emphasis on sport-specific training. Exercises, drills, and routines are chosen for their direct relevance to the athlete's sport. A football player, for instance, might focus on agility drills that mimic game scenarios, or a weightlifter might work on specific lifts that they'll perform in competitions.

- **Technique Refinement:** While the accumulation phase emphasizes mastering the basics, the transmutation phase is about refining those techniques to perfection. Minute adjustments in form, posture, or movement can lead to significant performance improvements. Athletes often work closely with coaches to analyze and perfect their techniques during this phase.

- **Energy System Targeting:** From a physiological perspective, the transmutation phase often targets specific energy systems relevant to the athlete's sport. For instance, a 400-meter sprinter might focus on training that targets the anaerobic glycolytic system, while a marathon runner would emphasize the aerobic system. This ensures that athletes are physiologically primed for their sport's unique demands.

- **Mental Conditioning:** As the training becomes more specialized and intense, there's also an emphasis on mental conditioning. Athletes might engage in visualization exercises, mental rehearsals, or even work with sports psychologists to ensure they are mentally resilient and focused.

In summary, the transmutation phase is a period of evolution and specialization. Athletes transition from broad, foundational training to a more focused and intense regimen that closely mirrors the demands of their sport. It's a time of fine-tuning, where every training session is purpose-driven, ensuring athletes are not just physically, but also mentally prepared for the challenges of high-level competition.

The Realization Phase

The realization phase is the apex of the block periodization model, where all the groundwork laid in the previous phases converges to prepare the athlete for maximal performance. This phase is all about optimization, ensuring that athletes are in their prime condition, both physically and mentally, for competition or key performance benchmarks. Let's explore the intricacies of the realization phase:

- **Maximal Intensity:** During the realization phase, training sessions reach their zenith in terms of intensity. Athletes are often working at or near their maximal capacities.

For weightlifters, this might mean attempting lifts at near-maximal weights. For sprinters, it could involve short bursts of speed at their absolute fastest.

- **Volume Minimization:** With the surge in intensity, there's a significant reduction in training volume. This is crucial to ensure that athletes are not overburdened and have ample time for recovery. The focus shifts from extensive training to intensive training, ensuring that while the sessions are challenging, they are also concise, allowing for optimal recuperation.

- **Tactical Training:** Beyond the physical aspects, the realization phase places a premium on tactical and strategic preparation. Athletes engage in scenario-based training sessions that mimic actual competition conditions. For example, a tennis player might play practice sets focusing on specific strategies they plan to employ in an upcoming match.

- **Fine-Tuning Techniques:** While technique change is a continuous process, the realization phase emphasizes precise details. It's about perfecting every movement, ensuring that each action is as efficient and effective as possible. This meticulous attention to detail can be the difference between success and failure in competitive scenarios.

- **Psychological Peak:** As the competition or performance day nears, there's a heightened focus on mental preparation. Athletes might engage in meditation, visualization exercises, or even work with sports psychologists to ensure they are mentally poised for the pressures of the big stage.

- **Nutrition and Hydration Focus:** The realization phase also sees a sharpened emphasis on nutrition and hydration. Athletes often follow specialized diets made for their specific needs, ensuring that their bodies are adequately fueled for optimal performance. Proper hydration is also paramount, especially for endurance athletes, to ensure optimal muscle function and recovery.

- **Rest and Active Recovery:** While active training is crucial, the realization phase also underscores the importance of rest and active recovery. Athletes might incorporate light exercises, stretching routines, and even therapeutic modalities like massage or cryotherapy to ensure their bodies are rejuvenated and ready for peak performance.

In essence, the realization phase is a masterclass in athletic optimization. Every aspect of an athlete's preparation, from physical training and technique refinement to mental conditioning and nutrition, is fine-tuned to perfection. It's a period of razor-sharp focus, ensuring that when the competition day arrives, the athlete is in the best possible shape, ready to showcase their skills and achieve their goals.

Who Stands to Benefit?

Block periodization, with its meticulous segmentation of training phases, is more than just a training model. It's a strategic approach to fitness and performance that can be directed to fit many goals and aspirations. Let's explore the diverse group of individuals and scenarios that can harness the power of this methodology:

Competitive Athletes

For athletes who immerse themselves in the competitive activity, every training session, every drill, and every rest day counts. Block periodization, with its structured and phased approach, emerges as a beacon, guiding them toward their peak potential. Here's a deeper exploration of how this methodology caters to competitive athletes:

- **The Essence of Seasonal Alignment:** Most competitive sports operate on a seasonal basis, with off-seasons, pre-seasons, and main competitive seasons. Block periodization seamlessly integrates with this cyclical nature. For instance, during the off-season, when the focus might be on recovery and building foundational skills, the accumulation phase of block periodization can be employed. This phase emphasizes volume, allowing athletes to work on their basic skills, strength, and conditioning without the pressure of imminent competition.

- **Event-Specific Design:** Not all competitions are created equal. An athlete might participate in multiple events throughout the year, but there will always be those one or two essential events – the ones they've been eyeing as their primary targets. Block periodization can be fine-tuned to ensure that the realization phase, where athletes are at their peak performance level, coincides with these major events. This ensures that they are in their best physical and mental shape when it matters the most.

- **Skill Refinement and Mastery:** The competitive world is dynamic, with ever-evolving techniques, strategies, and standards. During the specific preparation or transmutation phases of block periodization, athletes can focus on refining their techniques, adapting to new strategies, or even mastering a new skill that can give them an edge over their competitors.

- **Holistic Development:** While the primary focus might be on the physical aspect, competitive athletes also need to be mentally robust. Block periodization, with its structured approach, ensures that athletes are not just physically prepared, but also mentally conditioned. The varied phases allow athletes to experience different training intensities and volumes, helping them develop resilience, adaptability, and mental fortitude.

- **Feedback and Iteration:** One of the advantages of segmenting training into blocks is the opportunity for feedback. After each block, athletes and coaches can review performance, identify areas of improvement, and then direct the subsequent block to address these areas. This iterative process ensures continuous growth and adaptation.

In summary, for competitive athletes, block periodization is more than just a training model; it's a strategic tool. It provides a clear roadmap, guiding them through varied training landscapes, ensuring that they are always progressing, adapting, and inching closer to their competitive goals.

Athletes with Fluid Seasonal Objectives

For some athletes, the journey is characterized by evolving objectives that shift with the seasons or even within a single season. These athletes require a training approach that's as dynamic as their goals, and block periodization offers precisely that. Here's a closer look at how block periodization serves athletes with fluid seasonal objectives:

- **Diverse Training Focus:** Athletes with shifting goals often find themselves juggling multiple training focuses. For instance, a triathlete might prioritize swimming endurance in the spring, cycling strength in the summer, and running speed in the fall. Block periodization allows them to dedicate specific blocks to each discipline, ensuring concentrated and effective training.

- **Seamless Transition Between Objectives:** The structured nature of block periodization facilitates smooth transitions between different training focuses. After a block dedicated to strength building, an athlete can seamlessly move to a block focusing on agility or endurance. This ensures that while they're honing one skill, they're not neglecting others.

- **Optimal Resource Allocation:** Athletes with varied objectives need to be judicious about their time and energy. Block periodization, with its clear demarcation of phases, allows athletes to allocate their resources optimally. They can dedicate the most time and energy to the skills or attributes that are most crucial for their immediate goals.

- **Injury Prevention and Recovery:** Juggling multiple objectives can sometimes put athletes at risk of overtraining or injuries. However, the phased approach of block periodization inherently incorporates periods of recovery and reduced intensity. This ensures that athletes get the rest they need, even as they pursue diverse goals.

- **Performance Tracking Across Disciplines:** One of the advantages of block periodization for multi-disciplinary athletes is the ability to track performance across different areas. After each block, athletes can assess their progress in that specific discipline or skill set, making necessary adjustments for future blocks.

- **Mental Engagement and Motivation:** Continuously shifting goals can be both a challenge and a motivator. The varied focus keeps training fresh and engaging. With block periodization, athletes always have a new challenge on the horizon, keeping the flame of motivation burning.

In essence, for athletes whose goals are as varied as the seasons, block periodization offers a flexible yet structured approach. It ensures that they can pursue multiple objectives without spreading themselves too thin, achieving a balance that's crucial for long-term success and growth.

Fitness Aficionados with Diverse Aspirations

While the spotlight often shines on competitive athletes, there's a vast community of fitness enthusiasts who train with just as much passion and dedication, albeit with different objectives. These individuals might not be chasing medals, but they're certainly chasing personal milestones, better health, and holistic well-being. For them, block periodization offers a structured path to achieve diverse fitness goals. Here's how:

- **Personalized Goal Setting:** Fitness enthusiasts often have a spectrum of goals, from weight loss to muscle toning, from cardiovascular health to flexibility. Block periodization allows them to segment their training year, dedicating specific blocks to each of these objectives. This ensures concentrated effort and measurable progress in each area.

- **Structured Progression:** The fitness journey is not a sprint; it's a marathon. Block periodization offers a roadmap, guiding enthusiasts from foundational training (akin to the accumulation phase) where they build basic strength and endurance, to more advanced blocks where they might focus on specific skills or high-intensity training.

- **Balancing Intensity and Recovery:** Just like athletes, fitness enthusiasts are also at risk of overtraining or injuries. The phased nature of block periodization ensures that high-intensity training periods are balanced with adequate recovery, promoting sustainable and safe progress.

- **Skill Development and Mastery:** Beyond the physical attributes, many fitness enthusiasts also aim to master specific skills, be it a yoga pose, a dance move, or a weightlifting technique. Block periodization allows them to dedicate entire blocks to skill acquisition and refinement, ensuring they get the focused practice they need.

- **Motivation and Engagement:** One of the challenges of a fitness journey is maintaining motivation. The varied focus of block periodization ensures that training remains fresh and engaging. With each new block comes a new set of challenges and objectives, which keeps the enthusiasm alive.

- **Holistic Health and Well-being:** Fitness is not just about physical strength or endurance; it's also about mental well-being, flexibility, and overall health. Block periodization, with its comprehensive approach, ensures that enthusiasts get a well-rounded fitness regimen. They can dedicate blocks to meditation and mental health, flexibility training, or even nutritional education.

In conclusion, for fitness enthusiasts, block periodization is more than a training tool; it's a holistic approach to health and well-being. It offers a structured yet flexible framework, allowing them to navigate their fitness journey with clarity, purpose, and passion. Whether they're chasing a specific weight goal, aiming to master a skill, or simply seeking better health, block periodization provides the roadmap to get there.

In conclusion, the primary principle of Block periodization is the focus on sport-specific drills and skills. Similar to linear periodization, it starts low intensity-high volume and moves to high intensity-low volume. Unlike linear periodization, Block periodization uses high volume in phase 1, high sport specific in phase 2, and high intensity in phase 3, instead of maximizing sport and intensity in phase 3 like linear.

Block periodization stands as a testament to the importance of structured progression in fitness and athletic training. It's not just about the hours spent in the gym, on the track, or in the pool, but about how those hours are organized, optimized, and directed towards specific objectives.

The beauty of block periodization lies in its adaptability. Whether you're an elite athlete gearing up for international competitions or a fitness enthusiast aiming for personal milestones, this approach can fit your unique needs and aspirations. It ensures that every session, every rep, and every stride is purposeful by segmenting training into distinct blocks, each with a clear focus.

Moreover, block periodization recognizes the interconnectedness of various training aspects. Strength, endurance, skill acquisition, and recovery are not isolated elements but pieces of a larger puzzle. This approach, however, ensures holistic development by dedicating time to each aspect in a phased manner.

But beyond the physical gains, block periodization also addresses the mental and psychological facets of training. The varied focus keeps motivation high, challenges fresh, and goals attainable. It instills a sense of achievement as one block is completed and a sense of anticipation for the next.

In training methodologies, block periodization emerges as a method that combines science, strategy, and individualization. It's a reminder that success, whether on the athletic field or in personal fitness journeys, is often the result of meticulous planning, consistent effort, and a deep understanding of one's goals and capabilities.

Choosing the Right Periodization Model

Choosing the right periodization model is a crucial decision that can significantly influence an athlete's or fitness enthusiast's training outcomes. The selection isn't merely about picking a trendy model; it's about aligning the training approach with individual goals, circumstances, and preferences. Factors that should be considered when selecting a periodization model:

Training Experience

Every fitness journey athletes embark upon is uniquely woven with experiences, challenges, and milestones. This journey, rich and varied, profoundly influences their approach to training and periodization. Understanding one's position on this spectrum of training experience is pivotal in tailoring a periodization model that aligns with their needs and aspirations.

Novices in the Arena

- **Embarking on a New Voyage:** For those venturing into structured training for the first time, it can be both exciting and overwhelming. Their bodies are on the cusp of discovering new potentials, and their minds are eager to grasp the training.

- **The Need for Simplicity:** At this nascent stage, a straightforward, linear approach to periodization can be immensely beneficial. It offers a clear and uncomplicated path, allowing novices to focus on mastering the basics, from correct form to understanding their body's responses to different exercises.

- **Building a Robust Foundation:** The primary goal for beginners is to establish a solid base. This involves cultivating foundational strength, enhancing muscular endurance, and developing basic skills pertinent to their sport or fitness goals. A linear model, with its steady progression, ensures that they progressively challenge themselves without the risk of overtraining or injury.

Seasoned Warriors

- **A Rich Experience:** Those with years or even decades of training have rich experiences. They've tasted the exhilaration of surpassing goals, faced the frustration of plateaus, and have an understanding of their bodies and capabilities.

- **Craving Complexity and Challenge:** With a solid foundation in place, intermediate to advanced trainees often seek training regimens that introduce variability, challenge, and specificity. Models like block or undulating periodization cater to these evolved needs, offering phases or cycles that target different facets of fitness.

- **Breaking Boundaries:** For these seasoned athletes, training isn't just about maintenance; it's about pushing the envelope. They aim to shatter previous records, refine advanced skills, and perhaps even redefine what they believed was possible. Periodization models that introduce variability ensure that they are continually stimulated, both mentally and physically, propelling them toward these goals.

Therefore, the individual's history with training isn't just a chronological record; it's a rich narrative that offers insights into their needs, challenges, and aspirations. Recognizing and respecting this narrative is the first step in designing a periodization model that truly resonates and yields results.

Time Constraints

Time, often described as the most valuable resource, plays a pivotal role in shaping an individual's training regimen. In the realm of fitness and athletics, the amount of time one can dedicate to training isn't just a logistical consideration; it's a factor that can profoundly influence the effectiveness, sustainability, and outcomes of a training program. Let's delve deeper into how time constraints can guide the selection of a periodization model:

MUSCLE UNIVERSITY

The Impact Consistent Schedule

- **Predictable Patterns:** Some individuals have the privilege of a stable routine, where work, personal commitments, and other responsibilities follow a predictable pattern. This stability allows them to carve out dedicated slots for training, ensuring consistency.

- **Harnessing Block Periodization:** For those blessed with such consistency, block periodization emerges as a compelling choice. Given its structured nature, where each phase demands a specific focus and intensity, having a regular schedule ensures that they can fully immerse themselves in each block, reaping maximum benefits.

- **Optimal Recovery and Progression:** A stable routine also means that rest, recovery, and nutrition can be optimized around the training blocks. This holistic approach ensures that the body is adequately fueled, rested, and primed for each training session, paving the way for consistent progress.

The Challenge of Erratic Schedules

- **Juggling Multiple Hats:** Not everyone enjoys the luxury of a predictable routine. Many individuals grapple with fluctuating work hours, travel commitments, or personal responsibilities that make a consistent training schedule elusive.

- **The Flexibility of Undulating Periodization:** For such individuals, the dynamic nature of undulating periodization can be a boon. Given its inherent variability, where intensity and volume might change from one session to the next, it offers the flexibility to adapt to life's curveballs. Did you miss a high-intensity session due to an unexpected commitment? It can be rescheduled without disrupting the overall flow of the training cycle.

- **Maximizing Windows of Opportunity:** With erratic schedules, it's about making the most of available time. Undulating periodization ensures that each session, whether it's 30 minutes or 2 hours, is purposeful and contributes to the overarching training goals.

Competition or Performance Schedule

In sports and athletics, the calendar isn't just a measure of days, weeks, and months; it's a roadmap to key milestones, competitions, and performance benchmarks. The schedule of an athlete's training must be in harmony with this calendar, ensuring that they are at their peak when it truly counts. Let's explore how the competition or performance schedule can influence the choice of a periodization model:

The Precision of Specific Peak Times

- **The Countdown to D-Day:** For many athletes, there are specific dates circled in red on their calendars. It could be the date of a major championship, a marathon, or any other significant competition. The anticipation of these events dictates the flow and focus of their training.

- **The Strategic Use of Block Periodization:** When there's a clear target date, block periodization can be a powerful ally. This model allows athletes to segment their training into distinct phases, each building upon the last, culminating in a realization phase that aligns perfectly with the competition date. What's then the result? Athletes are physically and mentally primed to deliver their best performance when the spotlight is on them.

- **Micro and Macro Alignments:** While the broader blocks align with the competition schedule, micro-adjustments within each block can be made based on smaller competitions or trials leading up to the main event. This ensures continuous assessment and fine-tuning.

Navigating Multiple Competitions: The Marathon, Not Just the Sprint

- **A Year-Round Endeavor:** Some athletes face the challenge (and excitement) of multiple competitions spread throughout the year. Whether it's a tennis player participating in various tournaments or a track athlete with indoor and outdoor seasons, the training must cater to multiple peaks.

- **The Versatility of Undulating Periodization:** In such scenarios, undulating periodization shines brightly. Its dynamic nature, with frequent shifts in intensity and volume, allows athletes to peak for multiple events. Athletes can also ensure they are in top form for each competition, without the risk of burnout or overtraining by adjusting the microcycles.

- **Staying Competition-Ready:** The continuous variability also ensures that athletes remain in a state of readiness. They are always close to their peak, allowing them to seize opportunities, be it an unexpected competition invite or a sudden performance trial.

In the competitive arena, where seconds can separate the triumphant from the also-rans, the alignment of training with the competition calendar is paramount. It's a dance of preparation and performance, of buildup and climax. Choosing the right periodization model is akin to selecting the perfect dance partner, one that complements the athlete's rhythm, leading them gracefully to their moment of glory.

Personal Preferences and Motivation

Training is as much a mental endeavor as it is a physical one. The most meticulously designed training program can fall flat if it doesn't resonate with the individual's personal preferences and motivational drivers. Let's explore how these factors play a pivotal role in determining the choice of a periodization model:

The Thrill of Variety

- **The Quest for Novelty:** Some individuals are naturally inclined towards seeking new experiences and challenges. The monotony of a repetitive routine can quickly dampen their spirits. For them, every training session should feel like a new adventure, and a fresh challenge to conquer.

- **Undulating Periodization as the Answer:** The ever-changing undulating periodization can be a perfect match for these individuals. With its frequent shifts in intensity and volume, every week, or even every session, brings something new to the table. This constant flux can keep the training experience fresh, ensuring that motivation remains high and the flame of enthusiasm continues to burn brightly.

The Comfort of Structure

- **Predictability as a Strength:** On the other end of the spectrum, some find solace in structure and predictability. They thrive on routines and derive satisfaction from methodically working towards their goals. For them, knowing what lies ahead provides a sense of control and purpose.

- **Block Periodization or Linear Models as the Go-to:** These individuals might gravitate towards block periodization or linear models. The clear delineation of phases in block periodization provides a roadmap they can follow, with each block building on the previous one. Similarly, linear models, with their gradual and consistent progression, offer a straightforward path that aligns with their preference for a structured approach.

The Psychological Impact of Training Choices

- **Empowerment through Autonomy:** Giving individuals a say in their training approach can enhance their commitment and adherence. When they feel that the training resonates with their personal preferences, they are more likely to approach it with enthusiasm and dedication.

- **Feedback Loop:** Regularly checking in with individuals about their training experience can provide valuable insights. If they start to feel disengaged or demotivated, it might be a sign to re-evaluate and potentially switch to a different periodization model that aligns better with their evolving preferences.

Nevertheless, while science, strategy, and performance metrics are vital components of training, the human element cannot be overlooked. Personal preferences and motivation are the heartbeat of any training regimen. Recognizing and honoring these factors ensures not just effective training, but also a fulfilling and enriching training journey.

Specific Training Goals

Every individual embarks on their training journey with a set of goals in mind. These goals, whether they are short-term milestones or long-term aspirations, serve as the guiding star, shaping the direction and intensity of the training regimen. The periodization model chosen should be a reflection of these goals, acting as a designed blueprint to guide individuals toward their desired outcomes. Let's delve into how specific training goals influence the choice of a periodization model:

The Pursuit of Holistic Development

- **The Comprehensive Athlete:** Some individuals aim for a well-rounded fitness profile, seeking to excel in multiple areas such as strength, endurance, flexibility, and power. Their training regimen should be a balanced mix, ensuring that no aspect is neglected.

- **Block Periodization as a Comprehensive Tool:** For such all-rounders, block periodization can be an invaluable approach. By segmenting training into distinct blocks, each focusing on a specific aspect of fitness, it ensures a comprehensive development. For instance, one block might focus on building muscle mass (hypertrophy), followed by a block dedicated to enhancing cardiovascular endurance, and then a phase for power development.

Zooming in on Targeted Improvements

- **Specialized Goals:** Some individuals have laser-focused goals. A sprinter might be looking to shave off a few seconds from their 100m dash, or a weightlifter might be aiming to add a few kilograms to their clean and jerk. These specific objectives require an adequate approach.

191

- **Tailoring the Periodization Model:** In such cases, the periodization model should be aligned closely with these targeted improvements. If the goal is to maximize strength, the majority of the training might revolve around high-intensity, low-repetition exercises with ample recovery time. If the aim is to improve endurance, longer, sustained workouts with a focus on cardiovascular exercises might dominate the regimen.

The Flexibility to Pivot

- **Evolving Goals:** It's natural for goals to evolve over time. An individual who started with a goal of weight loss might transition to muscle building after achieving their desired weight. The training model should be adaptable enough to accommodate these shifting objectives.

- **Switching Gears with Periodization:** The beauty of periodization is its flexibility. As goals change, the focus of the training blocks or the intensity and volume of undulating periodization can be adjusted accordingly. This ensures that the training remains aligned with the individual's current objectives, providing a clear path towards achieving them.

In summary, specific training goals are the foundation upon which the entire training structure is built. The periodization model acts as the architecture, designed to transform these goals from mere aspirations into tangible achievements. By meticulously aligning the training approach with individual objectives, individuals are set on a trajectory of success, ensuring that every drop of sweat, every hour of effort, brings them one step closer to their dreams.

In conclusion, choosing the right periodization model is more than just a tactical decision; it's a strategic alignment of one's training philosophy with their overarching goals. This decision, while rooted in science, is also an art, requiring a deep understanding of one's body, aspirations, and the nuances of training methodologies.

The Interplay of Variables: The selection process isn't about isolating individual factors like training experience or competition schedule. Instead, it's about understanding how these variables interplay, and how one's daily life and long-term objectives weave together to form unique training needs.

Beyond the Gym: The implications of this choice extend beyond the confines of a gym or training ground. The right periodization model can influence motivation levels, mental well-being, and even one's outlook toward challenges and setbacks. It becomes a framework not just for physical training but also for mental fortitude and resilience.

A Dynamic Decision: It's essential to recognize that the choice of a periodization model isn't set in stone. As individuals evolve, as goals shift, and as new challenges emerge, there might be a need to re-evaluate and pivot. This adaptability ensures that the training remains relevant and effective, mirroring the ever-changing individual's fitness journey.

The Ultimate Aim: The decision to choose a particular periodization model boils down to one fundamental objective: optimizing results. Whether it's standing atop a podium, achieving a personal best, or simply feeling healthier and more vibrant, the right training approach is the catalyst that transforms effort into achievement.

In fitness and athletic training, periodization models are the threads that give structure and form to the narrative. By making an informed and thoughtful choice, individuals ensure that their training story is not just compelling but also triumphant. The journey toward fitness and athletic excellence is filled with challenges, but with the right periodization model, every step, every rep, and every drop of sweat becomes a purposeful stride toward success.

Implementing Periodization in Training Programs

Every individual embarks on their fitness journey with a unique set of attributes, aspirations, and challenges. Recognizing this uniqueness is the cornerstone of effective periodization. One can harness the full potential of periodization, ensuring optimal results and a safer training environment by tailoring the training program to the individual.

Assessing Individual Needs and Goals

Understanding the Starting Point: Before embarking on any journey, it's essential to know the starting point. In fitness and training, this involves a comprehensive understanding of one's current physical, mental, and emotional state. This foundational knowledge ensures that the subsequent training program is both effective and safe.

Self-Reflection and Introspection

- **Motivational Drivers:** Understanding what drives an individual can be instrumental in designing a training program that keeps them engaged and motivated. Is it a desire to compete, a health goal, or simply personal betterment? Pinpointing this can shape the training journey.

- **Perceived Limitations:** Recognizing any self-perceived barriers or limitations can help in addressing them head-on, ensuring they don't hinder progress. This could be anything from past injuries to mental blocks.

Diagnostic Assessments

- **Physical Evaluations:** Utilizing standardized fitness tests can provide a clear picture of one's current capabilities. This could include aerobic tests like the VO2 max, strength assessments, flexibility tests, and more.

- **Health Screenings:** Before starting any rigorous training program, it's wise to undergo health screenings. This can identify any underlying health conditions that might influence training decisions.

Goal Setting

- **SMART Goals:** Goals should be Specific, Measurable, Achievable, Relevant, and Time-bound. This framework ensures clarity and provides a tangible target to work towards.

- **Short-term versus Long-term:** While having a long-term vision is crucial, breaking it down into smaller, short-term goals can make the journey more manageable and provide frequent milestones to celebrate.

- **Documenting Goals:** Writing down goals or maintaining a training journal can serve as a constant reminder and a source of motivation. It also provides a record to look back on, tracking progress over time.

Feedback Mechanisms

- **Self-feedback:** This means regularly checking in with oneself, understanding how one feels after training sessions, and recognizing any persistent issues or challenges.

- **External Feedback:** It involves engaging with trainers, coaches, or peers to get an external perspective on one's performance and areas of improvement.

In summary, the assessment phase is a blend of introspection, objective measurement, and forward thinking. It sets the tone for the entire training journey, ensuring that every step taken aligns with the individual's unique needs and aspirations. One lays a solid foundation for a successful and fulfilling training experience by investing time and effort in this phase.

Setting Training Phases and Objectives

The Blueprint of Progress: Setting distinct training phases and objectives is similar to creating a roadmap for a journey. It provides direction, clarity, and structure, ensuring that every training session is purposeful and contributes to overarching goals. Here's a comprehensive look at how to effectively set and navigate through these phases:

Understanding the Training Cycle

- **Macrocycle:** This is the broadest phase, often spanning a year or an entire training season. It encompasses the overall training goal, be it preparing for a marathon, a bodybuilding competition, or simply achieving a certain fitness level.

- **Mesocycle:** Falling within the macrocycle, mesocycles are medium-length phases, typically lasting several weeks to a few months. Each mesocycle has a specific focus, such as building endurance, strength, or honing a particular skill.

- **Microcycle:** These are the shortest phases, usually spanning a week. They detail the day-to-day training activities, ensuring that each session aligns with the goals of the mesocycle and, by extension, the macrocycle.

Phased Objectives

- **Foundation Building:** It is especially crucial for beginners or those returning after a hiatus. This phase emphasizes general fitness, flexibility, and familiarization with exercises.

- **Skill and Strength Development:** As the name suggests, this phase focuses on enhancing specific skills and building strength. The exercises become more challenging, and there's a clear progression in intensity.

- **Performance Optimization:** This phase is about refining skills, improving efficiency, and preparing for any specific events or goals. It's the final push, where all the previous training comes together.

Re-evaluation and Flexibility

- **Mid-course Corrections:** Even with the best-laid plans, there might be a need for adjustments. Regularly reviewing progress and being open to tweaking the phases ensures that the training remains effective and relevant.

- **Adapting to External Factors:** Injuries, personal commitments, or even global events (like a pandemic) can disrupt training. Having the flexibility to adjust the training phases in response to such external factors is crucial.

In summary, setting training phases and objectives is a dynamic and iterative process. It's about having a clear vision, breaking it down into actionable steps, and being adaptable. Someone can navigate the training journey with purpose, clarity, and confidence by meticulously planning each phase and aligning it with individual goals.

Manipulating Training Variables

The Art and Science of Training Dynamics: Manipulating training variables is at the heart of periodization. It's the mechanism by which trainers and athletes can ensure continuous progress, adaptability, and reduced risk of stagnation. By understanding and effectively adjusting these variables, one can optimize training outcomes. Here's a comprehensive exploration of how to manipulate these variables for maximum benefit:

Understanding the Role of Each Variable

- **Intensity:** It dictates the level of effort or strain during an exercise. In weightlifting, it's often related to the percentage of one's one-repetition maximum (1RM). In cardiovascular training, it might be tied to heart rate zones or perceived exertion levels.

- **Volume:** This encompasses the total workload in a training session or phase. It's a product of sets, repetitions, and weight in resistance training or distance and time in endurance training.

- **Exercise Selection:** This involves choosing specific exercises that align with the goals of the training phase. The selection can target specific muscle groups, energy systems, or movement patterns.

- **Rest Periods:** The recovery time between sets or exercises can influence training outcomes, affecting factors like muscle recovery, lactic acid clearance, and energy system engagement.

- **Training Frequency:** This pertains to how often one trains, which can influence recovery, muscle protein synthesis, and overall adaptation.

Strategic Adjustments for Different Goals

- **Strength and Power Goals:** Intensity is often prioritized, with athletes lifting heavier weights (closer to their 1RM). Volume might be moderate, with longer rest periods to allow for maximal effort in each set.

- **Endurance and Stamina Goals:** Volume takes precedence, with longer runs, rides, or swim sessions. Intensity might be moderate, focusing on maintaining a steady pace. Rest periods, especially in interval training, might be shorter to challenge cardiovascular recovery.

- **Growth Goals:** A balance between volume and intensity is sought. Repetition ranges typically fall between 6-12 with weights that challenge the muscles to near failure by the last rep. Rest periods are moderate, allowing for both recovery and sustained muscle tension.

Periodic Re-assessment and Variation

- **Avoiding Plateaus:** The body is highly adaptive. If exposed to the same training stimulus repeatedly, it can lead to plateaus. Regularly adjusting training variables ensures that the body is continually challenged.

- **Incorporating Variation:** Introducing new exercises, adjusting rep schemes, or changing rest intervals can provide a fresh stimulus, keeping the training both effective and engaging.

Safety and Individual Considerations

- **Listening to the Body:** While manipulating variables, it's essential to be attuned to one's body. Signs of excessive fatigue, persistent soreness, or decreased performance can indicate a need for adjustment.

- **Personal Preferences:** Some individuals might prefer shorter, high-intensity sessions, while others might thrive on longer, moderate-intensity workouts. Personal preferences can play a role in how variables are adjusted.

In summary, manipulating training variables is both an art and a science. It requires a deep understanding of training principles, an awareness of individual needs and responses, and the flexibility to adapt. By strategically adjusting intensity, volume, exercise selection, rest periods, and frequency, one can craft a training program that is dynamic, effective, and designed to suit individual goals.

Monitoring and Adjustments

The Role of Continuous Feedback: Monitoring and making adjustments is akin to the feedback loop in any system. It ensures that the training program remains effective, relevant, and safe. Without regular monitoring, even the most meticulously planned program can fall short of its objectives or lead to unintended consequences like injuries. Here's a comprehensive exploration of the importance and methods of monitoring and making necessary adjustments.

The Importance of Monitoring:

- **Ensuring Progress:** Regular monitoring helps track whether the individual is moving closer to their goals. This could be in terms of strength gains, improved endurance, better skill proficiency, or any other specific objective.

- **Identifying Stagnation:** By keeping a close eye on performance metrics, one can quickly identify if they've hit a plateau, allowing for timely interventions.

- **Preventing Overtraining:** Continuous monitoring can help identify early signs of overtraining, such as persistent fatigue, mood changes, or decreased performance, allowing for necessary adjustments to prevent long-term setbacks.

- **Optimizing Recovery:** Monitoring can also provide insights into recovery rates, helping to adjust rest days or recovery techniques to ensure the body is adequately recuperating between sessions.

Methods of Monitoring

- **Performance Metrics:** These can include strength tests (like 1RM tests), endurance benchmarks (like time trials), or skill assessments.

- **Training Logs:** Keeping detailed logs of workouts, including exercises, weights, reps, sets, and rest periods, can provide valuable data for assessing progress and making adjustments.

- **Physiological Measures:** This might involve tracking heart rate, blood pressure, or even advanced metrics like VO2 max or lactate threshold for those with access to specialized equipment.

- **Subjective Feedback:** Listening to one's body is crucial. Tracking mood, energy levels, sleep quality, and general well-being can provide insights that objective metrics might miss.

- **Body Measurements:** For those with physique goals, regular measurements of body weight, body fat percentage, and specific body part dimensions can be useful.

Making Informed Adjustments

- **Tweaking Training Variables:** Based on monitoring feedback, one might need to adjust the intensity, volume, frequency, or exercise selection to better align with their goals.

- **Incorporating Deload or Recovery Weeks:** If signs of overtraining or excessive fatigue are noticed, incorporating a deload week (reduced training intensity and volume) can help the body recover.

- **Re-evaluating Goals:** Sometimes, the goals set at the beginning might need re-evaluation based on progress, changing circumstances, or new insights gained during training.

- **Seeking Expert Guidance:** If progress stalls or uncertainties arise, seeking the guidance of a coach, personal trainer, or sports scientist can provide expert insights and recommendations.

In conclusion, monitoring and adjustments are the heroes of a successful training program. They ensure that the plan remains dynamic, responsive, and directed to the evolving needs and circumstances of the individual. By embracing a proactive approach to monitoring and being flexible in making adjustments, one can navigate the challenges of training and steer their journey towards success.

Emphasis on Recovery and Injury Prevention

The Significance of Recovery: Recovery is an integral component of any training regimen. While the actual workouts stimulate growth and improvement, it's during the recovery periods that the body repairs, adapts, and grows stronger. Overlooking recovery can not only hinder progress but also increase the risk of injuries. Here's a detailed exploration of the importance of recovery and methods to ensure optimal recuperation:

Why Recovery Matters

- **Muscle Repair and Growth:** When we train, especially during resistance exercises, microscopic tears occur in our muscles. Recovery allows these tears to heal, leading to muscle growth and increased strength.

- **Replenishing Energy Stores:** Training depletes the body's energy stores, particularly glycogen. Adequate recovery ensures these stores are replenished, preparing the body for subsequent workouts.

- **Central Nervous System (CNS) Recovery:** Intense training can fatigue the CNS. Adequate rest ensures the CNS recovers, maintaining optimal neural function and muscle activation in future sessions.

- **Hormonal Balance:** Physical stress from training affects the body's hormonal balance. Recovery allows hormones like cortisol (a stress hormone) to return to baseline levels and promotes the release of growth-promoting hormones.

Methods to Enhance Recovery

- **Active Recovery:** This involves low-intensity, low-impact activities like walking, cycling, or swimming. Active recovery can boost blood circulation, facilitating nutrient delivery to muscles and speeding up the recovery process.

- **Sleep:** Quality sleep is paramount for recovery. It's during deep sleep that the body releases growth hormone, which plays a pivotal role in muscle repair and recovery.

- **Nutrition:** Consuming a balanced mix of proteins, carbohydrates, and fats after workouts can accelerate muscle repair and glycogen replenishment. Hydration is equally crucial, as even mild dehydration can impair recovery.

- **Stretching and Mobility Work:** Regular stretching and mobility exercises can alleviate muscle tightness, improve flexibility, and enhance overall recovery.

- **Massage and Foam Rolling:** These techniques can help in breaking down muscle knots and improving blood flow, which aids in faster recovery.

- **Cold and Heat Therapies:** Ice baths or contrast baths (alternating between hot and cold water) can reduce muscle soreness and inflammation, promoting quicker recovery.

Injury Prevention in Periodized Training: Injury prevention is paramount for sustained progress. An injury cannot only set back training but also have long-term implications. Here's how to minimize injury risks:

- **Proper Technique:** Ensuring correct form and technique during exercises is the first line of defense against injuries.

- **Gradual Progression:** You should allow the temptation to increase intensity or volume too quickly. Gradual progression allows the body to adapt without being overwhelmed.

- **Listening to the Body:** Pay attention to signs of fatigue, persistent pain, or any unusual discomfort. These could be early indicators of potential injuries.

- **Incorporating Rest Days:** Regular rest days give the body a chance to recover fully, reducing the risk of overuse injuries.

- **Cross-Training:** Engaging in different types of exercises or sports can prevent overuse injuries by distributing the stress of training across various muscle groups and joints.

In conclusion, recovery and injury prevention are as crucial, if not more so, than the actual workouts in a training program. Individuals can ensure consistent progress, longevity in their training endeavors, and overall well-being by prioritizing recovery and adopting a proactive approach to injury prevention.

Application Across Various Fitness Levels and Goals

The Universality of Periodization: Periodization, as a concept, is not exclusive to elite athletes or those with advanced training goals. Its principles can be applied across fitness levels, from novices to seasoned professionals. The adaptability of periodization makes it a valuable tool for anyone looking to structure their training for optimal results. Here's a closer look at how periodization can be tailored to various fitness levels and objectives:

Beginners and Novices

- **Foundation Building:** For those new to training, the initial phases of periodization would focus on building a solid foundation. This involves developing basic strength, endurance, and flexibility.

- **Skill Development:** Beginners also benefit from focusing on learning the correct techniques and forms for various exercises, ensuring safety and effectiveness as they progress.

- **Gradual Progression:** For novices, it's essential to progress slowly to avoid injury and ensure the body has adequate time to adapt to the new physical demands.

- **Motivation and Consistency:** Periodization can help beginners stay motivated by providing structured goals and milestones. Achieving these can boost confidence and encourage consistency.

Intermediate Trainees

- **Overcoming Plateaus:** Those with some training experience often encounter plateaus. Periodization, with its phased approach, can introduce the necessary variability to overcome these stagnation points.

- **Specialization:** Intermediate trainees might have specific goals, such as muscle growth or improved cardiovascular endurance. Periodization can be tailored to emphasize these areas during particular training phases.

- **Incorporating Advanced Techniques:** As trainees become more experienced, periodization can introduce advanced training techniques, such as supersets, drop sets, or interval training, to further challenge the body.

Advanced Athletes and Trainees

- **Peak Performance:** For those aiming for high-level competitions or specific performance benchmarks, periodization can be meticulously structured to ensure they peak at the right times.

- **Injury Prevention:** Advanced athletes often train at high intensities and volumes. Periodization can help manage these loads, ensuring adequate recovery and minimizing injury risks.

- **Tactical and Strategic Training:** Beyond physical training, advanced athletes can use periodization to incorporate tactical and strategic training relevant to their sport or discipline.

General Fitness Enthusiasts

- **Holistic Development:** Those training for general fitness and well-being can use periodization to ensure a balanced development across strength, flexibility, endurance, and other fitness components.

- **Adaptability:** Fitness enthusiasts often have varied goals that change over time. Periodization offers the flexibility to adapt the training program to these evolving objectives.

- **Sustainability:** By providing structure and variety, periodization can keep workouts fresh and engaging, promoting long-term adherence to a fitness regimen.

In summary, periodization is a versatile and adaptable training framework. Whether one's goal is to run a marathon, build muscle, lose weight, or simply stay fit, periodization can be customized to meet these objectives. By considering an individual's current fitness level, aspirations, and constraints, periodization offers a roadmap to success, ensuring that every workout is a step in the right direction.

MUSCLE UNIVERSITY

Crafting a Comprehensive Muscle Growth Blueprint

The Training, Nutrition, and Recovery: Building muscle is akin to crafting a masterpiece. It requires precision, dedication, and a harmonious blend of training, nutrition, and recovery. A personalized blueprint ensures that each note, each brushstroke, aligns perfectly with an individual's unique body, lifestyle, and aspirations, culminating in growth and transformation.

Starting with a Self-Audit and Vision Crafting

Baseline Measurements

- **Comprehensive Body Analysis:** Before embarking on the muscle-building journey, it's essential to have a clear understanding of your starting point. This involves a detailed body composition analysis, which can provide insights into muscle mass, body fat percentage, and even bone density.

- **Strength Benchmarks:** Determine your current strength levels across various exercises, from compound lifts like squats and deadlifts to isolation movements. This will not only give you a starting point but also help track progress over time.

- **Posture and Functional Assessments:** Often overlooked, posture and functional movement assessments can highlight imbalances or weaknesses that might need addressing. This ensures balanced muscle growth and reduces the risk of injuries.

- **Endurance and Flexibility Metrics:** While the primary focus is on muscle growth, understanding your cardiovascular endurance and flexibility can provide a holistic view of fitness. These metrics can influence the design of your warm-ups, cool-downs, and active recovery sessions.

Vision Crafting

- **Defining the Ideal Physique:** Visualization is a powerful tool. Create a clear mental image of your desired physique. This could be influenced by your role models, specific athletic goals, or personal aesthetic preferences.

- **Setting Quantifiable Targets:** While having a broad vision is great, breaking it down into specific, measurable goals can make the journey more tangible. This could be in terms of desired muscle measurements, body fat percentage, or even strength levels in specific lifts.

- **Short-term versus Long-term Goals:** While the ultimate vision might be long-term, setting intermediate milestones can keep motivation high. Celebrating these smaller victories can provide the necessary momentum to keep pushing forward.

- **Aligning with Lifestyle and Commitment:** It's essential to ensure that your muscle growth vision aligns with your lifestyle, time commitments, and even social considerations. Being realistic about how much time and effort you can dedicate will help in crafting a sustainable plan.

Feedback and Adjustments

- **Seek Expert Opinions:** Consider getting feedback on your goals and starting metrics from fitness professionals or coaches. They can provide valuable insights, highlight potential challenges, and even suggest adjustments to make your goals more achievable.

- **Personal Reflection:** Spend some time introspecting on why these goals matter to you. Understanding your 'why' can be a powerful motivator during challenging times or when faced with plateaus.

In essence, the initial self-audit and vision crafting phase is about laying a solid foundation for your muscle growth journey. It's about knowing where you stand, where you aim to go, and understanding the deeper motivations driving this desire. This clarity will serve as a guiding light, ensuring that every subsequent decision, from workout design to nutrition choices, aligns perfectly with your vision.

Strategic Workout Structuring with Periodization

Understanding the Role of Periodization

- **Foundation of Progression:** Periodization is a systematic approach to training that structures workouts in cycles, ensuring a balanced development and minimizing the risk of plateaus. For muscle growth, this structured approach is vital as it ensures that the body is continually challenged, adapting, and growing.

- **Avoiding Overtraining:** By cycling through different training focuses, periodization reduces the risk of overtraining a particular muscle group or energy system, which can hinder growth and lead to injuries.

Phases Tailored for Growth

- **Foundational Phase:** This phase focuses on building a solid base, emphasizing proper form, and increasing muscular endurance. It sets the stage for more intense training cycles.

- **Hypertrophy Phase:** The core of muscle-building, this phase emphasizes training that specifically promotes muscle size increase. It typically involves moderate weights with higher volume (sets and reps) to maximize muscle tension and induce growth.

- **Strength Phase:** While the primary goal is muscle size, increasing overall strength can aid growth in subsequent cycles. This phase involves lifting heavier weights with lower reps.

- **Active Recovery Phase:** This is a lighter training phase, allowing muscles to recover while still staying active. It might involve lighter weights, flexibility exercises, and cardiovascular training.

Cycling and Recurrence

- **Revisiting Phases:** After completing one cycle of the phases, the process begins anew, but with adjustments based on the progress made. This ensures continuous adaptation and growth.

- **Tweaking Based on Feedback:** As you progress, some phases might be extended, shortened, or intensified based on how your body is responding.

- **Integration with Other Training Goals**

- **Balancing Hypertrophy with Other Goals:** If you have other fitness objectives, like improving cardiovascular endurance or flexibility, periodization allows you to integrate these seamlessly. For instance, cardiovascular training can be incorporated more heavily during active recovery phases.

- **Sport-Specific Training:** For athletes, periodization can be tailored to ensure muscle growth while also developing skills and attributes necessary for their sport.

Consistency and Patience

- **Trust the Process:** Muscle growth is a gradual process, and the benefits of periodization become evident over time. It's essential to remain consistent, trust the structured approach, and resist the urge to make frequent changes.

- **Regular Re-evaluation:** At the end of each cycle, assess the progress made, and adjust the next cycle accordingly. This iterative approach ensures that the training remains aligned with evolving goals and capabilities.

In summary, integrating periodization into a muscle growth plan is about strategic progression. It's about understanding that muscle development isn't linear and that the body benefits from varied training stimuli. By cycling through different phases, each with a specific focus, you ensure that the muscles are continually challenged, leading to sustained growth while minimizing the risks of plateaus and injuries.

The Significance of Tracking Progress

- **Feedback Loop:** Monitoring provides immediate feedback on the effectiveness of the training and nutrition plan. It helps identify what's working and what might need adjustment.

- **Motivation and Accountability:** Seeing tangible progress can be a significant motivational boost. Regular check-ins can also instill a sense of accountability, ensuring adherence to the plan.

Methods of Monitoring Progress

- **Strength and Performance Metrics:** Tracking the weights lifted, repetitions performed, and overall workout performance provides insights into strength gains and muscle development.

- **Body Measurements:** Using a tape measure to track the size of key muscle groups (like arms, chest, and thighs) can give a direct indication of muscle growth.

- **Visual Assessments:** Periodic photos taken from multiple angles can offer a visual representation of changes in muscle definition and size over time.

- **Body Composition Analysis:** Techniques like DEXA scans, bioelectrical impedance, or skinfold calipers can provide data on muscle mass, body fat percentage, and overall body composition.

Interpreting the Data

- **Identifying Trends:** Instead of focusing on day-to-day fluctuations, look for consistent trends over weeks or months. This gives a more accurate picture of genuine progress.

- **Comparing with Baseline:** Regularly compare current metrics with baseline measurements (taken at the start) to gauge overall progress and growth.

Making Informed Adjustments:

- **Training Modifications:** If strength gains plateau or regress, it might be time to adjust the workout routine. This could involve changing exercises, rep ranges, or incorporating new training techniques.

- **Nutritional Tweaks:** If muscle growth seems stagnant despite consistent training, consider revisiting the nutrition plan. This might involve increasing caloric intake, adjusting macronutrient ratios, or optimizing nutrient timing.

- **Recovery and Rest:** If signs of overtraining or prolonged soreness appear, it might be necessary to increase rest days or incorporate more active recovery techniques.

Staying Flexible and Adaptable

- **Listening to the Body:** While data and metrics are valuable, it's equally important to listen to one's body. Factors like energy levels, mood, and sleep quality can provide insights into overall well-being and recovery.

- **Being Open to Change:** Muscle growth is a dynamic process, and what works at one stage might not be as effective later on. Being open to trying new approaches and adapting based on feedback is crucial for sustained progress.

In summary, the journey to muscle growth is not a static one. It requires continuous monitoring, reflection, and adjustments. By staying informed about one's progress and being willing to adapt based on feedback, individuals can navigate the path to muscle growth more effectively, ensuring that every effort in the gym and kitchen translates to tangible results.

Understanding the Role of Muscle Growth and Recovery:

- **Muscle Repair and Growth:** Contrary to popular belief, muscles don't grow during workouts. Instead, they grow during the recovery phase. When we exercise, especially during resistance training, microscopic tears occur in muscle fibers. The body repairs these tears during rest, making the fibers thicker and stronger in the process.

- **Central Nervous System (CNS) Recovery:** Intense workouts, especially strength training, place a significant demand on the CNS. Adequate rest ensures the CNS recovers, maintaining optimal performance in subsequent workouts.

- **Hormonal Balance:** Overtraining without sufficient recovery can lead to imbalances in hormones like cortisol (a stress hormone) and testosterone, which can hinder muscle growth and overall well-being.

Methods to Enhance Recovery

- **Sleep:** Often termed the best recovery tool, 7-9 hours of quality sleep is crucial for muscle repair, hormonal balance, and cognitive function.

- **Active Recovery:** This involves low-intensity activities like walking, cycling, or swimming, which increase blood flow to muscles without placing significant strain on them, aiding in faster recovery.

- **Stretching and Mobility Work:** Incorporating regular stretching and mobility exercises can alleviate muscle tightness, improve flexibility, and reduce the risk of injuries.

- **Hydration and Nutrition:** Drinking adequate water and consuming a balanced diet rich in proteins, vitamins, and minerals support muscle repair and growth.

Recognizing the Signs of Inadequate Recovery

- **Prolonged Muscle Soreness:** While some muscle soreness post-workout (known as DOMS) is normal, if it lasts for more than 72 hours, it might indicate inadequate recovery.

- **Decreased Performance:** A consistent decline in workout performance, despite proper nutrition and training, can be a sign of overtraining.

- **Mood Fluctuations and Fatigue:** Persistent feelings of fatigue, irritability, or mood swings can indicate that the body isn't recovering adequately between sessions.

Strategizing Rest Days

- **Scheduled Rest Days:** Incorporate at least 1-2 rest days per week in the training regimen, allowing muscles and the CNS to recover fully.

- **Deload Weeks:** Every 4-8 weeks, consider having a deload week where the intensity and volume of workouts are reduced, giving the body a more extended recovery period.

- **Listen to Your Body:** While structured rest days are essential, it's equally crucial to listen to one's body. If feeling overly fatigued or noticing signs of overtraining, it might be beneficial to take an unscheduled rest day.

Mental Recovery

- **Mental Break:** Rest days aren't just for physical recovery. Taking a break from the routine can also provide a mental refresh, ensuring motivation and focus remain high.

- **Mindfulness and Relaxation Techniques:** Practices like meditation, deep breathing exercises, and even hobbies can aid in mental recovery, ensuring a holistic approach to rest.

Building muscle is both a science and an art. It's about understanding the body's mechanics and also listening to its subtle cues. With a personalized muscle growth blueprint, one can navigate this journey with clarity, ensuring each step, each rep, and each set, is a purposeful stride toward the envisioned physique. Remember, it's a marathon, not a sprint. Celebrate the small victories, learn from the setbacks, and always keep the vision alive.

Conclusion--The Science of Periodization Programming

In this chapter, we studied periodization, a concept that stands as a pillar in athletic training and exercise physiology. Periodization is more than just a training schedule; it's a strategic approach that ensures every sweat drop counts, every muscle fiber is engaged, and every goal is within reach.

We began by understanding the essence of periodization, its foundational principles, and its paramount importance in optimizing training outcomes. The systematic division of training into distinct phases, each with a specific focus, ensures that athletes and fitness enthusiasts alike can continuously progress, overcome plateaus, and function at the right moments. This approach not only maximizes performance but also minimizes the risk of injuries, a balance that's crucial in sports and fitness.

The versatility of periodization was evident as we explored its various models, from the traditional linear approach to the dynamic undulating model and the targeted block periodization. Each model offers unique benefits, catering to different needs, goals, and training experiences. The choice of model becomes a reflection of one's objectives, competition schedules, and even personal preferences.

Implementing periodization is both an art and a science. While the principles are rooted in scientific research and understanding of human physiology, the application requires intuition, experience, and adaptability. When we tailor the program to individual needs, continuously monitor progress, and make necessary adjustments are all part of this intricate dance.

Lastly, we ventured into muscle growth, a goal many aspire to achieve. Building muscle is a multifaceted journey, intertwining the right training strategies with optimal nutrition and recovery. Periodization plays a pivotal role here, ensuring that training is structured, progressive, and aligned with muscle-building goals.

In conclusion, periodization is not just a training methodology; it's a philosophy. It embodies the belief that with the right plan, consistent effort, and a touch of adaptability, optimal performance is attainable. Whether you're an elite athlete gearing up for the world stage or a fitness enthusiast striving for personal bests, periodization offers a roadmap to success. As we close this chapter, remember that the journey of training is as important as the destination. Embrace the process, trust the plan, and let periodization guide you to your pinnacle of performance.

CHAPTER 7

◄◆►

SCIENTIFICALLY ORDERING EXERCISES, REPS, SETS, AND CARDIO

Fitness exercise comes with misconceptions and contradictions. Every athlete has a unique take on the "best" way to carry out their exercise. The questions that always come to mind are how many sets and reps are ideal for building muscle, and how does that change if you're aiming for endurance or strength? These questions are not just for gym chatter; they have real implications for the effectiveness of your workout and, ultimately, for achieving your fitness goals.

While personal preferences and anecdotal evidence have their place, they can't replace the value of scientific research in determining the most effective workout strategies. Science offers us a way to test hypotheses, compare outcomes, and arrive at conclusions that are more likely to be universally applicable, or at least, applicable to a broader range of people. This is crucial because what works for one person may not necessarily work for another due to some factors like age, sex, health conditions, and even genetic predispositions.

This chapter aims to provide you with a comprehensive, science-backed guide to structuring your workouts. A good knowledge of the physiology of exercise will help us understand how different types of activities affect our bodies. We'll also explore the science behind ordering exercises, the number of repetitions and sets, and the eternal debate between cardio and weights. By the end of this chapter, you'll have a solid foundation to not just understand but also implement a scientifically optimized workout routine targeted at solving your specific needs and goals.

Your present situation in the fitness world is not very important. This chapter will be your roadmap to a more effective, science-based approach to fitness.

The Science Behind Exercise Order

The sequence in which you perform exercises during a workout is not arbitrary; it's a crucial variable that can significantly impact your training outcomes. Whether you're a beginner or an experienced athlete, understanding the science behind exercise order can help you optimize muscle recruitment, energy utilization, and ultimately, the effectiveness of your workout.

Factors Influencing Exercise Order

Exercises can be categorized based on their complexity:

- **Complex Movements**: Complex movements often referred to as compound exercises, involve multiple muscle groups and joints working in tandem. They require a higher degree of coordination, balance, and strength. Examples: Squats, deadlifts, bench presses, pull-ups, and rows.

- **Simple Movements**: Simple movements commonly known as isolation exercises, target a specific muscle group and involve fewer joints. They are more straightforward and focus on isolating one muscle or muscle group. Examples: Bicep curls, tricep extensions, leg curls, calf raises, and lateral raises.

Generally, it is advisable to perform complex movements first when your neuromuscular system is fresh, which reduces the risk of injury and allows for better performance.

Muscle Group Size

- **Large Muscle Groups**: Exercises targeting large muscle groups like the chest, back, and legs should generally be performed before those targeting smaller muscle groups. The larger the muscle group and more joints involved, the earlier the order priority.

- **Small Muscle Groups**: Exercises for smaller muscle groups like the arms and shoulders can follow. Fewer joints equal later order.

The rationale is that exercises for larger muscle groups are more taxing and require more energy, so they should be performed when you're at your freshest.

Training Goals

Your specific training goals—whether they be strength, hypertrophy, or endurance can also influence the optimal order of exercises. For example, if your primary goal is to build leg strength, you might start with heavy squats even if your workout also includes upper-body exercises.

The Interplay of Energy Systems

As discussed in a previous section, your body relies on different energy systems for different types of activities. Knowing how these systems work can help you order your exercises for optimal performance.

- **Anaerobic Activities**: High-intensity, short-duration activities like weightlifting primarily use the phosphagen and glycolytic systems. These exercises are generally best performed at the beginning of a workout when these energy systems are at their peak.

- **Aerobic Activities**: Lower-intensity, longer-duration activities like running or cycling primarily use the aerobic system and can be placed later in the workout, especially if the primary goal is not cardiovascular endurance.

Practical Applications

1. **Warm-Up Appropriately**: Your warm-up should prepare you for the first exercise in your routine, activating the relevant muscle groups and energy systems.

2. **Prioritize Weaknesses**: If you have a weaker muscle group or a specific area you want to focus on, consider doing those exercises earlier in your workout when you have the most energy.

3. **Be Flexible**: While it's good to have a plan, be prepared to adjust your exercise order based on how you feel during the workout. Fatigue, soreness, or other factors may require you to modify your original plan.

The order in which you perform exercises is a critical yet often overlooked aspect of training. By understanding the factors that influence exercise order and how they align with your training goals, you can create a more effective and efficient workout routine.

Muscle Recruitment: The Foundation of Effective Workouts

Muscle recruitment refers to the activation of muscle fibers during exercise. When you lift a weight or perform any form of resistance training, your nervous system sends signals to your muscles to contract. Not all muscle fibers are activated at once; the number and type of fibers recruited depend on the intensity and type of the exercise. Understanding this concept is crucial for optimizing your workouts, as different exercises recruit muscles in varying degrees and patterns.

Compound Versus Isolation Exercises

- **Compound Exercises**: These are multi-joint movements that work for multiple muscle groups at the same time. Examples include squats, deadlifts, and bench presses. They are generally performed at the beginning of a workout when you have the most energy and focus. Scientific studies have shown that compound exercises are more effective for building strength and muscle mass.

- **Isolation Exercises**: These are single-joint movements that focus on one muscle group, like bicep curls or leg extensions. Isolation exercises are usually performed after compound exercises, as they require less overall energy but still benefit from a warmed-up body.

The Role of Fast-Twitch and Slow-Twitch Fibers

Muscle fibers can be broadly categorized into two types:

- **Type II - Fast-Twitch Fibers**: These fibers are responsible for quick, explosive movements and are primarily recruited during high-intensity, low-duration exercises like sprinting or heavy lifting.

- **Type I - Slow-Twitch Fibers**: These fibers are more endurance-oriented and are activated during low-intensity, long-duration exercises like distance running.

Knowing which type of muscle fiber you're aiming to engage can help you tailor your exercise order accordingly.

Practical Implications

1. **Start with Compound Exercises**: To maximize muscle recruitment, start your workout with compound exercises. This approach allows you to lift heavier weights, thereby engaging more muscle fibers.

2. **Isolation Exercises for Targeted Growth**: If you have specific muscles you want to focus on, isolation exercises are your best bet. However, they should generally follow compound exercises for optimal muscle recruitment.

3. **Consider Your Goals**: If you're training for a specific sport or activity, the order of exercises should mimic the muscle recruitment patterns needed for that activity.

4. **Listen to Your Body**: While scientific guidelines provide a solid foundation, individual differences in muscle recruitment patterns mean that you should also pay attention to how your body responds to different exercise orders.

Understanding muscle recruitment is not just an academic exercise; it has real-world implications for how you structure your workouts. By being mindful of which muscles are being engaged and in what order, you can create a more effective and efficient workout routine.

Energy Systems

The human body relies on three primary energy systems to perform various types of activities:

1. **Phosphagen System (ATP-PCrP)**: This system is used for very short-duration, high-intensity activities, lasting about 10 to 15 seconds. It's the primary energy system used for activities like sprinting or lifting heavy weights. The phosphagen system doesn't require oxygen and uses stored ATP (adenosine triphosphate) and CP (creatine phosphate) for immediate energy.

2. **Glycolytic System**: This system kicks in after the phosphagen system is depleted, providing energy for activities lasting around 30 seconds to 2 minutes. It breaks down carbohydrates, specifically glucose and glycogen, to produce ATP. This system can function with or without oxygen but is less efficient than the aerobic system.

3. **Oxidative System**: This is the most efficient but slowest system, providing energy for activities lasting longer than 2 minutes. It uses oxygen to convert carbohydrates, fats, and sometimes proteins into ATP. This system is primarily used during low-intensity, long-duration activities like jogging or swimming.

Balancing Energy Systems in Your Workout

Understanding these energy systems can help you structure your workout for maximum efficiency. For instance, if your workout involves both high-intensity weightlifting and low-intensity cardio, knowing which energy system to use first can make a significant difference in your performance.

- **High-Intensity First**: If your primary goal is to build strength or power, it's generally better to start with exercises that make use of the phosphagen and glycolytic systems. This allows you to perform these exercises when your energy stores are full.

- **Low-Intensity First**: If your focus is on endurance or fat loss, you might start with aerobic exercises. This approach can also serve as an extended warm-up for the muscles you'll engage in weightlifting.

The Importance of Nutrition

Your body's ability to utilize these energy systems is heavily influenced by your diet. Carbohydrates are crucial for the glycolytic and aerobic systems, while creatine supplementation can enhance the phosphagen system.

Practical Tips:

1. **Tailor Your Warm-Up**: Your warm-up should prepare the specific energy system you'll primarily use in your workout.

2. **Nutrient Timing**: Consuming the right nutrients before and after your workout can optimize the energy systems you're relying on.

3. **Rest and Recovery**: Different energy systems require different recovery times. Understanding this can help you optimize rest periods between sets and exercises.

Understanding your body's energy systems is like knowing the rules of a game; it equips you to play more effectively. By tailoring your workout to optimize these systems, you can improve both your performance and your results

Quality Over Quantity: The Importance of Form

While the number of reps and sets is crucial, the quality of each rep is equally important. Poor form can lead to ineffective workouts and even injuries. You should always prioritize proper technique over lifting heavier weights or performing more reps.

Practical Tips

1. **Progressive Overload**: To continue making progress, you need to gradually increase the weight, reps, or sets you're performing. This principle is known as progressive overload and is supported by extensive scientific research.

2. **Rest Periods**: Don't underestimate the importance of rest periods. They're not just a break but a crucial part of your training that affects muscle recovery and growth.

3. **Individual Variability**: Everyone's body responds differently to exercise. While these guidelines are based on scientific research, you may need to adjust the numbers slightly to fit your individual needs.

The science of reps and sets is more nuanced than simply lifting a weight as many times as you can. By understanding the relationship between reps, sets, and your fitness goals, you can create a more effective and safer workout routine.

Power Versus Hypertrophy Versus Strength Versus Endurance

Force-Velocity Relationship

The force-velocity relationship is a foundational concept in biomechanics and exercise physiology. It provides insights into how muscles produce force under varying conditions of speed and resistance. A good understanding of this relationship is crucial for athletes, coaches, and fitness enthusiasts aiming to optimize performance across different types of activities.

The Basic Principle

The force-velocity relationship illustrates an inverse relationship between the force a muscle can produce and the speed at which it contracts. In simpler terms, as the speed of a muscle contraction increases (velocity), the force it can produce decreases, and vice versa.

The Curve

When plotted on a graph, with force on the y-axis and velocity on the x-axis, the force-velocity relationship forms a descending curve. This curve represents the muscle's ability to produce force at various contraction speeds.

The curve starts at the top left, indicating maximum force at zero velocity (isometric contractions). As you move to the right, indicating faster contractions, the force capability decreases.

Implications for Training

- **Strength Training:** Strength is the maximization of force. When lifting heavy weights slowly (low velocity), the muscles generate a high force. This is why strength training exercises, like heavy squats or deadlifts, are performed at slower speeds. There are maximal amounts of myosin cross-bridges allowing high force but slow speed due to all the active binding sites being occupied.

- **Speed Training:** Speed is the maximization of velocity. Activities that prioritize speed, like running, involve fast muscle contractions. However, the force exerted by the muscles in such high-velocity movements is relatively low compared to strength training exercises. There are minimal amounts of myosin cross-bridges allowing low force but high speed due to many available active binding sites.

- **Power Training:** Power is best defined as explosiveness. It is the perfect force that propels velocity generation. Power exercises, such as plyometrics or Olympic lifts, require this balance of force and speed to achieve. Athletes must produce significant force in a very short time frame, making them sit at the mid-point of the force-velocity curve.

Real-World Applications

- **Athletic Performance:** Different sports and activities require athletes to operate at various points along the force-velocity curve. For instance, a shot putter needs to generate immense force rapidly, emphasizing the power region of the curve. In contrast, a marathon runner operates at a higher velocity, and a lower force end.

- **Injury Prevention:** Understanding the force-velocity relationship can help in designing training programs that balance force and speed, reducing the risk of injuries associated with excessive force or overly rapid movements.

- **Rehabilitation:** Post-injury, the force-velocity curve can guide the reintroduction of movement and resistance, ensuring that muscles are not overloaded too quickly.

The Role of Muscle Fiber Types

Different muscle fibers contribute differently to the force-velocity relationship. Fast-twitch fibers (Type II) are more suited for high-force, low-velocity movements, while slow-twitch fibers (Type I) are adapted for low-force, high-velocity activities.

Conclusion: The force-velocity relationship offers insights into speed and strength in muscular contractions. Trainers and athletes can tailor training regimens to specific goals, whether they're aiming for raw strength, explosive power, or rapid speed by understanding where different exercises and activities lie on the force-velocity curve. This knowledge not only enhances performance but also contributes to safer, more effective training practices.

Power

Power exercises are designed to improve your ability to exert force quickly. These exercises often involve explosive movements that require both strength and speed, such as kettlebell swings, power cleans, and plyometric jumps. Incorporating power exercises into your routine can enhance athletic performance, improve functional abilities, and add variety to your workouts.

When incorporating power exercises in your program, use:

- **Reps**: 3-6 per set
- **Sets**: 3-5
- **Rest**: 2-5 minutes between sets
- **Intensity**: Moderate to heavy weight (70-85% of your one-rep max)

Science Behind Power Exercises

The goal of power training is to increase your ability to produce force rapidly. Unlike strength training, which focuses solely on lifting the maximum amount of weight, or endurance training, which aims for prolonged performance, power training seeks to combine speed and strength. This type of training primarily employs fast-twitch muscle fibers, which are responsible for quick, explosive movements.

Neurological Benefits

These exercises also have a neurological component, improving the efficiency and speed of the signals sent from your brain to your muscles. This can enhance your reaction times and coordination.

Types of Power Exercises

1. **Olympic Lifts**: Exercises like the snatch and the clean and jerk are classic examples of power training.

2. **Plyometrics**: These include various types of jumps, such as box jumps or squat jumps.

3. **Ballistic Exercises**: Movements like kettlebell swings and medicine ball throws fall under this category.

4. **Sprints**: Short bursts of running at maximum effort can also be considered a form of power training.

Incorporating Power Exercises into Your Routine

- **Placement**: Due to their intense nature, power exercises are often best performed at the beginning of a workout when you're fresh.

- **Volume and Intensity**: These exercises are typically performed at high intensity but low volume to minimize fatigue and maximize power output.

- **Rest Periods**: Longer rest periods (2-5 minutes) are generally recommended to allow for full recovery between sets.

- **Progressive Overload**: Just like with strength and muscle enlargement training, it's important to gradually increase the intensity of your power exercises to continue making progress.

Practical Tips

1. **Prioritize Form**: Given the explosive nature of power exercises, maintaining proper form is crucial to prevent injury. Consider working with a certified trainer when you're first learning these movements.

2. **Quality Over Quantity**: Power training is not about how many reps you can do; it's about the quality and speed of each rep. Focus on executing each movement with maximum force and speed.

3. **Warm-Up Appropriately**: A thorough warm-up is essential before engaging in power exercises. Dynamic stretches and low-intensity versions of the movements you'll be performing can prepare your muscles and nervous system for the workout.

4. **Use Compound Movements**: Exercises that engage multiple muscle groups, like power cleans or kettlebell swings, are generally more effective for power training.

5. **Rest and Recover**: Due to the high intensity of power training, adequate rest between sets and workouts is crucial. This allows your neuromuscular system to recover, enabling you to perform at your best in each set.

6. **Nutrition**: Consuming a balanced meal or snack rich in protein and carbohydrates before your workout can provide the energy needed for these high-intensity movements.

Power training is a specialized form of exercise that requires a unique approach to reps, sets, rest periods, and intensity. By understanding these variables and how they differ from other forms of training, you can effectively incorporate power exercises into your routine to improve both athletic performance and functional fitness.

Strength

Strength training aims to increase the maximum amount of force your muscles can produce. Lifting heavy weights for fewer reps recruits more fast-twitch muscle fibers, which are responsible for generating power. Longer rest periods allow for complete recovery of the ATP-CP energy system, which enables maximum performance in each set.

When incorporating strength exercises into your program, use:

- **Reps**: 1-6 per set
- **Sets**: 3-5
- **Rest**: 2-5 minutes between sets
- **Intensity**: Heavyweight (75-90% of your one-rep max)

Neural Adaptations

When you first start strength training, the initial gains in strength are largely due to neural adaptations. Your nervous system becomes more efficient at recruiting muscle fibers, especially the fast-twitch ones, and coordinating their contractions.

Over time, with consistent training, there's an increase in the synchronization of motor units (a motor neuron and the muscle fibers it controls), allowing for more forceful contractions.

Hormonal Responses

Strength training stimulates the release of various hormones, including testosterone and growth hormone, both of which play pivotal roles in muscle growth and repair.

Energy Systems

The ATP-CP system, or the phosphagen system, is the primary energy source during high-intensity, short-duration activities like strength training. This system provides immediate energy by donating a phosphate molecule to ADP to form ATP, the body's energy currency.

The longer rest periods in strength training ensure that the ATP-CP system is fully replenished, allowing for maximum force production in subsequent sets.

Practical Tips

- **Compound Movements:** Exercises like squats, deadlifts, and bench presses are foundational to strength training. They engage multiple muscle groups, allowing for the lifting of heavier weights and promoting functional strength.
- **Periodization:** Varying your training routine over time, in terms of intensity, volume, and exercise selection, can prevent plateaus. This systematic variation keeps the muscles adapting and growing.
- **Safety First:** Proper form and technique are paramount in strength training to prevent injuries given the heavyweights involved. It's beneficial to work with a certified trainer, especially as a beginner.

- **Recovery:** Ensure you're giving your muscles adequate time to recover between sessions. This not only prevents overtraining but also ensures that muscles repair and grow effectively.

- **Nutrition:** Consuming protein-rich meals post-workout can aid in muscle repair and growth. Additionally, carbohydrates can help replenish glycogen stores, preparing you for your next session.

Strength training is a dynamic interplay of neural, muscular, and hormonal responses, all working in tandem to enhance your power and muscle size. By understanding the science behind it and incorporating the practical tips, you can optimize your training regimen, ensuring not just gains in strength but also in overall health and fitness.

Hypertrophy: Building Muscle Mass

The goal of hypertrophy training is to increase muscle size. Research shows that performing exercises in the 6-12 rep range stimulates the maximum release of muscle-building hormones like testosterone and growth hormone. The moderate rest periods and moderate intensity are designed to create the optimal level of muscle tension and metabolic stress, which are key factors in muscle growth.

When incorporating hypertrophy exercises into your program, use:

- **Reps**: 6-12 per set
- **Sets**: 3-5
- **Rest**: 60-90 seconds between sets
- **Intensity**: Moderate weight (60-75% of your one-rep max)

Science Behind Hypertrophy Training

Muscle hypertrophy refers to the process where muscle fibers increase in size, primarily as a response to resistance training. The physiological mechanisms behind hypertrophy are multifaceted:

- **Mechanical Tension:** Lifting weights creates mechanical tension in the muscles. This tension, especially when sustained over time, signals the muscle cells to grow and strengthen.

- **Metabolic Stress:** When you lift weights, especially in the 6-12 rep range, you create metabolic stress or a buildup of metabolites like lactate. This stress is believed to contribute to muscle growth by increasing the release of anabolic hormones and promoting cell swelling.

- **Muscle Damage:** The soreness you feel a day or two after a workout is a result of microscopic damage to muscle fibers. This damage signals the body to repair and rebuild the fibers, making them larger and stronger in the process.

- **Hormonal Responses:** Hypertrophy training stimulates the release of anabolic hormones like testosterone and growth hormone, which play pivotal roles in muscle protein synthesis and muscle growth.

Practical Tips

- **Variety:** Incorporate a mix of compound and isolation exercises to target different muscle groups comprehensively.

- **Eccentric Focus:** Emphasize the eccentric (lengthening) phase of exercises. Slow down during this phase, as controlled eccentric movements have been shown to cause more muscle damage, leading to greater hypertrophy.

- **Progressive Overload:** Gradually increase the weight or resistance over time to continually challenge your muscles and stimulate growth.

- **Nutrition:** Ensure you're consuming adequate protein to support muscle repair and growth. Post-workout protein intake can optimize muscle protein synthesis.

- **Recovery:** While it's essential to challenge your muscles, it's equally crucial to give them time to recover and grow. Ensure you're getting adequate rest between workouts targeting the same muscle group.

Endurance

Endurance training focuses on improving your muscles' ability to sustain prolonged periods of work. This type of training primarily, which is more resistant to fatigue is slow-twitch muscle fibers. The higher rep ranges and shorter rest periods increase the time under tension, improving muscle stamina.

When incorporating endurance exercises into your program, use:

- **Reps**: 12-20 per set

- **Sets**: 2-4

- **Rest**: 30-60 seconds between sets

- **Intensity**: Lightweight (40-60% of your one-rep max)

Science Behind Endurance Training

Endurance training, (muscular or cardiovascular), is designed to enhance the body's ability to sustain prolonged physical activity. The physiological adaptations from this type of training are multifaceted:

1. **Mitochondrial Adaptations:** Mitochondria are the energy-producing structures in cells. Endurance training increases both the number and efficiency of mitochondria in muscle cells, enhancing the muscles' ability to produce energy through aerobic metabolism.

2. **Capillary Density:** With consistent endurance training, there's an increase in the number of capillaries surrounding muscle fibers. This allows for better oxygen and nutrient delivery to the muscles and more efficient removal of waste products, aiding in prolonged muscle function.

3. **Oxidative Enzyme Increase:** Enzymes that support aerobic metabolism become more abundant and efficient, allowing muscles to produce more energy for longer durations.

4. **Muscle Fiber Type Shift:** While endurance training primarily employs slow-twitch fibers, there can be a shift in some fast-twitch fibers to take on the characteristics of slow-twitch fibers, making them more fatigue-resistant.

5. **Enhanced Fat Metabolism:** The body becomes more efficient at using fat as a fuel source during prolonged exercise, conserving glycogen stores.

6. **Improved Cardiovascular Function:** Endurance training strengthens the heart, allowing it to pump more blood (and therefore oxygen) to working muscles. This is crucial for prolonged activities.

Practical Tips

- **Consistent Training:** For endurance adaptations to occur, consistent and progressive training is essential. Increase the duration or intensity of your workouts over time gradually.

- **Cross-Training:** Incorporate different forms of endurance exercises (e.g., cycling, swimming, running) to challenge different muscle groups and prevent overuse injuries.

- **Nutrition:** Ensure you're consuming adequate carbohydrates, as they are the primary fuel source for endurance activities. Consider electrolyte replenishment during longer workouts.

- **Recovery:** While endurance training can be less tasking on the muscles compared to high-intensity workouts, recovery is still vital. Incorporate rest days and consider active recovery activities like walking or yoga.

Endurance training is a cornerstone for many athletic endeavors and general fitness goals. By understanding the underlying science, you can optimize your training regimen to maximize stamina and overall endurance. Whether you're training for a marathon, looking to improve your cardiovascular health, or simply wanting to increase your daily energy levels, endurance training, when done correctly, offers a plethora of benefits.

Goal	% of 1RM	Reps	Rest
Power	50-80	2-5	2-5 Min
Strength	≥85	2-6	2-5 Min
Hypertrophy	70-80	8-12	30-90 Sec
Endurance	≤65	15+	≤30 Sec

The Importance of Rest Periods

Rest periods are the intervals of time you take to recover between sets during a workout. Rest periods play a critical role in determining the effectiveness of your exercise routine. The length and quality of your rest periods can significantly impact muscle recovery, hormone regulation, and overall workout performance.

The Science Behind Rest Periods

Muscle Recovery

- **Microtrauma Repair:** When we exercise, especially during resistance training, we create microscopic tears in our muscle fibers. These tears might sound harmful, but they're actually a natural part of the muscle-building process. During rest periods, the body initiates repair mechanisms to mend these tears.

- **Muscle Protein Synthesis:** The repair process involves muscle protein synthesis, where new proteins are formed to replace damaged ones. This synthesis, when combined with adequate nutrition, leads to muscle growth.

- **Prevention of Overtraining:** Continuous training without adequate rest can lead to overtraining syndrome, characterized by fatigue, decreased performance, and increased risk of injury. Rest periods help prevent this risk.

Energy Replenishment

- **ATP Restoration:** Adenosine triphosphate (ATP) is the primary energy molecule used during short, intense exercise. During rest, ATP stores in the muscle are replenished, allowing for sustained performance in subsequent sets or exercises.

- **Phosphocreatine (PCr) Recovery:** PCr is another energy molecule that helps rapidly regenerate ATP during high-intensity activities. Rest periods allow PCr levels to be restored, ensuring that the ATP-PCr energy system functions optimally in subsequent efforts.

Lactic Acid Clearance

- **Metabolic Byproduct:** During anaerobic exercise, like weightlifting or sprinting, the body produces lactic acid as a metabolic byproduct. Accumulation of lactic acid can lead to a burning sensation in the muscles and contribute to fatigue.

- **Buffering and Removal:** The body has mechanisms to buffer and remove lactic acid, and rest periods facilitate this process. As lactic acid is cleared from the muscles, the pH balance is restored, reducing muscle discomfort and preparing the body for the next exercise.

Hormonal Balance

- **Testosterone and Growth Hormone:** These are anabolic hormones that play a crucial role in muscle growth and repair. Intense exercise can stimulate their release, and adequate rest ensures that the body can utilize these hormones effectively.

- **Cortisol Regulation:** Cortisol, a catabolic hormone, breaks down muscle tissue. While some cortisol release is natural during exercise, prolonged, intense workouts without adequate rest can lead to excessive cortisol levels, counteracting muscle growth. Rest periods help regulate cortisol release, ensuring a favorable anabolic-to-catabolic balance.

Directing Rest Periods to Your Goals

Hypertrophy (Muscle Growth)

The primary goal of hypertrophy training is to increase muscle size. This involves creating enough muscle tension and metabolic stress to stimulate muscle protein synthesis.

Rest Period Duration: 60-90 seconds.

- **Rationale:** A moderate rest period between allowing muscles to recover and maintaining a level of muscle engagement that promotes growth. Shorter rest intervals can heighten metabolic stress, leading to an increased release of muscle-building hormones like growth hormone and IGF-1.

- **Additional Tip:** During these rest intervals, it's beneficial to stay active by doing light stretches or mobility exercises, which can further enhance blood flow and nutrient delivery to the muscles.

Strength

Strength training aims to increase the maximum force a muscle or muscle group can produce. It typically involves lifting heavier weights for fewer repetitions.

Rest Period Duration: 2-5 minutes.

- **Rationale:** Longer rest periods are essential for complete recovery of the ATP-CP energy system, which fuels short, high-intensity efforts like heavy lifting. This ensures that you can exert maximum force in subsequent sets, leading to optimal strength gains.

- **Additional Tip:** During these longer rest intervals, focus on deep breathing and mental preparation for the next set. Visualization techniques can also be beneficial.

Endurance

Endurance training focuses on improving the muscles' ability to sustain activity over prolonged periods. It often involves lighter weights and higher repetitions.

Rest Period Duration: 30-60 seconds.

- **Rationale:** Shorter rest periods challenge the muscles to recover quickly, enhancing their ability to resist fatigue over time. This trains the aerobic energy system and improves muscle stamina.

- **Additional Tip:** To further challenge endurance, consider incorporating circuit training or supersets, where you move from one exercise to another with minimal rest.

Exercise Order in Programing
1. Power – Olympic, plyometric, sprint
2. Core Lifts – bench, squat, deadlift
3. Compound joint groups
4. Single joint lifts
5. Endurance lifts
6. Cardio

Practical Tips for Optimizing Rest Periods

Rest periods can be fine-tuned in various ways to enhance your workout's effectiveness. These are some practical strategies to make the most of your rest intervals:

Use a Timer

- **Why It's Important:** It's easy to get distracted or lose track of time during rest periods. Without a timer, you might rest too long, reducing the workout's intensity, or too little, compromising recovery and future performance.

- **How to Implement:** Many fitness apps and smartwatches come with built-in interval timers. Alternatively, a simple stopwatch or even your smartphone can do the trick. Set the timer for your desired rest period as soon as you finish a set to ensure consistency.

Active Versus Passive Rest

- **Active Rest:** This involves doing low-intensity activities during your rest periods, such as walking, light stretching, or even performing a different exercise that doesn't target the same muscle group.

- **Benefits:** Active rest can help maintain an elevated heart rate, promoting cardiovascular fitness and potentially enhancing calorie burn. It also facilitates blood flow, aiding in the removal of waste products from muscles.

- **Passive Rest:** This is when you take a complete break, sitting or standing still.

- **Benefits:** Passive rest allows for maximum recovery, especially after high-intensity sets. It's particularly beneficial for strength training where the focus is on lifting heavy weights.

- **How to Choose:** Your choice between active and passive rest largely depends on your workout goals and current fitness level. If you're doing a high-intensity interval training (HIIT) session or circuit training, active rest might be more appropriate. On the other hand, for heavy strength training, passive rest is usually recommended.

Listen to Your Body

- **Why it's important:** Everyone's body is unique. Factors like your fitness level, age, nutrition, sleep quality, and even stress can influence how quickly you recover between sets.

- **How to Implement:** Pay attention to how you feel. If your breathing hasn't normalized or your muscles feel excessively fatigued, consider extending your rest period slightly. Conversely, if you feel fully recovered before the timer goes off, you might be able to shorten your rest intervals or increase the intensity of your workouts.

- **Additional Tip:** Keeping a workout journal can help you track how different rest periods affect your performance. Over time, this can provide insights into what works best for you.

Rest periods play a pivotal role in determining the effectiveness of your workouts. By using these practical tips, you can ensure that your rest intervals are not just passive breaks but strategic components of your training regimen, targeted at optimizing performance and recovery.

Should Cardio Be Performed Before or After Weights?

One of the most hotly debated topics in the fitness community is whether to perform cardio before or after weightlifting. Scientific research provides valuable insights into how the order can affect different aspects of fitness, such as muscle growth, endurance, and overall caloric burn.

Factors to Consider

Energy Expenditure

- **Cardio First**: Doing cardio first can serve as a warm-up and may increase overall energy expenditure if the cardio is high-intensity.

- **Weights First**: Weightlifting first allows you to expend more energy during resistance training, as you'll be able to lift heavier weights.

Muscle Fatigue

- **Cardio First**: Prolonged cardio can fatigue your muscles, potentially affecting your performance in subsequent weightlifting exercises.

- **Weights First**: Lifting weights first can also lead to muscle fatigue but is less likely to affect your cardio performance, especially if the cardio is low to moderate intensity.

Glycogen Stores: Your muscles store carbohydrates in the form of glycogen, which serves as a key energy source during exercise.

- **Cardio First**: Intense cardio can deplete glycogen stores, which might compromise your ability to lift heavy weights.

- **Weights First**: Starting with weightlifting preserves your glycogen stores for more strenuous anaerobic activities.

The Cardio-First Debate: Pros and Cons of Starting with Cardiovascular Exercise

Warming Up the Body

One of the primary arguments for doing cardio first is that it serves as an effective warm-up. A moderate-intensity cardio session can increase your heart rate, warm up your muscles, and improve blood flow, preparing your body for the more strenuous activity of weightlifting.

Priming the Aerobic System

Starting with cardio can also prime your aerobic system, enhancing your body's ability to utilize oxygen throughout the workout. This can be particularly beneficial if your workout routine includes high-repetition, lower-weight resistance exercises that use aerobic metabolism.

Enhancing Fat Loss

Some proponents argue that doing cardio first may help with fat loss. The idea is that cardio can deplete glycogen stores, forcing your body to use fat as a primary fuel source during subsequent weightlifting. However, this theory is still a subject of debate among experts.

The Drawbacks of Cardio First

Depleting Glycogen Stores

While cardio can serve as an effective warm-up, it can also deplete your muscle glycogen stores if performed at high intensity or for an extended period. Glycogen is the primary energy source for anaerobic activities like weightlifting. Starting with cardio could compromise your ability to lift heavy weights, affecting muscle growth and strength gains.

Risk of Overtraining

If you start with an intense cardio session, your cardiovascular system might get weak, leading to decreased performance in your weightlifting exercises. Over time, this could increase the risk of overtraining and injury.

Potential for Muscle Catabolism

Performing cardio first, especially for extended periods, could potentially lead to muscle catabolism, where the body breaks down muscle tissue for energy. This is generally undesirable if muscle preservation or growth is your goal.

Scientific Insights

Research on the topic is mixed, with some studies suggesting that the order may not significantly impact overall fitness gains. However, most experts agree that if your primary goal is muscle growth or maximal strength development, it's generally better to perform weightlifting exercises first.

Conclusion

The "Cardio-First Debate" is complex, with valid arguments on both sides. The optimal choice depends on various factors, including your specific fitness goals, the type of cardio, its intensity, and duration, as well as your overall workout plan. Understanding these can help you make an informed decision that aligns with your objectives and maximizes the effectiveness of your workout routine. However, one thing is clear-cardio first depletes your glycogen energy stores.

The Weights-First Argument

Maximizing Muscle Recruitment

Starting with weightlifting allows you to perform at your peak when your muscles are fresh. This is particularly important for exercises that require high levels of strength and coordination, such as squats, deadlifts, and bench presses. Maximizing muscle recruitment can lead to better strength gains and muscle growth over time.

Preserving Glycogen Stores

Weightlifting primarily relies on anaerobic energy systems, which use glycogen as a primary fuel source. By starting with weights, you ensure that your glycogen stores are intact, allowing you to lift heavier and perform more reps, thereby maximizing the effectiveness of your resistance training.

Focused Technique

When you start with weightlifting, you're more likely to maintain proper form and technique, reducing the risk of injury. As fatigue sets in later in the workout, maintaining form during cardio exercises like running or cycling is generally less complex than during weightlifting movements.

The Drawbacks of Weights First

Potential for Cardiovascular Underperformance

If you get tired during weightlifting, your subsequent cardio performance might suffer. This could be a concern if your fitness goals are more oriented toward cardiovascular endurance or weight loss.

Inadequate Warm-Up

Starting directly with heavy lifting without a proper warm-up can increase the risk of injury. However, this can be avoided by the use of a targeted warm-up that prepares the specific muscles you'll be working on.

Energy Imbalance

If you're aiming for a balanced workout that includes both anaerobic and aerobic elements, starting with weights might leave you too fatigued to perform well in aerobic exercises, potentially leading to an imbalance in your fitness regimen.

Scientific Insights

Research generally supports the idea of doing weightlifting first if your primary goal is to increase strength or muscle mass. Studies have shown that strength performance tends to be higher when resistance training is performed before aerobic exercise, particularly for high-intensity, short-duration activities.

Conclusion

The "Weights-First Argument" has strong merits, especially for those focused on strength training or muscle building. However, like the "Cardio-First Debate", the optimal order is not one-size-fits-all. It depends on your specific fitness goals, the types of exercises included in your routine, and your body's physiological responses to those exercises. By understanding the advantages and disadvantages of starting with weightlifting, you can direct your workout to better meet your objectives.

The Verdict: Personalizing Your Approach for Optimal Results

The Importance of Individual Goals

The decision to start with cardio or weights should be primarily influenced by your specific fitness goals. If muscle growth and strength are your main objectives, then beginning with weightlifting is generally more advantageous. On the other hand, if your focus is on improving cardiovascular health, endurance, or weight loss, starting with cardio may offer benefits.

The Role of Exercise Intensity and Duration

The intensity and duration of each component— cardio, and weights also play a significant role in determining the optimal order. High-intensity, short-duration cardio is more likely to deplete glycogen stores and fatigue muscles, making it less ideal before weightlifting. Conversely, low-to-moderate intensity cardio can serve as an effective warm-up without significantly impacting your weightlifting performance.

Flexibility and Adaptability

It's essential to remain flexible and willing to adapt your workout routine based on how you feel on a given day. Factors like sleep quality, nutrition, and stress levels can all impact your performance and may necessitate adjustments to your planned exercise order.

Scientific Consensus

Individual studies offer varying conclusions, however, the general scientific consensus leans toward performing weightlifting first for muscle hypertrophy and strength gains. However, the impact on general fitness, endurance, and weight loss is less clear-cut. Conversely, there is an unclear result on cardio's benefit of being first but clear scientific evidence to the loss of glycogen, when in doubt, weights before cardio.

Practical Tips for Your Personal Fitness

Trial and Error

- **Experiment with Both**: If you're new to combining cardio and weights in a single workout, consider trying both orders for a few weeks each. Track your performance, how you feel during and after the workout, and any changes in your fitness metrics.

- **Adjust Based on Feedback**: Listen to your body and make adjustments based on how you feel. If you find that one order consistently leaves you too fatigued to perform well in the second part of your workout, it might be worth switching things up.

Hybrid Models

- **Circuit Training**: This involves a series of exercises performed one after the other with little to no rest in between. You can mix cardio exercises like jumping jacks with weightlifting exercises like squats for a balanced workout.

- **Supersets**: Pair a cardio exercise with a weightlifting exercise and perform them back-to-back with no rest in between. This approach can save time and keep your heart rate elevated throughout the workout.

Consult a Professional

- **Fitness Assessment**: A certified fitness trainer can assess your current fitness level and help you engage in a program that aligns with your goals.

- **Nutritional Guidance**: A registered dietitian can help you optimize your pre-workout and post-workout meals to support your exercise routine.

Warm-Up and Cool-Down

- **Targeted Warm-Up**: Regardless of the order you choose, make sure to include a warm-up that prepares your body for the specific exercises you'll be doing.

- **Cool-Down**: Don't neglect a cool-down phase, which can include stretching and low-intensity cardio to help your body recover.

Monitor Your Progress

- **Keep a Workout Log**: Documenting your workouts, including the order of exercises, weights lifted, and how you felt, can provide valuable insights into what's working and what needs adjustment.

- **Regular Check-Ins**: Periodically review your progress toward your fitness goals and adjust your workout routine as needed.

Rest and Recovery

- **Adequate Rest**: Make sure to include rest days in your routine, especially if you're doing intense workouts that combine both cardio and weights.

- **Active Recovery**: On rest days, consider light activities like walking or swimming that allow your muscles to recover without adding additional strain.

Listen to Your Body

- **Adaptability**: Your energy levels can vary from day to day due to factors like sleep, stress, and nutrition. Be prepared to adapt your workout plan accordingly.

- **Signs of Overtraining**: Keep an eye out for symptoms like persistent fatigue, decreased performance, or increased injury risk, which could indicate overtraining.

The optimal order of cardio and weights is not set in stone and can vary based on individual goals, fitness levels, and preferences. These practical tips offer a roadmap to help you manage your personal fitness journey, allowing you to make informed decisions that align with your objectives.

Conclusion: The Art and Science of Structuring Your Workout

Optimal fitness is a complex interplay of various factors ranging from the types of exercises you choose and the order in which you perform them, to the energy systems you engage and the rest periods you take. As we've studied so far, each of these elements is supported by a wealth of scientific research and practical experience, offering valuable insights into how to maximize your workout effectiveness.

Key Takeaways

1. **Individual Goals Matter**: Whether your aim is muscle growth, strength gains, endurance, or a combination, your specific goals should be the cornerstone upon which your workout routine is built.

2. **Quality Over Quantity**: The number of reps and sets is important, but the quality of each repetition is crucial. Proper form and technique can make a significant difference in your results and help prevent injuries.

3. **Energy Systems**: Understanding the body's different energy systems can help you channel your workout for maximum efficiency. Whether it's the phosphagen system for short bursts of strength or the aerobic system for prolonged endurance, knowing how to tap into these systems can enhance your performance.

4. **Rest Periods**: Rest periods are integral to muscle recovery and overall workout effectiveness. The length and quality of your rest can significantly impact your training outcomes.

5. **Exercise Order**: The sequence in which you perform exercises can affect your workout's efficiency and effectiveness. Whether it's weights before cardio or vice versa, the choice can have implications for muscle growth, strength, and endurance.

6. **Practical Tips**: From experimenting with exercise orders to consulting professionals and keeping a workout log, practical strategies can help you go through the complexities of workout planning.

Final Thoughts

While science provides us with general guidelines and principles, it's essential to remember that each individual's response to exercise is unique. Flexibility, adaptability, and a willingness to listen to your body are crucial for long-term success. By combining scientific insights with practical experience, you can create a workout routine that is not only effective but also sustainable and enjoyable.

So, as you lace up your workout shoes and step into the gym or onto the track, remember that you're not just following a set of exercises; you're engaging in a well-researched, finely-tuned regimen designed to help you reach your fullest potential.

CHAPTER 8

DEVELOPING A PERSONALIZED MUSCLE GROWTH PLAN

Studying muscle growth necessitates a clear understanding of one's current fitness standing. The primary purpose of this assessment is not just to set a benchmark but to create a roadmap to individual needs. By pinpointing the exact starting point, individuals can effectively measure their progress, celebrate their achievements, and make necessary adjustments to their strategies when required.

However, while muscle growth might be the central focus, it's important to approach fitness holistically. This comprehensive perspective encompasses various facets of fitness, including strength, endurance, flexibility, and even mental well-being. Each of these elements intertwines to ensure that the individual is not merely building muscle but also enhancing their overall health and functionality.

One of the often-overlooked benefits of recognizing one's fitness level is the motivational boost it provides. Observing tangible improvements over time can serve as a powerful catalyst for commitment and determination to overcome challenges. Moreover, a proper assessment acts as a safety net, ensuring that individuals don't prematurely dive into advanced exercises. This paced progression is pivotal in reducing injury risks, ensuring that the journey is not just about pushing limits but also about progressing safely and sustainably.

Physical Fitness Assessment

Physical fitness is a multifaceted domain that encompasses various aspects of health and performance. An effective physical fitness assessment provides a comprehensive overview of an individual's current fitness level, acting as a roadmap to guide training decisions and track progress over time. By understanding one's strengths and areas of improvement, training programs can be developed to achieve specific fitness goals.

Strength Assessment: Strength is the foundation of many physical activities, from lifting groceries to performing a heavy deadlift. Assessing strength provides insights into an individual's ability to generate force against resistance.

- **One-Repetition Maximum (1RM) Test:** This test is the gold standard for measuring maximal strength. The 1RM determines the maximum amount of weight an individual can lift in a single repetition of a specific exercise. Common exercises used for this test include squats, bench presses, and deadlifts. To conduct the test, the individual starts with a warm-up set using a manageable weight. The weight is gradually increased in subsequent sets with adequate rest in between until the individual reaches a weight they can lift only once with proper form. While the actual 1RM can be directly tested, it's often estimated for safety reasons using submaximal lifts. For example, an individual might lift a weight they can manage for 5 repetitions, and then a formula is used to estimate their 1RM. This method reduces the risk of injury that can come from lifting maximal loads.

- **Isometric Strength Tests:** These tests measure the maximum force an individual can produce when a muscle contracts without changing its length. Unlike dynamic movements like lifting or pulling, isometric contractions involve exerting force without any visible movement. A common example of this test is the handgrip dynamometer test, where an individual squeezes a device as hard as possible, and the device measures the force of the grip. Another example is pushing or pulling against an immovable object, such as a wall, with maximum effort for a few seconds. The force exerted is then measured using specialized equipment. These tests are particularly useful for assessing strength in individuals where dynamic movements might be risky or for specific rehabilitation settings.

By incorporating these detailed strength assessments, individuals can gain a comprehensive understanding of their maximal and isometric strength capabilities. This data is invaluable for strength training programs, setting benchmarks, and tracking progress over time.

Endurance Assessment: Muscular endurance refers to the ability of a muscle or group of muscles to sustain repeated contractions against resistance for an extended period.

- **Push-Up Test:** This classic test measures upper body endurance, specifically targeting the chest, triceps, and anterior deltoids. The individual begins in a plank position with arms fully extended and hands positioned slightly wider than shoulder-width apart. Keeping the body in a straight line from head to heels, the individual lowers their body until the chest nearly touches the ground and then pushes back up to the starting position. The goal is to perform as many push-ups as possible without rest, maintaining proper form. The test ends when the individual can no longer maintain proper form or becomes fatigued.

- **Sit-Up Test:** This test evaluates core muscular endurance, focusing on the rectus abdominis and oblique muscles. The individual starts by lying on their back with knees bent and feet flat on the ground. Arms can be crossed over the chest or placed behind the head. The individual lifts their upper body off the ground towards the knees and then lowers back down without letting the shoulders touch the ground. The objective is to perform as many sit-ups as possible in a minute while maintaining consistent form. The test concludes at the end of the minute or when the individual can no longer maintain the correct form.

- **Step-Up Test:** This test evaluates lower body endurance, particularly the quadriceps and calves. The individual steps up and down on a platform or bench at a set pace for a specified time, usually around 3 minutes. The heart rate is then measured immediately after the test to gauge cardiovascular and muscular endurance. The faster the heart rate returns to its resting state, the better the individual's endurance level.

Body Composition Assessment: Body composition provides a more detailed look at one's fitness than body weight alone. It breaks down weight into fat mass and lean mass, offering insights into muscle development and overall health.

- **Skinfold Calipers:** Skinfold calipers are handheld devices used to pinch and measure the thickness of skinfolds at various standardized sites on the body. Common measurement sites include the triceps, suprailiac, and thigh. By assessing the thickness of these skinfolds, professionals can estimate the subcutaneous fat layer, which is then used to derive an estimate of total body fat percentage. The sum of the measurements from the various sites is compared to reference charts or used in equations to estimate body fat. While this method is cost-effective and widely used, it requires a skilled technician to ensure accuracy and consistency in measurements.

- **Bioelectrical Impedance Analysis (BIA):** BIA devices measure the resistance or impedance of body tissues to a low-level electrical current. Since fat and lean tissues conduct electricity differently, the resistance measured by the device can be used to estimate body fat percentage. The individual typically stands on a scale-like device with footpads or holds onto handheld electrodes. The device then sends a harmless electrical current through the body. The speed at which the current travels can determine the amount of water in the body, which can then be used to estimate lean body mass and body fat. Factors like hydration levels can influence the results, so it's essential to follow pre-test guidelines, such as avoiding exercise or large meals before testing.

- **Dual-Energy X-ray Absorptiometry (DEXA) Scans:** DEXA scans use two different low-dose X-rays to measure body composition. The individual lies on a scanning table while the machine scans over them, providing detailed images of the body's composition. The scan breaks down the body into fat, lean muscle, and bone, giving a comprehensive view of body composition. DEXA can also provide regional body fat measurements, such as trunk versus limbs, and even assess bone density. While DEXA is considered one of the most accurate methods for body composition assessment, it is more expensive and less accessible than other methods.

- **Bod Pod:** The Bod Pod is a cutting-edge body composition tool that uses the principle of air displacement plethysmography. The individual sits inside an egg-shaped chamber wearing minimal clothing and a swim cap. As the chamber is sealed, the device measures the volume of air displaced by the person's body. By comparing the volume of air inside the chamber with and without the person, the Bod Pod can determine body volume. This volume, along with body weight, is then used to calculate body density, from which body fat and lean body mass percentages are derived. The Bod Pod is known for its accuracy, consistency, and quick testing time. It's a non-invasive method that is becoming increasingly popular in both clinical and research settings due to its precision.

Each of these body composition assessment methods offers unique advantages and considerations. The choice of method often depends on the individual's goals, the available resources, and the level of precision required. By understanding body composition, individuals can channel their fitness and nutrition strategies more effectively, tracking changes over time and adjusting their approach as needed.

Functional Movement Assessment

Functional movement patterns are the foundation of our daily activities. From the simple act of standing up from a chair to more complex movements like lifting heavy objects, our body relies on muscles working in harmony. However, not all of us have perfect movement patterns. Muscle imbalances, mobility limitations, or movement dysfunctions can arise from various factors, including sedentary lifestyles, previous injuries, or even just habitual poor posture.

The importance of assessing functional movement cannot be overstated. It's not just about optimizing performance in the gym; it's about ensuring that our bodies function efficiently in everyday life. By identifying and addressing these movement issues, individuals can prevent potential injuries, improve their exercise efficiency, and even enhance their quality of life.

Functional movement assessments typically involve a series of tests that challenge the body's foundational movement patterns. Common tests include:

- **Squat Test:** The squat is a foundational movement that engages multiple muscle groups and joints. When performing the squat test, individuals are typically asked to stand with feet shoulder-width apart and then lower their body as if sitting in a chair, keeping their heels on the ground and chest up. The depth and form of the squat can provide insights into the strength and flexibility of the lower body. A deep, controlled squat indicates good quadriceps, hamstring, and glute strength, as well as adequate flexibility in the ankles and hips. Additionally, the squat can reveal information about core stability and hip mobility. For instance, knees caving inwards might suggest weak hip abductors, while a forward lean could indicate tight hip flexors or weak core muscles.

- **Lunge Test:** The lunge is a unilateral movement that assesses the strength and stability of each leg individually. To perform the test, individuals step forward into a lunge position, ensuring the front knee is aligned with the ankle and not extending past the toes. The depth and stability of the lunge can gauge the balance, strength, and flexibility of the leg muscles. A stable lunge indicates good quadriceps, hamstring, and glute strength on the leading leg, as well as adequate flexibility in the hip flexors of the trailing leg. The lunge test can also highlight any asymmetries between the left and right sides, which could be indicative of muscle imbalances or previous injuries.

- **Overhead Press Test:** The overhead press movement evaluates the strength and mobility of the shoulders and upper back. Individuals are typically asked to press weight or resistance overhead while maintaining a neutral spine. The range of motion, control, and form during this movement can provide insights into shoulder mobility, scapular stability, and upper body strength. Difficulty in achieving a full range of motion might indicate tightness in the shoulder muscles or restrictions in the shoulder joint. Weakness or instability during the press can suggest underactive muscles supporting the shoulder girdle, such as the deltoids or rotator cuff.

- **Single-Leg Balance Test:** Balance and stability are essential for many daily activities and athletic movements. In the single-leg balance test, individuals stand on one leg, keeping the other foot off the ground, and try to maintain balance for a set duration. The ability to hold this position without excessive wobbling or needing to touch down the other foot can reveal a lot about an individual's proprioception, ankle stability, and strength imbalances between the legs. Difficulty in maintaining balance might suggest weak stabilizing muscles in the ankle or hip or challenges in proprioceptive feedback, which is the body's ability to sense its position in space.

Each of these functional movement tests offers valuable insights into an individual's movement patterns, strengths, and areas that might need attention. By assessing these movements, professionals can design targeted interventions to improve functional performance, reduce the risk of injury, and enhance overall movement quality.

Goal Setting

Goal setting is a fundamental step in any fitness journey. Through clear, and measurable objectives, individuals can stay motivated, track their progress, and achieve their desired outcomes more effectively. Proper goal setting involves more than just stating a desire; it requires a systematic approach to ensure that the goals are both challenging and achievable. Key points of the goal-setting process:

1. **Specificity:** Goals should be clear and specific. Instead of setting a vague goal like "I want to get fit", aim for something more precise, such as "I want to increase my bench press weight by 20 pounds in the next three months". Specific goals provide a clear direction and make it easier to measure progress.

2. **Measurability:** Every goal should have a metric attached to it. Whether it's a certain weight, a specific number of repetitions, a particular body fat percentage, or a race time, having a measurable outcome helps in tracking progress and determining whether the goal has been achieved.

3. **Attainability:** While goals should be challenging, they should also be realistic. Setting unattainable goals can lead to frustration and demotivation. It's essential to assess one's current abilities, resources, and constraints before setting a goal.

4. **Relevance:** The goals set should align with broader life objectives and values. If someone values cardiovascular health due to a family history of heart disease, a

relevant goal might be to run a half-marathon. Ensuring relevance keeps individuals committed and passionate about their goals.

5. **Time-Bound:** Setting a deadline creates a sense of urgency and commitment. Whether it's a short-term goal over a few weeks or a long-term goal running into several months or years, having a timeframe helps in planning and prioritizing efforts.

6. **Break Down Larger Goals:** Sometimes, the end goal can seem overwhelming. In such cases, breaking it down into smaller, more manageable milestones can make it more approachable. For instance, if the goal is to lose 50 pounds in a year, one could aim for roughly 4 pounds a month.

7. **Visualize Success:** Taking the time to visualize achieving the goal can be a powerful motivator. It helps in reinforcing belief in oneself and the importance of the goal. Visualization techniques can range from simple daydreaming to more structured practices like guided imagery.

8. **Regularly Review and Adjust:** Goals aren't set in stone. As one progresses, it might become evident that adjustments are needed. Maybe the goal was too easy and needs to be made more challenging, or perhaps unforeseen challenges have made it necessary to extend the timeframe. Regularly reviewing goals ensures they remain relevant and challenging.

9. **Accountability:** Sharing goals with friends, family, or a workout partner can provide an added layer of motivation. Knowing that someone else is aware of your objectives and might check in on your progress can be a powerful incentive to stay on track.

10. **Celebrate Achievements:** Every time a milestone is reached or a goal is achieved, take the time to celebrate. Recognizing and rewarding efforts, no matter how small, boosts morale and motivation for the next challenge.

Therefore, goal setting is more than just stating a desire to achieve something. It's a structured process that, when done correctly, can provide direction, motivation, and a clear path to success in any fitness journey.

Individual Preferences

Everyone is unique, and what works for one person might not necessarily work for another. By understanding and respecting personal inclinations, individuals can create a workout regimen that not only meets their goals but also aligns with their lifestyle, values, and enjoyment factors. Here's a comprehensive look at the role of individual preferences in fitness planning:

Exercise Selection

- **Type of Exercise:** Some people might prefer weightlifting, while others gravitate towards cardio exercises like running or cycling. Still, others might find joy in group classes, yoga, or dance. It's essential to choose exercises that one enjoys and looks forward to.

- **Intensity:** While some thrive on high-intensity interval training (HIIT) sessions, others might prefer steady-state cardio or moderate weightlifting sessions. Understanding one's comfort and challenge zones can help in directing the intensity.

Training Environment

- **Location:** Some individuals love the equipment variety of a gym, while others prefer the comfort of home workouts. Outdoor enthusiasts might opt for runs, hikes, or outdoor boot camps.

- **Social Aspect:** While some find motivation in group classes or having a workout buddy, others might prefer solitude during their workouts, using it as 'me-time.'

Time Commitment

- **Duration:** Some can dedicate an hour or more daily, while others might only have 20-30 minutes. It's crucial to design workouts that fit within these time constraints but are still effective.

- **Frequency:** The number of days one prefers to work out in a week can vary. Some might prefer shorter daily routines, while others might opt for longer sessions a few days a week.

Equipment Preferences

- Some enjoy using various gym equipment such as resistance machines and free weights. In contrast, others might prefer bodyweight exercises or minimal equipment workouts using bands or dumbbells.

Motivational Factors

- **Tracking and Metrics:** Some individuals are motivated by tracking their progress, be it through wearable tech, apps, or old-fashioned workout logs.

- **External Motivation:** This could come from personal trainers, workout videos, or motivational music playlists. Knowing what gets you pumped can make a significant difference.

Dietary Preferences

- If muscle growth is the goal, nutrition plays a pivotal role. However, dietary choices can vary widely based on personal preferences, dietary restrictions, or ethical considerations. Whether one is vegan, vegetarian, pescatarian, or omnivorous can influence their nutritional approach to muscle growth.

Recovery and Rest

- **Active Recovery:** Some might prefer active recovery days involving light activities like walking or yoga.

- **Rest Days:** Others might opt for complete rest days, focusing on relaxation and perhaps activities like reading or meditation.

Feedback and Adjustments

- Some individuals appreciate regular feedback and thrive on adjusting their routines based on results. Others might prefer setting a routine and sticking to it for more extended periods before making changes.

Learning Preferences

- **Self-guided:** Some prefer researching and crafting their workout plans.

- **Guided Instruction:** Others might want structured guidance from personal trainers, fitness apps, or workout programs.

Incorporating individual preferences ensures that the fitness journey remains enjoyable, sustainable, and aligned with one's personal values and lifestyle. It's a reminder that fitness is not a one-size-fits-all endeavor but a deeply personal journey according to each individual.

Professional Guidance

Seeking professional guidance in fitness and muscle growth can be a game-changer. Professionals bring a wealth of knowledge, experience, and expertise that can help individuals go through their fitness journeys more effectively and safely. Here's an in-depth exploration of the importance and benefits of seeking professional guidance:

1. **Expertise and Knowledge:** Certified fitness professionals have undergone rigorous training and education to understand the human body, exercise physiology, and nutrition. They are often required to participate in continuing education to stay updated with the latest research and trends in the fitness industry.

2. **Personalized Assessment:** A fitness professional can conduct a comprehensive assessment to gauge an individual's current fitness level, strengths, weaknesses, and potential areas of concern. Based on this assessment, they can design a program specifically suitable to an individual's goals, needs, and preferences.

3. **Safety and Injury Prevention:** One of the primary roles of fitness professionals is to ensure exercises are performed in the correct form, minimizing the risk of injury. For those with medical conditions or past injuries, a fitness professional can recommend modifications or alternative exercises.

4. **Motivation and Accountability:** Having someone to push and encourage can make challenging workouts more manageable. Scheduled sessions with a trainer or regular check-ins can motivate individuals to stick to their routines.

5. **Nutritional Guidance:** Many fitness professionals have knowledge of nutrition and can provide general dietary advice or collaborate with registered dietitians to create meal plans. They can offer insights into beneficial supplements that align with fitness goals, ensuring individuals avoid potentially harmful products.

6. **Advanced Techniques and Strategies:** Professionals can introduce new exercises or techniques to keep workouts fresh and challenging. They can guide individuals through periodized training cycles, optimizing results by manipulating intensity, volume, and type of exercise over time.

7. **Mental and Emotional Support:** When progress stalls, a fitness professional can provide strategies and tweaks to overcome plateaus. They can help boost an individual's confidence in the gym, ensuring they feel competent and comfortable with various exercises and equipment.

8. **Access to Resources and Tools:** Professionals often have access to the latest fitness equipment and can introduce clients to new tools that they might not have encountered before. They can refer individuals to other professionals, such as physiotherapists, dietitians, or sports psychologists, if specialized assistance is needed.

9. **Feedback and Progress Tracking:** Scheduled assessments can track progress in strength, endurance, body composition, and other metrics. Based on feedback, professionals can make necessary adjustments to the training program, ensuring it remains effective and aligned with evolving goals.

In conclusion, the guidance of a qualified professional can accelerate progress, ensure safety, and provide a well-rounded, holistic approach to health and muscle growth. Whether it's through personal training sessions, consultations, or group classes, professional guidance can be an invaluable asset on the path to achieving fitness goals.

Monitoring Progress and Making Adjustments

The journey to achieving fitness goals is not a straight path but rather a series of trials, errors, successes, and adjustments. As individuals embark on their fitness endeavors, it's not enough to merely follow a program; it's equally vital to monitor progress and make necessary changes along the way. This continuous feedback loop ensures that the training remains effective, reduces the risk of plateaus, and aligns the program with evolving goals and circumstances.

Monitoring progress goes beyond just tracking the weights lifted or the miles run. It encompasses a holistic view of one's fitness journey, taking into account physical, mental, and even emotional indicators of progress. By paying attention to these signs, individuals can make informed decisions about their training, nutrition, and recovery strategies.

Furthermore, the importance of adjustments cannot be overstated. No training program, no matter how well-designed, will remain optimal forever. As the body adapts, goals shift, and life situations change, the need to recalibrate becomes evident. Adjustments ensure that the training remains challenging, relevant, and in harmony with one's current state and aspirations.

In the subsequent sections, we will delve deeper into the various methods of monitoring progress, the indicators to watch out for, and the strategies to effectively make adjustments to keep the momentum going and inch closer to one's fitness goals.

Performance Measurements

Performance measurements serve as tangible indicators of one's progress in their fitness journey. They provide a clear picture of where an individual started, where they currently stand, and how far they've come. These metrics are crucial not only for motivation but also for making informed decisions about training adjustments. Here's a deeper look into the significance and methods of performance measurements:

Importance of Tracking Performance

- **Progress Validation**: Regularly measuring performance validates the effectiveness of a training program. Seeing improvements over time can be a significant morale booster.

- **Identifying Plateaus**: By tracking performance, one can quickly identify when they've hit a plateau, signaling that it might be time to adjust the training regimen.

- **Customization**: Performance metrics help in channeling the training program to an individual's unique strengths and weaknesses.

Common Performance Metrics

- **Strength Metrics**: This includes tracking the amount of weight lifted in exercises like squats, deadlifts, and bench presses. By noting down the weight and repetitions for each set, one can gauge improvements in strength over time.

- **Endurance Metrics**: This could involve tracking the time taken to run a specific distance or the number of repetitions of a particular exercise over a set duration. Improvements in these metrics indicate enhanced cardiovascular or muscular endurance.

- **Flexibility Metrics**: Recording the range of motion in exercises or stretches can help gauge improvements in flexibility. For instance, noting how close one's hands are in a seated forward bend can indicate progress in hamstring flexibility.

Tools and Methods

- **Workout Logs**: Keeping a detailed log of each workout, including exercises, sets, reps, and weights, can provide a clear picture of progress over weeks and months.

- **Fitness Apps**: Numerous apps allow users to input their workout details, track their progress graphically, and even provide insights based on the data.

- **Benchmark Workouts**: Periodically performing standardized workouts can serve as benchmarks. By repeating these workouts every few months, one can measure performance improvements.

Interpreting Data

- **Trends Over Time**: Instead of focusing on day-to-day fluctuations, it's more beneficial to observe trends over weeks or months. This provides a more accurate representation of genuine progress.

- **Contextual Factors**: It's essential to consider external factors that might affect performance, such as sleep, nutrition, stress, or even the time of day the workout was performed. These factors can influence individual workout performances and should be taken into account when interpreting data.

In conclusion, performance measurements are a cornerstone of effective training. They provide the feedback loop necessary to validate one's efforts, motivate for future workouts, and make the necessary adjustments to ensure continuous progress.

Body Composition Analysis

Body composition analysis provides a comprehensive understanding of the distribution of fat, muscle, and bone within the body. Unlike traditional weight scales that only provide a singular number, body composition analysis offers a more detailed view of one's physical makeup. This information is invaluable for those seeking to optimize their fitness, health, and overall well-being. Here's a deeper exploration of body composition analysis:

Significance of Body Composition

- **Beyond the Scale**: While weight can give a general idea about one's health, it doesn't distinguish between muscle, fat, and bone. Two individuals with the same weight might have vastly different muscle-to-fat ratios.

- **Health Implications**: High body fat percentages, especially visceral fat around the organs, can increase the risk of various health issues, including cardiovascular diseases, diabetes, and more.

- **Training Optimization**: Understanding one's body composition can help training programs target specific goals, such as muscle gain or fat loss.

Methods of Analysis

- **Skinfold Calipers**: This method involves pinching the skin and subcutaneous fat in specific areas of the body. The thickness of these pinches can be used to estimate overall body fat percentage.

- **Bioelectrical Impedance Analysis (BIA)**: BIA devices send a low-level electrical current through the body. Since muscle and fat conduct electricity differently, the resistance measured can be used to estimate body fat percentage.

- **Dual-Energy X-ray Absorptiometry (DEXA) Scans**: DEXA provides a detailed breakdown of bone density, fat distribution, and muscle mass. It uses X-rays of two different energies to scan the body, making it one of the most accurate methods available.

- **Bod Pod**: This method uses air displacement plethysmography to measure body volume. The Bod Pod can accurately estimate body density and, subsequently, body composition by determining the volume of air displaced by the individual inside the chamber,

Factors Affecting Body Composition

- **Diet**: The quality and quantity of one's diet play a significant role in determining body composition. Diets high in processed foods and sugars can lead to increased fat storage.

- **Physical Activity**: Regular exercise, especially strength training, can increase muscle mass and reduce body fat percentage.

- **Genetics**: Genetic factors can influence how and where the body stores fat, as well as one's natural muscle-building potential.

- **Hormonal Balance**: Hormones like testosterone, estrogen, and cortisol can influence muscle growth, fat storage, and overall body composition.

Interpreting Results

- **Individual Variation**: It's essential to understand that "ideal" body composition numbers can vary based on factors like age, gender, and genetics. What's optimal for one person might not be for another.

- **Trends Over Time**: Similar to performance measurements, it's more beneficial to observe body composition trends over time rather than focusing on individual readings.

- **Comprehensive View**: Body composition should be considered alongside other health metrics, such as cardiovascular fitness, strength levels, and metabolic markers, to get a comprehensive view of one's health.

In conclusion, body composition analysis offers a more detailed and insightful view of one's physical health than traditional weight measurements. By understanding the intricacies of one's body makeup, individuals can make informed decisions about their diet, exercise, and lifestyle to achieve their health and fitness goals.

Subjective Feedback

Subjective feedback, while often overlooked in favor of more quantifiable metrics, plays a pivotal role in understanding an individual's overall well-being, progress, and response to a training regimen. It encompasses personal perceptions, feelings, and experiences related to physical activity, recovery, and overall health. Importance of subjective feedback:

Understanding Subjective Feedback

Subjective feedback is an individual's personal interpretation of their experiences, feelings, and perceptions related to various aspects of their training and overall health.

Unlike objective data, which is quantifiable and measurable, subjective feedback is more about personal sensations, emotions, and interpretations. Understanding subjective feedback involves:

- **Nature of Subjectivity**: Every individual has a unique way of perceiving their body, performance, and experiences. What might feel strenuous for one person might be moderate for another. This inherent subjectivity makes personal feedback crucial in engaging in training regimens.

- **Physical Sensations and Their Interpretations**: After a workout, an individual might feel muscle soreness, fatigue, or even exhilaration. These sensations can vary in intensity and duration from one session to another and can offer insights into recovery needs, workout intensity, or potential areas of concern.

- **Emotional Responses to Training**: Emotions play a significant role in one's fitness journey. Feelings of accomplishment, frustration, motivation, or even apprehension can influence an individual's approach to training, consistency, and overall commitment.

- **Mental State and Training**: An individual's mental state, including their focus, clarity, and mindfulness, can impact their performance, form, and even their risk of injury. For instance, feeling distracted or mentally fatigued might affect the quality of a training session.

- **Influence of External Factors**: External factors such as personal life events, work stress, or even weather can influence one's subjective feedback. Recognizing these influences can help in understanding fluctuations in performance or mood-related to training.

Importance of Tracking Subjective Feedback

- Paying attention to subjective feedback is a pivotal aspect of a holistic approach to fitness and well-being. While objective metrics provide quantifiable data, subjective feedback offers a deeper understanding of an individual's personal experiences, feelings, and perceptions. Here's why tracking subjective feedback is essential:

- **Personalized Training Adjustments**: By listening to how one feels after specific exercises or routines, adjustments can be made to better suit individual needs. For instance, if a particular exercise consistently leads to excessive soreness or discomfort, it might be worth revisiting the technique or considering an alternative.

- **Mental Well-being and Motivation**: Recognizing feelings of accomplishment, enthusiasm, or even periods of demotivation can help with appropriate motivational strategies. Celebrating small victories or addressing sources of discouragement can significantly impact long-term adherence to a fitness regimen.

- **Injury Prevention**: Often, the body provides subtle hints before an injury manifests. By paying attention to unusual discomfort, twinges, or persistent pain, one can take proactive measures, such as rest or seeking professional advice, to prevent potential injuries.

- **Optimizing Recovery**: Recovery isn't just physical; it's also mental. Understanding feelings of mental fatigue, stress, or burnout can signal the need for rest days, relaxation techniques, or even activities like meditation to ensure comprehensive recovery.

- **Holistic Health Insights**: Beyond just physical training, subjective feedback can offer insights into other aspects of health, such as sleep quality, dietary responses, or even reactions to supplements or medications.

- **Enhanced Communication with Professionals**: When working with fitness trainers, physiotherapists, or nutritionists, sharing subjective feedback can provide them with a more comprehensive view of their experiences, aiding in more personalized guidance.

Recognizing and Addressing Signs of Overtraining and Fatigue

- **Overtraining**, often referred to as overtraining syndrome (OTS), occurs when there is an imbalance between training and recovery: when the training intensity and/or volume exceeds the body's ability to recover. Recognizing and addressing the signs of overtraining is crucial for long-term fitness success, health, and well-being. Here's a deeper dive into understanding and managing overtraining:

- **Symptoms of Overtraining**: The signs of overtraining can be both physical and psychological. Physical symptoms might include persistent soreness, decreased performance, increased susceptibility to injuries, and prolonged recovery times. On the psychological front, one might experience mood swings, irritability, depression, loss of motivation, or even insomnia.

- **Hormonal and Immune System Impacts**: Overtraining can lead to hormonal imbalances. For instance, chronic overtraining can result in decreased testosterone and increased cortisol levels, which can hinder muscle growth and recovery. More so, a compromised immune system might lead to frequent illnesses or infections.

252

- **Importance of Rest and Recovery**: Recovery isn't merely the absence of training; it's an active process. This includes quality sleep, proper nutrition, hydration, and even techniques like foam rolling, stretching, or engaging in low-impact activities like walking or swimming.

- **Listening to the Body**: It's essential to observe one's body and recognize when it's asking for a break. If performance is stagnating or regressing, or if fatigue becomes a constant companion, it might be time to reassess the training regimen.

- **Scheduled Deload Weeks**: Incorporating deload weeks, where the intensity and volume of training are intentionally reduced, can be a proactive measure to prevent overtraining. These periods allow the body and mind to recover fully, setting the stage for subsequent progress.

- **Holistic Wellness Practices**: Integrating practices like meditation, deep breathing exercises, and even hobbies outside of fitness can provide mental relaxation and reduce the stress that might exacerbate overtraining symptoms.

- **Consultation with Professionals**: If symptoms of overtraining persist, it's advisable to consult with fitness professionals or healthcare providers. They can offer professional guidance on adjusting training regimens, provide recovery techniques, or address any underlying health concerns.

Adjusting Training Variables Based on Feedback

- Training is not a one-size-fits-all endeavor. As individuals progress in their fitness journey, it's essential to adjust training variables based on feedback from the body and performance metrics. This ensures that the training remains effective, reduces the risk, and caters to the evolving needs of the individual. Here's a comprehensive look at how to adjust training variables based on feedback:

- **Understanding the Feedback Loop**: The feedback loop in training involves monitoring performance, gathering data (like strength levels, endurance capacity, or even subjective feelings of fatigue), and then making informed adjustments to the training regimen.

- **Volume Adjustments**: Volume refers to the total amount of work done, usually calculated as sets multiplied by repetitions. If recovery is optimal but progress has stalled, increasing the volume can stimulate further muscle growth or strength gains. Conversely, if signs of overtraining appear, reducing volume temporarily can aid recovery.

- **Intensity Modifications**: Intensity relates to the weight lifted or the resistance used in exercises. If strength gains are the goal but progress is slow, increasing the intensity while possibly reducing volume can be effective. For those feeling overly fatigued, a temporary reduction in intensity can be beneficial.

- **Exercise Selection**: Over time, the body can adapt to specific movements. Introducing new exercises or variations can challenge the muscles in different ways, promoting growth and preventing adaptation. For instance, if traditional squats have been a staple, one might try front squats or Bulgarian split squats for variation.

- **Training Frequency**: This refers to how often one trains. If recovery is good and one feels energetic, increasing the frequency of training sessions can accelerate progress. However, if fatigue sets in or performance drops, it might be wise to reduce the number of sessions per week and focus on quality over quantity.

- **Rest Periods**: The time taken to rest between sets can significantly impact training outcomes. For strength gains, longer rest might be beneficial, while shorter rest periods can boost endurance and metabolic conditioning. Adjusting rest based on goals and how one feels can optimize training sessions.

- **Periodization Reassessment**: Periodization involves cycling through different training phases to optimize results and prevent overtraining. If progress stalls in a particular phase, it might be time to transition to a new phase or adjust the current one.

- **Incorporating Feedback from Technology**: With the advent of wearable tech and fitness apps, individuals have access to a plethora of data about their performance, sleep, heart rate, and more. Using this data can provide insights into when to push harder and when to pull back.

- **Staying Flexible and Adaptable**: While structured training plans are valuable, it's essential to remain adaptable. If something isn't working or if an individual's goals shift, the training plan should evolve accordingly.

In conclusion, subjective feedback provides invaluable insights into an individual's physical, mental, and emotional responses to their training regimen. By paying attention to these personal perceptions and experiences, individuals can make informed decisions, direct their training, and ensure a balanced and holistic approach to their health and fitness journey.

Adjusting Training Variables for Optimal Results

The process of adjusting training variables is a cornerstone of effective fitness programming. By fine-tuning these variables, individuals can ensure that they are continually progressing, avoiding plateaus, and reducing the risk of injury. More about adjusting training variables:

Understanding the Importance

Training variables are the specific components of a workout that can be manipulated to achieve desired outcomes. These include volume, intensity, exercise selection, training frequency, and rest periods.

Regularly adjusting these variables ensures that the body is continually challenged, preventing adaptation and ensuring consistent progress.

Volume Adjustments

Volume typically refers to the total number of repetitions and sets performed for a particular exercise or workout. Increasing volume can stimulate muscle growth and endurance, but it's essential to balance this with adequate recovery to prevent overtraining. Conversely, if an individual is feeling overly fatigued or is at risk of injury, reducing volume temporarily can be beneficial.

Intensity Modifications

Intensity relates to the level of effort relative to one's maximum capability, often reflected in the weight or resistance used. For strength gains, increasing intensity is crucial. However, it's essential to ensure that the form is not compromised. Periodically reducing intensity, known as "deloading" can help with recovery and prevent burnout.

Exercise Selection and Variation

The body can adapt to specific exercises over time. It's beneficial to rotate exercises or introduce new ones to prevent this adaptation and continue challenging the muscles. Variations of standard exercises can target muscles differently, thereby offering a fresh stimulus. For instance, transitioning from a standard bench press to an incline bench press can shift the emphasis to the upper pectorals.

Training Frequency

This refers to how often specific muscles or muscle groups are trained. Overtraining a muscle group can lead to fatigue and increased injury risk. Conversely, undertraining can result in suboptimal gains. It's essential to find a balance, ensuring that each muscle group receives adequate stimulation and recovery.

255

Rest and Recovery Periods

Rest periods between sets can impact the training outcome. Shorter rests can increase metabolic stress, beneficial for hypertrophy, while longer rests are essential for maximal strength training. Beyond in-session rest, ensuring adequate days of recovery between intense workouts is crucial for muscle repair and growth.

Incorporating Advanced Techniques

As individuals become more advanced in their training, they might benefit from advanced techniques like drop sets, supersets, or pyramid sets. These can introduce a new stimulus and further challenge the muscles.

Listening to the Body

While structured plans and guidelines are beneficial, it's equally important to listen to one's body. If fatigue, soreness, or signs of overtraining appear, it might be time to adjust the variables accordingly.

In conclusion, adjusting training variables lies in understanding the body's responses and manipulating workouts to align with specific goals. Regular assessment and a willingness to adapt are key to long-term success and continuous improvement in one's fitness journey.

Nutritional Adjustments for Enhanced Training Outcomes

Nutrition is a pivotal component of any fitness journey. As the saying goes, "You can't out-train a bad diet". As individuals progress in their training, their nutritional needs may evolve as well. Making timely and appropriate adjustments to one's diet can significantly impact training outcomes, recovery, and overall health. Importance of nutritional adjustments and how to implement them:

The Role of Nutrition in Training

Nutrition provides the fuel for workouts and the building blocks for muscle repair and growth.Proper nutrition can enhance performance, reduce recovery time, and help prevent injuries.

Macronutrient Ratios

As training goals shift, so might the optimal balance of proteins, carbohydrates, and fats. For instance, during heavy strength training phases, protein intake might need to increase to support muscle repair. Conversely, endurance athletes might prioritize carbohydrates to enhance longer training sessions.

Caloric Intake

Training intensity and volume can influence caloric needs. As training volume or intensity increases, caloric needs might also rise. It's essential to balance caloric intake with expenditure to support training goals, whether that's muscle gain, fat loss, or maintenance.

Nutrient Timing

The timing of nutrient intake can influence training and recovery. Consuming protein and carbohydrates post-workout, for instance, can enhance muscle protein synthesis and glycogen replenishment. Pre-workout meals or snacks can provide the necessary energy for optimal performance.

Hydration

Training intensity, duration, and environmental factors can influence hydration needs. Staying adequately hydrated can improve performance and recovery. Electrolyte balance, especially during prolonged or intense sessions, is crucial to prevent cramps and optimize muscle function.

Supplementation

As training demands increase, some individuals might benefit from supplements like protein powders, branched-chain amino acids (BCAAs), or creatine. However, it's essential to consult with a healthcare professional before starting any supplementation. Remember, supplements should complement a balanced diet, not replace it.

Dietary Restrictions and Preferences

Individuals following specific diets (e.g., vegan, ketogenic, intermittent fasting) might need to make additional adjustments to ensure they're meeting their nutritional needs while supporting their training goals.

Monitoring and Feedback

Regularly track dietary intake, energy levels, performance, and recovery to gauge the effectiveness of nutritional strategies. Adjustments might be needed based on feedback. For instance, if energy levels are consistently low, it might indicate insufficient caloric or carbohydrate intake.

Consultation with Professionals

A registered dietitian or nutritionist, especially one specialized in sports nutrition, can provide personalized guidance, ensuring that dietary strategies align with training goals and individual needs.

In conclusion, as training progresses and evolves, so should nutritional strategies. Also, individuals can ensure they propel their bodies effectively, optimizing performance, and supporting overall health and well-being by making informed and timely adjustments to their diet.

Seeking Professional Guidance for Training Optimization

Physical fitness and muscle growth can be complex and multifaceted. While many individuals embark on this journey independently, leveraging the expertise of professionals can significantly enhance outcomes, prevent injuries, and provide clarity during overwhelming information. Importance of seeking professional guidance and the various avenues available:

The Value of Expertise

Professionals, whether they're personal trainers, physiotherapists, or sports nutritionists, bring years of education and practical experience to the table. Their knowledge can help demystify the complexities of training and nutrition. They can provide evidence-based recommendations, ensuring that individuals are not swayed by fitness fads or misinformation.

Personalized Training Programs

A one-size-fits-all approach rarely works in fitness. Professionals can design training programs appropriately to fit an individual's goals, fitness level, and any specific challenges or limitations they might have. This personalized program can lead to more efficient results and reduce the risk of injuries.

Nutritional Counseling

Registered dietitians or sports nutritionists can guide dietary choices, ensuring that individuals are maintaining their bodies effectively for their training regimen. They can also offer insights into supplementation, helping individuals navigate the vast and often confusing world of vitamins, minerals, and performance-enhancing supplements.

Injury Prevention and Rehabilitation

Physiotherapists or sports therapists can offer strategies to prevent injuries, especially if an individual has pre-existing conditions or is engaging in intense training. In the event of injuries, these professionals can guide rehabilitation, ensuring a safe and efficient return to training.

Mental and Psychological Support

The physical journey is often intertwined with the mental. Sports psychologists or counselors can provide strategies to enhance motivation, deal with performance anxiety, or navigate the psychological challenges that might arise during training. They can also offer techniques for visualization, goal-setting, and building a growth mindset, all of which can enhance training outcomes.

Continuous Monitoring and Feedback

Regular check-ins with professionals can provide a platform for feedback, allowing for timely adjustments to training or nutrition plans. This continuous monitoring can ensure that individuals remain on track toward their goals and can adapt to any challenges or changes in circumstances.

Education and Empowerment

Beyond providing advice, professionals can also educate individuals on the principles of training, nutrition, and recovery. This knowledge empowers individuals to make informed decisions even outside the guidance sessions. Workshops, seminars, or courses offered by these experts can further deepen one's understanding of fitness and health.

Networking and Community Building

Professionals often have networks within the fitness and health community. They can introduce individuals to group classes, training camps, or other experts, fostering a sense of community and shared purpose.

In conclusion, while the journey of fitness and muscle growth is deeply personal, it doesn't have to be solitary. Individuals can enhance their training outcomes, navigate challenges with confidence, and embark on a path of continuous learning and growth in their fitness journey just by seeking the guidance of professionals.

Conclusion

The journey of muscle growth is a comprehensive process that goes beyond just lifting weights. It's a blend of understanding one's current fitness level, setting clear and realistic goals, incorporating structured training methods like periodization, and ensuring proper nutrition. Monitoring progress and making necessary adjustments, both in training and nutrition, are crucial for continuous improvement. Throughout this journey, the guidance of professionals can be invaluable, providing expertise, personalized recommendations, and support.

From assessing one's starting point to understanding training variables, we've examined the science and art of muscle growth. We've also explored the importance of periodization, the role of nutrition, and the significance of regular monitoring and feedback. Each section has been a building block, guiding you toward a holistic understanding of what it takes to achieve your muscle growth goals.

But the journey doesn't end here. As we've often reiterated, the mind and body are deeply interconnected. In our next chapter, we will look at the mind-muscle connection. How can mental focus enhance muscle activation? How does visualization play a role in performance? And how can mindfulness practices complement your physical training? Stay connected as we explore these intriguing aspects, bridging the gap between the physical and the mental, and unveiling another dimension of your muscle growth journey.

CHAPTER 9

THE MIND-MUSCLE CONNECTION

The mind-muscle connection is a concept that emphasizes the importance of neural activation and conscious focus during exercise. It involves enhancing the communication between your mind and the specific muscles you are targeting, resulting in greater muscle recruitment, activation, and ultimately, better muscle growth.

Developing a strong mind-muscle connection can significantly enhance your training experience and maximize the effectiveness of your workouts. Here, we delve into the fundamentals of neuromuscular control and how to harness the power of the mind-muscle connection for optimal muscle growth.

Emphasis on Neural Activation During Exercise

A significant aspect of neuromuscular control is the emphasis on neural activation during exercise. Neural activation is the process by which our nervous system activates specific muscle fibers, leading to muscle contraction. The role it plays in exercise is paramount. By ensuring efficient and effective muscle contractions, neural activation directly impacts the quality of the workout and the results one can achieve. Several factors influence this activation. Mental focus and attention during exercise, maintaining proper form and technique, and an adequate warm-up to prepare the nervous system are all crucial. When neural activation is optimized, the benefits are manifold. There's a greater recruitment of muscle fibers, which paves the way for better muscle growth potential. Additionally, exercise performance is improved, and the risk of injury is significantly reduced. This optimization also means that workouts become more efficient, allowing individuals to achieve more in less time.

Enhanced Communication Between Mind and Muscles

This refers to the conscious effort one makes to focus on the working muscle during exercise. It's this mental connection that allows an individual to truly "feel" the muscle working, ensuring that the targeted muscle is effectively engaged and reducing the involvement of secondary or compensatory muscle groups. Several strategies can enhance this mind-muscle communication. Visualization techniques, where one mentally "sees" the muscle working, can be particularly effective. More so, practicing mindful exercise execution, where attention is paid to every phase of the movement, can significantly enhance this connection. Regular feedback, whether through self-assessment or with the guidance of a trainer, ensures that muscle engagement is proper and effective. The benefits of this enhanced communication are profound. Not only is there improved muscle activation, which leads to better results, but there's also a reduced risk of imbalances or overuse injuries. Moreover, workouts become a more immersive and focused experience, adding another dimension to the exercise regimen.

In essence, understanding and harnessing the power of neuromuscular control, through neural activation and the mind-muscle connection, can revolutionize one's approach to exercise, leading to better outcomes and a more enriching training experience.

Understanding Neuromuscular Control

Neuromuscular control is a fascinating and intricate system that underpins our every movement, from the simplest gestures to the most complex athletic feats. To truly grasp its significance, one must delve into the mechanics and relationships that form its foundation.

Coordinated Interaction Between Nervous and Muscular Systems

At the heart of neuromuscular control is the coordinated interaction between the nervous and muscular systems. This interaction is likened to, where the nervous system acts as the conductor, guiding and directing the muscular system, to produce harmonious movements. The nervous system sends signals, in the form of electrical impulses, to the muscles, instructing them when to contract and relax. This communication is continuous and dynamic, adjusting in real-time to the demands placed on the body. Whether you're lifting a heavy weight, sprinting, or simply reaching for an object, this coordinated interaction ensures that the right muscles activate in the correct sequence and intensity. The beauty of this system is its adaptability. With training and repetition, the communication between the nervous and muscular systems becomes more efficient, leading to improved performance and reduced risk of injury.

Role of Motor Units in Muscle Contractions

Central to this system's functionality is the role of motor units in muscle contractions. A motor unit consists of a single motor neuron and all the muscle fibers it innervates. Let's think of it as a team, with the motor neuron being the team leader, directing its group of muscle fibers. When a motor neuron receives a signal from the brain, it transmits this signal to its associated muscle fibers, causing them to contract. The strength and type of contraction depend on the number and size of motor units activated. For instance, lifting a light object might only require the activation of a few small motor units, while lifting a heavy weight would engage many more, including larger motor units with more muscle fibers. The recruitment of these motor units is hierarchical, with smaller units (controlling fewer muscle fibers) being activated before larger ones. This ensures that the body uses only the energy and force necessary for a given task, optimizing efficiency. Over time, with consistent training, the body becomes adept at recruiting the necessary motor units more quickly and effectively, leading to stronger and more controlled muscle contractions.

In conclusion, neuromuscular control is a testament to the body's incredible design and adaptability. We can better appreciate the complexity of our movements and the potential for growth and improvement by understanding their mechanisms, such as the coordinated interaction between the nervous and muscular systems and the role of motor units.

Developing the Mind-Muscle Connection

The mind-muscle connection is more than just a buzzword in the fitness community; it's a fundamental principle that can significantly amplify the results of any training regimen. This connection is the bridge between mental intention and physical action, ensuring that exercises are performed with maximum efficiency and effectiveness.

Importance of Active Engagement During Exercise

Understanding the importance of active engagement during exercise is the first step in harnessing the power of the mind-muscle connection. Active engagement means being mentally present during each repetition, feeling the muscle stretch and contract, and visualizing its movement. This heightened awareness ensures that the targeted muscle is doing the majority of the work, minimizing the involvement of secondary muscles and reducing the risk of injury. Moreover, by actively engaging the mind, you can recruit a greater number of muscle fibers, leading to more effective muscle contractions and, ultimately, better muscle growth.

However, recognizing the importance of the mind-muscle connection is just the beginning. To truly develop and strengthen this connection, one must employ specific strategies:

Concentration and Focus: This is the foundation of the mind-muscle connection. By zeroing in on the muscle you're working on, you can direct your mental energy towards feeling it contract and relax. This focus not only enhances muscle activation but also minimizes distractions, ensuring that each repetition is purposeful and effective.

Slow and Controlled Movements: Speed often sacrifices form. By slowing down, you allow yourself to feel every bit of the movement. This deliberate pace emphasizes both the eccentric (lowering) and concentric (lifting) phases of an exercise, allowing for better muscle engagement and a deeper connection with the targeted muscle.

Proper Form and Technique: Without the correct form, even the most focused mind-muscle connection can be rendered ineffective. Proper technique ensures that the target muscle is being engaged fully and reduces the risk of injury. It's always beneficial to occasionally check in with a fitness professional to ensure that your form is on point.

Mindful Breathing: Breathing is the rhythm of exercise. By focusing on deep, controlled breaths, you can enhance relaxation, reduce unnecessary tension, and improve the overall mind-muscle connection. This practice not only helps in oxygenating the muscles but also in centering the mind.

Visualization: This technique takes the mind-muscle connection to a deeper level. By mentally picturing the muscle working, growing, and achieving the desired outcome, you can enhance the neural drive to that muscle. This mental rehearsal can significantly improve muscle activation and engagement.

Incorporating these strategies into your training regimen can transform your workouts from mere physical exertions to holistic experiences that engage both mind and body. Over time, with consistent practice, the mind-muscle connection can become a potent tool in your fitness arsenal, leading to improved performance, enhanced muscle growth, and a deeper understanding of your body's capabilities.

Benefits of the Mind-Muscle Connection

The mind-muscle connection, while often discussed in fitness circles, is more than just a trendy concept. It's a fundamental approach that offers tangible benefits, enhancing the quality and results of one's training. By consciously focusing on the muscles being worked during exercise, individuals can tap into a range of benefits that go beyond mere muscle growth.

Increased Muscle Activation: One of the primary advantages of the mind-muscle connection is the heightened activation of targeted muscles. When you mentally focus on a specific muscle or muscle group during exercise, you're essentially directing more neural drive to that area. This increased neural drive means that a greater number of muscle fibers are recruited during each contraction. The result however will be more effective muscle contractions and a higher potential for muscle growth. Over time, this can lead to more pronounced muscle definition and strength gains.

Improved Muscle Control: The mind-muscle connection also plays a pivotal role in enhancing muscle control. By being mentally present during each repetition and truly feeling the muscle work, individuals can achieve more precise and controlled movements. This improved control is particularly beneficial for exercises that require a high degree of coordination or for movements that target smaller muscle groups, which might otherwise be challenging to engage.

Enhanced Mindful Training: Mindfulness, or the act of being fully present in the moment, has been shown to offer many benefits, from reduced stress to improved focus. By cultivating a strong mind-muscle connection, individuals inherently practice mindfulness during their workouts. This enhanced mindful training can increase the overall enjoyment and effectiveness of exercise sessions. It allows individuals to connect deeply with their bodies, understand each sensation, and make real-time adjustments to optimize their training.

Prevention of Compensation: One common issue many face during training is the tendency for stronger muscle groups to compensate for weaker or underactive ones. This compensation can lead to imbalances, reduced effectiveness of exercises, and even injuries. The mind-muscle connection acts as a safeguard against this. By mentally focusing on the target muscle, individuals can ensure that it's doing the majority of the work, reducing the likelihood of other muscles jumping in to compensate. Over time, this focused training can help correct muscle imbalances, leading to a more balanced physique and reduced risk of injury.

In conclusion, the mind-muscle connection is a powerful tool in fitness. It bridges the gap between mental intention and physical action, ensuring that exercises are not just movements but purposeful engagements that maximize muscle growth and overall training effectiveness.

Application in Workouts

The concept of the mind-muscle connection is not just theoretical; it has practical applications that can transform the way we approach our workouts. By integrating the principles of the mind-muscle connection into our training routines, we can optimize muscle growth, improve technique, and elevate the overall training experience.

Emphasis on Target Muscle: Every exercise in a workout routine is designed to target specific muscles or muscle groups. However, without a conscious effort to engage the intended muscle, other dominant muscles might take over, leading to suboptimal results. By emphasizing the target muscle, we mean mentally focusing on that muscle during the exercise. This mental focus ensures that the muscle is actively engaged and working to its fullest potential. For instance, during a bicep curl, one should mentally concentrate on the bicep contracting and relaxing with each repetition. This conscious effort ensures that the bicep, rather than other muscles, bears the brunt of the work, leading to more effective muscle activation and growth.

Techniques and Strategies for Enhancement: While the basic principle of the mind-muscle connection is to mentally focus on the working muscle, several techniques and strategies can further enhance this connection:

- **Visualization**: Before and during the exercise, visualize the target muscle working. Imagine the muscle fibers contracting and relaxing, and mentally "see" the muscle going through the motions. This mental imagery can significantly enhance muscle engagement.

- **Tactile Feedback**: Sometimes, physically touching or tapping the muscle you're working on can enhance the mind-muscle connection. For instance, placing a hand on your obliques during side crunches can help you feel the muscles working more intensely.

- **Tempo Adjustments**: Slowing down the tempo of your repetitions, especially during the eccentric (or lowering) phase, can give you more time to focus on the muscle and feel it working. This slower pace can lead to better muscle engagement and more effective workouts.

- **Isolation Exercises**: Incorporating isolation exercises, which target a single muscle group, can be beneficial. These exercises reduce the involvement of secondary muscles, allowing for a more focused engagement of the target muscle.

- **Mindful Breathing**: Breathing plays a crucial role in exercise. By focusing on deep, rhythmic breathing, you can stay more connected to the exercise and enhance the mind-muscle connection. Proper breathing can also improve oxygen delivery to the muscles, supporting better performance.

Incorporating the mind-muscle connection into your workouts might require some practice initially, but the benefits are well worth the effort. Over time, this focused approach becomes second nature, leading to more effective workouts, better muscle growth, and an enhanced training experience.

Visualization and Muscle Activation

Role of Visualization: Beyond Just Seeing

- **Neurological Foundations:** At its core, every movement we make is a result of electrical impulses traveling from our brain to our muscles. Visualization strengthens these neural pathways, making the connection between thought and action more efficient. It's like fine-tuning a musical instrument, ensuring that every note (or movement) is pitch-perfect.

- **Psychological Benefits:** Visualization isn't just about physical performance. It's a powerful tool for mental well-being. By mentally rehearsing success, athletes can combat self-doubt, build self-efficacy, and foster a growth mindset.

Imagining Movements and Desired Outcomes

- **Detailed Scripting:** Effective visualization goes beyond mere imagery. Athletes are often encouraged to script detailed scenarios, encompassing every twist, turn, and nuance of their performance. This meticulous mental rehearsal prepares them for every eventuality, ensuring they're not caught off guard during an actual performance.

- **Emotional Anchoring:** By visualizing past successes or imagining future victories, athletes can anchor positive emotions to their performance. This emotional anchoring can be a source of motivation during challenging times, acting as a mental reservoir of strength and resilience.

- **Feedback Loop:** Visualization creates a feedback loop. The more an athlete visualizes success, the more confident they become. This increased confidence, in turn, enhances their actual performance, which then feeds back into more positive visualization. It's a virtuous cycle of continuous improvement.

The Science Behind Visualization

- **Brain Plasticity:** Our brains are not static; they're dynamic and ever-changing. Visualization taps into this ever-changing nature of the brain. By repeatedly visualizing a movement, we can create and strengthen neural pathways, making the actual execution of that movement more efficient.

- **Mirror Neurons:** These are neurons that fire both when we perform an action and when we see someone else perform that action. Visualization activates these mirror neurons, further blurring the line between imagined and actual performance.

Practical Applications

- **Rehabilitation:** Visualization isn't just for elite athletes. It's a valuable tool in injury rehabilitation. By mentally rehearsing movements, patients can maintain neural pathways even when the actual movement is not possible due to injury.

- **Skill Acquisition:** For those learning a new skill, be it a dance move, a tennis stroke, or a yoga pose, visualization can accelerate the learning process. By mentally rehearsing the skill, learners can refine their technique even outside of actual practice sessions.

In conclusion, visualization is a potent tool in the athlete's toolkit. It bridges the gap between mental intent and physical execution, proving that during performance, the mind and body are inextricably linked.

Enhancing Neural Pathways

The Neural Landscape: An Introduction

Before diving deep into the specifics, it's essential to understand the neural landscape. Neurons are the primary cells of the nervous system, responsible for transmitting information throughout the body. These cells communicate through intricate networks, forming pathways that dictate everything from reflex actions to complex cognitive tasks. The strength and efficiency of these pathways can be influenced by various factors, including repetition, experience, and, as we'll explore, mental rehearsal.

Mental Rehearsal of Exercises: The Power of the Mind's Eye

- **Cognitive Simulation:** Mental rehearsal is a cognitive simulation. When an athlete visualizes an exercise or movement, they're not just passively daydreaming. They're actively engaging the same brain regions that would be involved if they were performing the action in reality. This mental "practice" can be as effective as physical practice in refining and reinforcing motor skills.

- **Sensory Engagement:** Effective mental rehearsal goes beyond mere visualization. It encompasses all senses. An athlete might imagine the feel of equipment in their hands, the sound of their feet hitting the ground, or even the smell of the gym. This multisensory engagement creates a more holistic and immersive rehearsal experience, further enhancing neural pathways.

- **Emotional and Psychological Components:** Beyond the physical, mental rehearsal also involves emotional and psychological aspects of performance. By visualizing success and positive outcomes, athletes can build confidence, reduce performance anxiety, and foster a more resilient mindset.

Activation of Neural Pathways: The Science of Synaptic Strengthening

- **Hebbian Theory:** Coined by Donald Hebb, the phrase "neurons that fire together, wire together" encapsulates the essence of synaptic strengthening. When two neurons are activated simultaneously, the connection between them – the synapse strengthens. Mental rehearsal repeatedly activates specific neural pathways, reinforcing these connections and making the subsequent physical performance more efficient and precise.

- **Role of Neurotransmitters:** Neurotransmitters are chemical messengers that facilitate communication between neurons. Mental rehearsal can influence the release of certain neurotransmitters, enhancing the efficiency of neural communication. For instance, dopamine, often associated with reward and motivation, can be released during positive visualization, further reinforcing the desired neural pathways.

- **Mirror Neurons:** As previously mentioned, mirror neurons play a pivotal role in the link between visualization and action. These neurons fire both when we perform an action and when we observe (or imagine) that action being performed. By mentally rehearsing exercises, we activate these mirror neurons, further blurring the line between imagined and actual performance.

- **Plasticity and Adaptability:** The brain's ability to reorganize and adapt, known as plasticity, is central to the concept of enhancing neural pathways. With each mental rehearsal, the brain fine-tunes its neural networks, adapting to better suit the demands of the task at hand.

Enhancing neural pathways through mental rehearsal is a testament to the incredible adaptability and sophistication of the human brain. It underscores the profound interplay between thought and action, cognition and physicality. Whether for elite athletes aiming for gold or individuals rehabilitating from injury, the power of the mind's eye offers a potent tool for optimizing performance and outcomes.

Improved Motor Learning: The Brain and Muscle

The Essence of Motor Learning

Motor learning is a fascinating and intricate process that involves acquiring and refining skills through practice. It's the reason we can ride a bike, play an instrument, or perfect a tennis serve. At the heart of motor learning lies the dynamic interplay between the brain and muscles, a relationship that is continually evolving and adapting.

Reinforcement of Brain-Muscle Connection

- **The Motor Cortex:** Located in the brain's frontal lobe, the motor cortex plays a pivotal role in planning, controlling, and executing voluntary movements. Every time we practice a movement, whether physically or mentally, the motor cortex is actively engaged, sending signals to the relevant muscles.

- **Muscle Memory:** This is a somewhat misleading term, as the memory isn't stored in the muscles but rather in the brain. As we repeat a movement, the brain starts to automate the process, reducing the need for conscious thought. This "memory" allows for smoother, more efficient movement over time.

- **Feedback Loops:** As we perform a movement, our body provides feedback to the brain. This feedback, through sensory organs and the peripheral nervous system, informs the brain about the movement's accuracy, allowing for real-time adjustments. Over time, this continuous feedback refines the brain-muscle connection, enhancing precision and efficiency.

- **Emotional and Cognitive Components:** The brain-muscle connection isn't just about mechanics. Emotions, motivation, and cognition play crucial roles. Positive emotions and motivation can enhance the connection, making learning more effective. Conversely, stress or anxiety can hinder the process.

Strengthening of Neural Pathways: Building the Highways of Communication

- **Repetition and Synaptic Plasticity:** Every time a movement is practiced, the neural pathway responsible for that movement is activated. Repetition strengthens this pathway, a phenomenon known as synaptic plasticity. The more frequently a pathway is used, the stronger and more efficient it becomes.

- **Role of Neurotransmitters:** As with mental rehearsal, neurotransmitters play a crucial role in motor learning. Chemicals like dopamine, associated with reward and motivation, can enhance the learning process. When we achieve a movement correctly and feel a sense of accomplishment, the release of dopamine reinforces the neural pathway, making it more likely we'll perform the movement correctly in the future.

- **Neural Pruning:** An equally important aspect of strengthening neural pathways is the elimination of unnecessary or redundant connections, a process known as neural pruning. As we refine a movement, the brain "prunes" less efficient pathways, streamlining the process and ensuring that only the most effective pathways remain.

- **Incorporation of New Skills:** As we learn and incorporate new movements or skills, the brain creates new neural pathways. This adaptability ensures that we can continually learn and refine skills throughout our lives.

Improved motor learning, through the reinforcement of the brain-muscle connection and the strengthening of neural pathways, is a testament to the body's incredible adaptability and resilience. It underscores the profound relationship between thought, action, and adaptation. Whether for a professional dancer perfecting a routine or an individual learning to walk again after an injury, the principles of motor learning offer insights into human movement and potential.

Direct Attention to Specific Muscles: The Spotlight Effect

- **Selective Attention:** Just as a spotlight illuminates a specific area on a stage, our mind can "shine" its focus on particular muscles or muscle groups. This selective attention ensures that we're not just going through the motions but are deeply connected to the specific muscles we're targeting.

- **Sensory Awareness:** Directing attention to specific muscles enhances our sensory awareness. We become more attuned to the sensations in that muscle – the stretch, the contraction, and even the subtlest twitch. This heightened awareness allows for better control and more effective muscle engagement.

- **Feedback and Adjustment:** With increased focus, we can better detect when a muscle isn't activating as it should or when our form starts to falter. This immediate feedback loop allows for on-the-spot adjustments, ensuring optimal performance and reducing the risk of injury.

- **Enhanced Learning:** When we direct our attention to specific muscles, we're not just improving our performance at the moment; we're also facilitating long-term learning. The focused practice reinforces the neural pathways associated with that movement, leading to better muscle memory and more efficient future performance.

Visualization for Muscle Fiber Activation: The Mind's Eye in Training

- **The Science of Visualization:** Visualization, or mental rehearsal, isn't just a psychological trick. Studies have shown that visualizing a movement can activate the same areas of the brain as physically performing that movement. This mental activation can prime the muscles for action, even before they move.

- **Micro-Level Engagement:** By visualizing the muscle fibers contracting and relaxing, we can achieve a deeper level of muscle engagement. It's like tuning into the individual instruments in an orchestra, appreciating each one's role in creating the movement or beat.

- **Enhancing Muscle Recruitment:** Effective visualization can lead to better muscle fiber recruitment. Instead of just the dominant muscle fibers doing the heavy lifting, visualization can help engage a broader range of fibers, distributing the load more evenly and enhancing overall muscle performance.

- **Emotional and Motivational Boost:** Visualization isn't just about the mechanics of movement. Imagining a successful lift, a perfect sprint, or any other desired outcome can provide a significant emotional and motivational boost. This positive mindset can further enhance the mind-muscle connection, driving better results.

The journey of physical training is as much a mental endeavor as it is a physical one. The increased focus and mind-muscle connection serve as bridges, linking intention with action, and thought with movement. Athletes, trainers, and fitness enthusiasts can unlock new levels of performance, ensuring that every drop of sweat and every ounce of effort is channeled effectively and efficiently by understanding and harnessing these principles.

Technique Improvement

Technique, in physical training and sports, is the bedrock upon which performance is built. Proper technique not only ensures that movements are efficient and effective but also minimizes the risk of injury. The mind plays a pivotal role in honing technique, and this is where mental rehearsal and the reinforcement of motor patterns come into play.

Mental Rehearsal of Proper Form

- **The Power of Visualization**: Before even lifting a weight or taking a step, athletes and fitness enthusiasts can mentally rehearse the movement. By visualizing the correct form, from the positioning of the feet to the posture of the spine, individuals can create a mental blueprint of the ideal movement.

- **Benefits of Mental Practice**: Studies have shown that mentally rehearsing a movement can activate the same brain regions as physically performing it. This means that by just thinking about a movement, one can strengthen the neural connections associated with it. Over time, this mental practice can translate to better execution during actual performance.

- **Consistency in Thought and Action**: Regularly visualizing the correct technique ensures that when it's time to perform, the body can more naturally fall into the correct form. It's like having a mental checklist that the body automatically follows.

Reinforcement of Motor Patterns

- **Neurological Foundations**: Every movement we make, from the simple act of tying a shoelace to executing a perfect jump shot in basketball, involves a specific pattern of neural activation. These patterns, known as motor patterns or engrams, are the brain's way of encoding movement.

- **Repetition and Refinement**: Each time a movement is practiced, its associated motor pattern is reinforced. However, if the technique is flawed, the brain reinforces an incorrect pattern. This is why it's crucial to ensure that the technique is correct from the outset. By mentally rehearsing the proper form and then physically practicing it, individuals can solidify the correct motor patterns in their neural architecture.

- **Feedback Loop**: As one continues to practice and mentally focus on the technique, the brain receives continuous feedback from the muscles and joints. This feedback allows for micro-adjustments, fine-tuning the movement over time. The more refined the motor pattern, the more automatic and efficient the movement becomes.

- **Long-term Benefits**: Over time, as the correct motor patterns are reinforced, they become the default. This means that even under pressure or fatigue, the chances of maintaining proper technique are higher. This not only optimizes performance but also reduces the risk of injuries that can arise from poor form.

In conclusion, the technique is not just a physical endeavor but a mental one as well. By harnessing the power of the mind through mental rehearsal and by consistently reinforcing correct motor patterns, individuals can elevate their performance, ensure safety, and achieve their fitness or athletic goals with greater precision.

Mental Rehearsal for Success

Success in sports and fitness is not just about physical prowess; it's equally about mental fortitude. The mind's power to influence performance is profound, and one of the most effective tools at an athlete's or fitness enthusiast's disposal is mental rehearsal. By visualizing success and building confidence through this visualization, individuals can significantly enhance their performance and outcomes.

Imagining Successful Workouts

The Power of Positive Imagery: When individuals close their eyes and vividly imagine themselves executing a flawless workout, hitting every rep, and feeling strong and energized, they are essentially programming their minds for success. This mental imagery serves as a precursor to the actual physical act, setting the stage for a positive outcome.

Neurological Impacts: Neuroscientific research has shown that imagining a movement can activate the same brain regions as physically performing the movement. This means that by visualizing a successful workout, individuals are, in a way, practicing it in their minds, making the actual execution more familiar and attainable.

Overcoming Challenges: Mental rehearsal allows individuals to anticipate potential challenges and mentally strategize ways to overcome them. Whether it's pushing through the last few reps of a challenging set or maintaining focus during a long run, visualizing these scenarios and their successful outcomes equips individuals with the mental tools to handle them in reality.

Building Confidence Through Visualization

Reinforcing Self-belief: By repeatedly visualizing success, individuals reinforce their belief in their abilities. This self-belief acts as a shield against doubts and negative thoughts that can hinder performance.

Emotional Regulation: Visualization can also evoke the positive emotions associated with success, such as pride, joy, and satisfaction. Experiencing these emotions in the mind can help regulate anxiety and stress, making individuals more emotionally resilient during their workouts or competitions.

The Ripple Effect: Confidence is not just about the immediate task at hand. When individuals visualize and then experience success, it creates a positive feedback loop. This success breeds more confidence, which in turn leads to more success, creating a virtuous cycle that can extend beyond the gym or the sports field into other areas of life.

Enhanced Motivation: Confidence and motivation are closely linked. When individuals believe in their abilities and visualize their successes, they are more motivated to train harder, stay committed, and push their boundaries.

In summary, mental rehearsal for success is a potent tool that goes beyond mere daydreaming. It's a deliberate and focused exercise that harnesses the mind's power to influence performance. Individuals can unlock higher levels of performance, resilience, and overall well-being by imagining successful workouts and building confidence through visualization.

Incorporating Visualization in Training

Visualization, while often associated with elite athletes, is a tool that can benefit anyone, regardless of their fitness level or athletic prowess. It's a mental technique that, when integrated into training routines, can amplify results, enhance focus, and foster a deeper connection between the mind and body. Here's how one can seamlessly incorporate visualization into their training regimen:

Pre-Workout Ritual

Mental Warm-Up: Just as physical warm-ups prepare the body for exercise, a mental warm-up using visualization can set the stage for a successful workout. Before starting the physical activity, take a few moments to close your eyes and vividly imagine the upcoming workout. Visualize each exercise, the movements, and the sensations.

Anticipate Success: Envision yourself performing each exercise with perfect form, feeling strong, and completing the set with confidence. This not only mentally prepares you for the workout but also instills a sense of anticipation and positivity.

Intention Setting

Clarify Your Goals: Before going into the workout, set clear intentions. Ask yourself what you aim to achieve in this session. Is it to improve stamina, increase strength, or perhaps perfect a particular technique?

Visualize the Outcome: Once the intention is clearly set, visualize it being achieved. If the goal is to run a certain distance, imagine crossing that finish line. If it's lifting a particular weight, visualize the triumphant moment when you achieve that lift.

Focus on Muscle Engagement

Mind-Muscle Connection: During the workout, use visualization to enhance the mind-muscle connection. For instance, when doing a bicep curl, visualize the bicep muscle fibers contracting and then relaxing. This deepens the engagement and can lead to more effective muscle activation.

Enhance Sensations: Pay attention to the sensations in the muscles. Imagine the blood flowing into the muscle, nourishing it, and the feeling of the muscle working hard. This not only enhances the workout experience but can also improve technique and reduce the risk of injury.

Use of Imagery Cue Words

Simplifying Visualization: Sometimes, during a challenging workout, it might be hard to maintain a detailed visualization. This is where cue words can help. These are simple words or short phrases that evoke a particular image or feeling. For example, "strong" could be a cue word to remind you of your strength during a lift, or "fluid" could evoke the image of a seamless and smooth running stride.

Reinforce Positive Actions: Cue words can also be used to reinforce positive actions or correct techniques. For instance, if you tend to hunch your shoulders during a particular exercise, a cue word like "open" can remind you to open up your chest and maintain proper posture.

Incorporating visualization into training is like adding a secret weapon to your fitness arsenal. It not only enhances the physical aspects of training but also fortifies the mental and emotional components, leading to a holistic and enriched training experience.

Mindfulness and Muscle Growth

Understanding Mindfulness: Mindfulness is about being fully present. It's about anchoring oneself in the current moment, observing thoughts, feelings, and sensations without judgment. Derived from ancient Buddhist practices, mindfulness has transcended its spiritual origins to become a widely accepted tool for mental well-being in modern psychology and neuroscience.

Beyond Mental Well-being: While mindfulness is often associated with meditation and stress reduction, its applications extend far beyond. When applied to physical activities like exercise, mindfulness can transform the experience, making it more effective and enjoyable.

Application in Muscle Growth

Deepening the Mind-Muscle Connection: One can achieve a deeper mind-muscle connection by being fully present during a workout. This means truly feeling each contraction and relaxation of the muscle, understanding the range of motion, and being acutely aware of one's form. Such a connection can lead to more effective muscle activation, potentially accelerating muscle growth.

Enhancing Workout Quality: Mindfulness can improve the quality of workouts. Instead of merely going through the motions, a mindful approach ensures that each rep, set, and exercise is done with intention and focus. This can lead to better results in the long run.

Reducing Risk of Injury: A mindful approach to training means being fully attuned to one's body. This heightened awareness can help in recognizing when a particular movement feels off or when the body signals that it's time to rest, thereby reducing the risk of injuries.

Emotional Benefits: Mindfulness in training also offers emotional benefits. By being present, one can find joy in the process of exercising and muscle-building, rather than just focusing on the end goal. This can lead to a more sustainable and long-term commitment to fitness.

In summary, integrating mindfulness into muscle growth and training routines can offer a holistic approach to fitness. It's not just about building physical strength but also about cultivating mental resilience, focus, and a deeper connection with one's body.

Present-Moment Awareness

The Essence of Being Present: Being fully present during exercise means immersing oneself entirely in the activity, free from distractions and external thoughts. It's about experiencing every breath, every bead of sweat, and every muscle contraction in real-time.

Distraction-Free Zone: In today's digital age, distractions are everywhere. From smartphones buzzing with notifications to thoughts about daily chores, it's easy to be physically present but mentally elsewhere. However, dedicating oneself to the act of exercising, by creating a distraction-free zone, can elevate the quality of the workout. This might mean putting the phone on airplane mode, finding a quiet space, or even closing one's eyes during certain exercises to truly focus.

Benefits of Full Presence: By being wholly present, one can go into a deeper level of concentration and awareness. This not only enhances the effectiveness of each movement but also turns the workout into a form of active meditation, offering mental relaxation and clarity.

Enhanced Mind-Muscle Connection

Understanding the Connection: The mind-muscle connection is the conscious, focused effort to engage specific muscles during exercise. It's not just about moving weights or completing reps; it's about mentally directing and feeling the targeted muscle work through its entire range of motion.

The Role of Awareness: Present-moment awareness plays a pivotal role in enhancing this connection. By directing one's full attention to the muscle being worked, one can better isolate and engage it, leading to more effective contractions and, over time, better muscle development.

Benefits of a Strong Connection: A robust mind-muscle connection can lead to several benefits:

- **Improved Muscle Activation**: By focusing on the muscle, one can ensure it's activated to its fullest potential, leading to more efficient workouts.

- **Better Technique**: Being mindful of each movement can help in maintaining proper form, ensuring exercises are done correctly, and reducing the risk of injury.

- **Faster Results**: With improved muscle activation and technique, results can be achieved more quickly, be it muscle growth, strength gains, or enhanced muscle definition.

Therefore, present-moment awareness in exercise is not just a mental tool but a bridge that connects the mind and body, amplifying the benefits of physical activity and paving the way for holistic well-being.

Greater Body Awareness

Tuning into the Body: Body awareness, often referred to as proprioception, is the sense of how our body parts are oriented in space. By cultivating mindfulness during workouts, individuals can heighten their sensitivity to each movement, understanding the positioning and alignment of various body parts.

Feedback Loop: As one becomes more attuned to their body, one can feel the nuances of each exercise more distinctly. This heightened sensation acts as a feedback loop, allowing individuals to adjust and refine their movements in real-time. For instance, if a certain posture feels off, being in tune with one's body can help in identifying and rectifying it immediately.

Deepening the Exercise Experience: Greater body awareness not only improves technique but also enriches the overall exercise experience. It transforms workouts from mere physical exertion to a dance of awareness, where every movement is felt deeply and appreciated.

Correction of Imbalances

Identifying Weak Spots: Everyone has imbalances, whether due to daily habits, past injuries, or natural predispositions. Mindfulness in training can help in recognizing these imbalances. For instance, if one leg tends to take on more weight during a squat, a mindful approach can help identify and correct this discrepancy.

Prevention and Rehabilitation: Recognizing and addressing imbalances is crucial not just for achieving symmetrical muscle development but also for preventing potential injuries. Over time, unchecked imbalances can lead to strain and injury. By correcting them early on, one can ensure a safer and more effective training journey.

Tailored Training: With the knowledge of one's imbalances, training can be targeted to address specific needs. For example, if an individual notices a weaker left arm, they can incorporate unilateral exercises to strengthen it, ensuring balanced development.

In conclusion, integrating mindfulness into training can be a game-changer. It not only ensures that exercises are performed with optimal technique and form but also paves the way for a deeper understanding of one's body, leading to more personalized and effective workouts.

Enhancing Sensory Perception

Tuning into the Subtle: Mindfulness encourages individuals to become acutely aware of even the most subtle physical sensations during exercise. This could range from the stretch of a muscle during a particular movement to the slight shift of weight from one foot to another.

Deepening the Experience: By paying close attention to these sensations, individuals can deepen their connection to the exercise. It's no longer just about lifting a weight or completing a set; it's about feeling every fiber of the muscle engage, stretch, and relax. This heightened awareness can transform a routine workout into a profoundly sensory experience.

Body's Natural Barometer: The body often communicates its limits and needs through sensations. A sharp pain might indicate a wrong posture, while a burning sensation in the muscles might signify that they are being effectively worked. Being attuned to these signals allows individuals to train in harmony with their body's capabilities and needs.

Adjustments Based on Body Feedback

Real-time Refinements: As individuals become more aware of their body's feedback, they can make real-time adjustments to their form and technique. For instance, if they feel an undue strain in their lower back during a deadlift, they can immediately correct their posture to prevent injury.

Personalized Pacing: Mindfulness allows individuals to adjust the pace of their workouts based on how their body feels. On days when they feel energetic and strong, they might push themselves a bit more, while on days when they feel fatigued, they might opt for a lighter workout.

Optimizing Rest and Recovery: By being in tune with their body's feedback, individuals can also gauge when to rest and when to push through. If a particular muscle group feels sore or overworked, it might be a sign to give it a day or two of rest. This ensures that muscles recover adequately, reducing the risk of overtraining and injury.

So, enhancing sensory perception through mindfulness offers a more holistic approach to training. It's not just about the external goals of lifting heavier or running faster; it's about understanding and respecting the body's signals, leading to a more balanced and sustainable fitness journey.

Stress Reduction Techniques

Mindful Breathing: One of the foundational practices of mindfulness, focused breathing exercises can significantly reduce stress. By concentrating on each inhalation and exhalation, individuals can divert their attention from stressors, calming the mind and body. This practice can be particularly beneficial before or after intense workouts to center oneself.

Progressive Muscle Relaxation: This technique involves tensing and then relaxing different muscle groups in the body. By doing so, individuals can become more aware of physical sensations and release tension stored in the muscles. After exercise, this can aid in relaxation and recovery.

Guided Imagery: This involves visualizing peaceful and calming scenarios, such as a serene beach or a tranquil forest. Such visualization can lower cortisol levels (the stress hormone) and promote a state of relaxation, which is conducive to recovery.

Meditation: Regular meditation sessions, even if they're short, can help in managing stress. By training the mind to focus on the present and let go of anxieties, meditation can create a serene mental environment, complementing physical training.

Promotion of Muscle Growth Environment

Optimal Hormonal Balance: Chronic stress can elevate cortisol levels, which can be detrimental to muscle growth. By managing stress through mindfulness techniques, one can maintain a more favorable hormonal environment, where testosterone and growth hormone levels are optimized for muscle repair and growth.

Enhanced Sleep Quality: Stress is a common culprit behind sleep disturbances. As sleep is a critical component of muscle recovery, managing stress can indirectly promote muscle growth by ensuring restful and restorative sleep.

Improved Nutrient Absorption: Chronic stress can impact digestive health, potentially hindering the absorption of vital nutrients necessary for muscle repair and growth. By reducing stress, one can ensure that the body efficiently utilizes the nutrients consumed, aiding in muscle development.

Increased Blood Flow: Stress reduction can lead to better circulation and increased blood flow to the muscles. This not only delivers essential nutrients to the muscles but also helps in the removal of waste products, facilitating quicker recovery.

In summary, while physical training is a crucial aspect of muscle growth, the mental and emotional states play an equally vital role. By managing stress and creating an environment conducive to recovery, individuals can significantly enhance their muscle growth potential. Mindfulness practices offer tools to achieve this balance, making them indispensable in the holistic approach to fitness and health.

Applying Mindfulness Throughout the Day

Morning Meditation: Starting the day with a brief meditation session can set a positive and focused tone for the entire day. Even just 10 minutes of concentrated breathing and centering can make a noticeable difference in one's mindset and approach to daily challenges.

Mindful Eating: Instead of rushing through meals or eating while distracted, take the time to savor each bite. Pay attention to the textures, flavors, and sensations of the food. This not only enhances the enjoyment of the meal but can also aid in digestion and ensure that one is attuned to their body's hunger and fullness cues.

Mindful Movement: Whether it's a workout, a walk, or simply stretching, being fully present during physical activity can enhance its benefits. By paying attention to each movement and listening to the body, one can prevent injuries and get the most out of the activity.

Gratitude Journaling: At the end of the day, take a few minutes to jot down three things you're grateful for. This simple act can shift the focus from daily stressors to positive aspects, promoting a sense of contentment and well-being.

Body Scan: Before sleeping, perform a mental scan of your body from head to toe. Notice any areas of tension or discomfort and mentally send relaxation to those areas. This practice can promote relaxation and improve sleep quality.

Holistic Approach for Muscle Growth

Mind-Body Connection: By applying mindfulness throughout the day, one can strengthen the mind-body connection. This heightened awareness can lead to better workouts as individuals become more attuned to their body's needs, capabilities, and limitations.

Stress Management: Chronic stress can hinder muscle growth by affecting hormonal balance and recovery. By incorporating daily mindfulness practices, one can manage and reduce stress, creating an optimal environment for muscle growth.

Improved Recovery: Mindfulness can enhance the quality of sleep and promote relaxation, both of which are crucial for muscle recovery. By being mindful of your body signals, you can also ensure they're giving you adequate rest between workouts.

Nutritional Awareness: Mindful eating can lead to better nutritional choices. By being fully present during meals, individuals are less likely to overeat and more likely to choose nutrient-dense foods that support muscle growth.

In essence, while the physical aspects of training are undeniably crucial for muscle growth, the mental and emotional components are equally vital. We can adopt a holistic approach that supports not only muscle growth but overall well-being by integrating mindfulness practices throughout the day.

Techniques for Mindful Training

Mindful Breathing

Mindful breathing is the foundation of many mindfulness practices. It helps anchor the mind to the present moment, reduces stress, and can enhance focus during workouts.

How to Practice:

- Begin by finding a comfortable seated or standing position.

- Close your eyes and take a deep breath through the nose, feeling the air fill your lungs.

- Exhale slowly through the mouth, being aware of the sensation of the breath leaving your body.

- Continue this pattern, focusing solely on your breathing. If your mind wanders, gently bring it back to the breath.

- Incorporate this technique before starting a workout, between sets, or during rest periods to maintain focus and calmness.

Body Scan

The body scan technique helps in developing a deeper connection with one's body, recognizing areas of tension, and promoting relaxation.

How to Practice:

- Start at the top of your head and mentally scan down through your body.

- Notice any areas of tension, discomfort, or warmth.

- As you identify these areas, imagine sending your breath to them, promoting relaxation and release.

- This technique can be especially useful during warm-ups to identify any tightness or during cool-downs to promote relaxation.

Visualization

Visualization can enhance performance, improve technique, and boost confidence by mentally rehearsing movements or visualizing successful outcomes.

How to Practice:

- Close your eyes and imagine yourself in a specific scenario – it could be performing a perfect squat, running with ease, or achieving a personal best.

- Engage all your senses in this visualization. What do you see, feel, hear, or even smell?

- The more vivid and detailed the visualization, the more effective it can be in reinforcing positive outcomes and techniques.

Affirmations

Affirmations are positive statements that can help overcome self-sabotaging thoughts, boost self-confidence, and reinforce a positive mindset.

How to Practice:

- Choose or create a positive statement that resonates with you. It could be something like "I am strong and capable" or "Every workout brings me closer to my goals."

- Repeat this affirmation to yourself, either silently or out loud, especially during challenging parts of your workout.

- You can also write down these affirmations and place them where you'll see them regularly, like on your mirror or gym locker.

Incorporating these mindful training techniques can significantly enhance the quality of workouts, improve the mind-muscle connection, and foster a positive and focused mindset. By being present and intentional in every movement, individuals can optimize their training outcomes and enjoy a more holistic and fulfilling fitness journey.

Recap of the Mind-Muscle Connection

In the journey of physical transformation and athletic prowess, the power of the mind is often overshadowed by the emphasis on physical exertion. However, as we've explored in this chapter, the mind plays an indispensable role in optimizing our workouts and achieving our fitness goals. The mind-muscle connection isn't just a catchy phrase; it's a fundamental principle that bridges our mental intentions with physical actions. By harnessing techniques like visualization, mindfulness, and focused attention, we can enhance our training sessions, improve technique, and foster a deeper connection with our bodies. This holistic approach ensures that our workouts are not just about lifting weights or clocking miles but about a comprehensive understanding and synergy between mind and body.

Teaser for the Importance of Recovery in Muscle Growth

While the mind-muscle connection lays the foundation for effective workouts, another crucial component that often goes unnoticed is recovery. Think of your body as a finely tuned machine. Just as a car needs regular maintenance and downtime after a long journey, our muscles need time to repair, rebuild, and grow after intense workouts. But what exactly happens during this recovery phase? And why is it so important for muscle growth? In the next chapter, we'll delve deep into the science of recovery, exploring its multifaceted importance and providing insights on how to maximize this crucial aspect of the fitness journey. Prepare to uncover the secrets behind muscle regeneration, the role of sleep, and the nutritional strategies that can amplify your gains.

CHAPTER 10

—••—

RECOVERY AND MUSCLE GROWTH

Every time we engage in strenuous physical activity, especially resistance training, our muscles undergo a series of microscopic damages or micro-tears. Though damaging, it's a natural and essential part of muscle growth. These tiny tears are a result of the force exerted on the muscle fibers during exercises like weightlifting, sprinting, or even intense yoga sessions. The body recognizes these micro-tears as minor injuries and thus triggers an inflammatory response, signaling the body to start the repair process. This repair mechanism is the foundation upon which stronger and bigger muscles are built.

Process of Muscle Protein Synthesis

Muscle protein synthesis (MPS) is the body's way of repairing and rebuilding these micro-tears. It's a complex biochemical process where new proteins are formed to replace the damaged ones. After a workout, the rate of MPS increases, reaching its peak around 24-48 hours post-exercise. This is why the soreness you feel after a rigorous workout, known as delayed onset muscle soreness (DOMS), is most pronounced a day or two after the exercise. During MPS, amino acids – the building blocks of proteins are used to reconstruct and fortify muscle fibers, making them thicker and more resilient. This entire process, when coupled with adequate nutrients and rest, leads to muscle enlargement or growth.

Importance of Nutrients in Muscle Repair

Nutrition plays a pivotal role in the muscle repair process. Just as a car requires fuel to run, our muscles need nutrients, especially proteins and amino acids, to repair and grow. After a workout, there's a window of opportunity, often referred to as the "anabolic window" where the muscles are primed to absorb nutrients. Consuming a balanced meal or a protein during this period can significantly enhance the repair process.

Proteins provide the essential amino acids required for MPS. However, other nutrients like carbohydrates are equally crucial. Carbohydrates replenish the muscle glycogen stores that are depleted during exercise. Moreover, carbohydrates stimulate the release of insulin, a hormone that helps transport amino acids into the muscle cells, further aiding the repair process. Additionally, fats, vitamins, and minerals play supportive roles, ensuring that the muscle recovery process is efficient and comprehensive.

In essence, rest and recovery aren't just about taking a break; they're about giving the body the time and resources it needs to rebuild, strengthen, and grow. Proper understanding and implementation of these principles can significantly enhance one's fitness journey, ensuring sustainable and optimal muscle growth.

Preventing Overtraining

Overtraining, often referred to as overtraining syndrome (OTS), occurs when there is an imbalance between training and recovery — when the training intensity and/or volume exceeds the body's ability to recover. It's essentially the result of pushing the body too hard for too long without providing it adequate time to heal and recover.

Symptoms of overtraining can manifest in various ways and can be both physical and psychological. Common physical symptoms include:

- Persistent muscle soreness that doesn't alleviate with rest.
- A decline in performance despite increased training intensity or volume.
- Increased susceptibility to injuries.
- Chronic fatigue and tiredness.
- Disturbed sleep patterns.
- Frequent illnesses due to a compromised immune system.

On the psychological front, symptoms might include:

- Mood swings and irritability.
- Loss of motivation and enthusiasm for training.
- Increased perception of effort during workouts.
- Persistent feelings of being drained or burned out.

Impact on Muscle Growth and Overall Health

Overtraining not only hampers muscle growth but can also have detrimental effects on overall health. When the body is overstrained, the muscle protein breakdown exceeds the muscle protein synthesis, leading to muscle loss rather than growth. The continuous strain on the muscles without adequate recovery can lead to chronic injuries, which might sideline an individual for extended periods.

Furthermore, overtraining can lead to hormonal imbalances. Chronic overtraining can elevate cortisol levels, a stress hormone, which in high amounts can lead to muscle breakdown and inhibit growth. Simultaneously, it can suppress the production of anabolic hormones like testosterone, which play a pivotal role in muscle building.

The immune system also takes a hit with overtraining. A compromised immune system means a higher susceptibility to infections, leading to frequent illnesses that can further disrupt training schedules.

Strategies to Prevent Overtraining

Preventing overtraining is crucial for sustained muscle growth and overall well-being. Here are some strategies to ensure you don't fall into the overtraining trap:

- **Listen to Your Body:** Pay attention to signs of fatigue, persistent soreness, and any other symptoms mentioned above. If you notice these signs, it might be time to scale back and rest.

- **Incorporate Rest Days:** Ensure you have at least 1-2 rest days a week where you either don't exercise or engage in light, restorative activities.

- **Vary Your Routine:** Periodization, or changing up your workout routine every few weeks, can prevent overuse injuries and give specific muscle groups time to recover.

- **Stay Hydrated and Well-Nourished:** Proper nutrition and hydration can fasten recovery and reduce the risk of overtraining.

- **Prioritize Sleep:** Sleep is the body's prime recovery time. Ensure you're getting 7-9 hours of quality sleep each night.

- **Active Recovery:** On rest days, consider activities like walking, yoga, or swimming, which are low-intensity but can enhance blood flow and aid recovery.

- **Seek Expert Guidance:** For beginners, especially working with a personal trainer or coach can help in designing a balanced workout routine that promotes growth while preventing overtraining.

In conclusion, while pushing one's limits can lead to growth, it's equally essential to recognize the importance of rest and recovery. Striking the right balance ensures not only muscle growth but also long-term health and well-being.

Hormonal Balance

Role of Cortisol in Muscle Growth

Cortisol, often labeled as the "stress hormone" is produced by the adrenal glands in response to stress and low blood glucose. Its relationship with muscle growth is particularly noteworthy in addition to regulating metabolism, reducing inflammation, and controlling the sleep-wake cycle.

When we engage in intense physical activity, cortisol levels rise. This is a natural and immediate response to the stress placed on the body. In the short term, this spike in cortisol can actually be beneficial, helping to regulate energy, reduce inflammation, and even aid in fat metabolism.

However, chronically elevated cortisol levels can be detrimental to muscle growth for several reasons:

- **Muscle Protein Breakdown:** High cortisol levels can increase the rate of muscle protein breakdown, which can hinder muscle growth and repair.

- **Inhibits Testosterone Production:** Cortisol can suppress the secretion of anabolic hormones like testosterone, which are crucial for muscle development.

- **Impairs Nutrient Uptake:** Elevated cortisol can interfere with the transport and uptake of amino acids into the muscle cells, slowing down the repair and growth process.

Importance of Testosterone in Muscle Development

Testosterone is a primary male sex hormone, though it's present in both men and women. It plays a pivotal role in muscle development, among other functions. Here's how testosterone promotes muscle growth:

- **Stimulates Muscle Protein Synthesis:** Testosterone enhances the body's ability to synthesize proteins, which are the building blocks of muscles.

- **Increases Bone Density:** A higher bone density can support stronger and larger muscles.

- **Enhances Muscle Recovery:** Testosterone can improve the rate at which muscles repair and grow post-exercise.

- **Promotes Fat Burning:** Higher testosterone levels can lead to an increased metabolic rate, helping in reducing body fat, which in turn can accentuate muscle definition.

Impact of Sleep on Hormonal Balance

Sleep is a cornerstone of recovery and hormonal balance. The deep stages of sleep, in particular, are when the body undergoes most of its repair, recovery, and growth. Here's how sleep impacts hormonal balance:

- **Testosterone Production:** The majority of daily testosterone release in men occurs during sleep, indicating the importance of adequate rest for maintaining optimal testosterone levels.

- **Regulation of Cortisol:** A good night's sleep can help in regulating cortisol levels. Chronic sleep deprivation can lead to consistently elevated cortisol levels, which, as discussed, can be detrimental to muscle growth.

- **Growth Hormone Release:** Sleep triggers the release of growth hormone, another vital player in muscle repair and growth. Growth hormone also plays a role in fat metabolism, helping in fat loss and muscle definition.

In summary, hormonal balance is intricately linked with muscle growth and overall well-being. Factors like stress, nutrition, exercise, and especially sleep play a significant role in maintaining this balance. For those looking to optimize muscle growth, understanding and managing these factors can make a whole lot of difference.

Injury Prevention

Common Overuse Injuries

Overuse injuries, as the name suggests, occur when a particular part of the body is subjected to repeated stress without adequate time for recovery. These injuries are common among athletes and fitness enthusiasts who push their limits without allowing sufficient rest. Some prevalent overuse injuries include:

- **Tendinitis:** This is the inflammation of a tendon, the fibrous tissue that connects muscles to bones. Common areas affected include the Achilles tendon, wrist, and elbow.

- **Stress Fractures:** These are tiny cracks in a bone that result from repetitive force, often from activities like running or jumping.

- **Shin Splints:** Medically known as medial tibial stress syndrome, shin splints cause pain along the inner edge of the shinbone. They often occur in runners or those new to exercise.

- **Runner's Knee:** Also known as patellofemoral pain syndrome, this condition is characterized by pain around the kneecap. It's common in runners but can affect anyone.

- **Rotator Cuff Syndrome:** This affects the group of muscles and tendons that surround the shoulder joint, leading to pain and reduced range of motion.

Importance of Rest in Preventing Injuries

Rest is not just about muscle recovery; it's a crucial component in injury prevention. Here's why:

- **Muscle Recovery:** Muscles that are fatigued and not fully recovered are more susceptible to strains and tears. Rest allows muscles to repair and strengthen, reducing the risk of injury.

- **Joint Health:** Continuous training without adequate rest can put undue stress on joints, leading to conditions like tendinitis or even arthritis in the long run.

- **Connective Tissue Recovery:** Tendons and ligaments, which connect muscles to bones and bones to each other, respectively, also need time to recover from the stresses of exercise.

- **Mental Refreshment:** Mental fatigue can lead to a lack of focus during workouts, increasing the risk of injuries due to poor form or misjudged movements.

Role of Proper Form and Technique

Maintaining proper form and technique during exercises is paramount in injury prevention. Here's why:

- **Target the Right Muscles:** Proper form ensures that the right muscles are engaged during an exercise, reducing the risk of straining non-target muscles.

- **Protects Joints:** Incorrect technique can place undue stress on joints, leading to acute injuries or long-term damage.

- **Efficient Movement:** Proper form ensures that movements are biomechanically efficient, reducing the risk of overuse injuries.

- **Enhances Performance:** Beyond injury prevention, proper technique can also improve performance, ensuring that exercises are effective and goals are achieved faster.

In conclusion, while pushing one's limits in training can lead to impressive gains, it's essential to balance this with proper rest, technique, and awareness of one's body. This holistic approach not only prevents injuries but also ensures sustainable and long-term progress in one's fitness endeavors.

Optimizing Performance

Role of Glycogen Stores in Performance

Glycogen is the primary storage form of glucose in our bodies and plays a pivotal role in sustaining prolonged physical activity. Stored mainly in the liver and muscles, glycogen acts as a readily available energy reserve for the body. Here's how it influences performance:

- **Immediate Energy Source:** During short bursts of high-intensity activity, the body taps into muscle glycogen stores to fuel the effort. This is especially crucial in activities like weightlifting, sprinting, or high-intensity interval training.

- **Endurance Fuel:** For prolonged, lower-intensity activities like marathons or long cycling events, the body relies on a mix of fat and glycogen for energy. As the activity continues and fat metabolism becomes slower, the body increasingly depends on glycogen.

- **Post-Exercise Recovery:** After exercise, replenishing glycogen stores is essential for muscle recovery and preparation for the next workout session. Carbohydrate consumption after a workout can aid in faster glycogen synthesis.

- **Muscle Preservation:** In the absence of adequate glycogen, the body might resort to breaking down muscle protein for energy, which is counterproductive for athletes and fitness enthusiasts aiming for muscle growth.

Impact of Mental Focus and Motivation

The mind plays an equally, if not more, significant role in performance than the body. Here's how:

- **Drive and Determination:** A strong mental focus can push an individual to train harder, persevere through challenging workouts, and achieve their fitness goals.

- **Overcoming Plateaus:** When physical progress stalls, motivation, and a positive mindset can be the catalysts that drive an individual to tweak their training regimen, seek guidance, and break through barriers.

- **Enhancing Skill Acquisition:** In sports or activities that require skill, mental focus is crucial for mastering techniques, strategies, and movements.

- **Stress Management:** A calm and focused mind can better handle the pressures of competition, preventing performance anxiety and ensuring optimal output during crucial moments.

Strategies for Peak Performance

Achieving peak performance requires a blend of physical preparation and mental fortitude. Here are some strategies:

- **Tapering:** This involves reducing training volume and intensity as one approaches a competition or performance day, ensuring the body is well-rested and primed for peak output.

- **Nutritional Timing:** Consuming the right nutrients at the right times, especially around workouts, can optimize energy levels, muscle recovery, and overall performance.

- **Mental Imagery:** Visualizing successful performance scenarios can boost confidence and prepare the mind for the actual event.

- **Rest and Sleep:** Ensuring adequate rest and quality sleep is crucial for muscle recovery, cognitive functions, and overall well-being.

- **Continuous Learning:** Regularly updating training techniques, staying abreast of the latest research, and seeking expert advice can lead to incremental improvements in performance.

In summary, optimizing performance is a multifaceted endeavor, requiring attention to both the body's physiological needs and the mind's psychological demands. When these elements are in harmony, peak performance is not just possible; it's inevitable.

Strategies for Effective Rest and Recovery

Physical Restoration: Sleep is the prime time for the body to undergo repair and regeneration. During the deeper stages of sleep, blood flow to the muscles increases, facilitating the repair of tissues and bones and promoting the release of growth hormone, essential for muscle growth.

Cognitive Recovery: A good night's sleep enhances cognitive functions like memory, decision-making, and reaction times, all of which are important for athletes and individuals engaged in physical training.

Mood Regulation: Sleep plays a pivotal role in regulating mood. Adequate rest can prevent irritability, mood swings, and mental fatigue, ensuring a positive mindset for training sessions.

Immune Function: Regular sleep boosts the immune system, reducing the risk of illnesses that can interrupt training schedules.

Role of Active Recovery

Enhanced Blood Flow: Engaging in low-intensity activities on rest days, like walking or light cycling, can promote blood circulation, aiding in the delivery of nutrients essential for muscle repair.

Lactic Acid Reduction: Active recovery can help in flushing out lactic acid, which might accumulate in muscles after intense workouts, reducing soreness and stiffness.

Maintaining Mobility: Gentle stretching or yoga during active recovery can help maintain flexibility and range of motion.

Nutritional Considerations

Protein Intake: Consuming adequate protein after a workout aids in muscle repair and growth. Sources include lean meats, dairy, eggs, and plant-based options like lentils and chickpeas.

Carbohydrates: Replenishing glycogen stores post-exercise is crucial, including complex carbs like whole grains, fruits, and vegetables can aid in this.

Hydration: Water plays a vital role in recovery by aiding in nutrient transport and waste removal from the body.

Micronutrients: Vitamins and minerals, especially antioxidants like vitamins C and E, can combat exercise-induced oxidative stress.

Stress Management Techniques

Mindfulness and Meditation: Regular meditation can reduce cortisol levels, promoting a conducive environment for muscle growth and recovery.

Deep Breathing: Techniques like diaphragmatic breathing can activate the body's relaxation response, aiding in recovery.

Time Management: Organizing one's day and setting aside dedicated "me-time" can reduce daily stressors that might impede recovery.

Recovery Modalities

Cold Compressions and Ice Baths: These can reduce muscle inflammation and soreness after exercise.

Massage: Regular massages can improve blood flow, reduce muscle tension, and promote relaxation.

Foam Rolling: This self-myofascial release technique can alleviate muscle tightness and improve flexibility.

Compression Garments: Wearing compression clothing post-exercise can enhance blood circulation and reduce muscle soreness.

So, effective rest and recovery are as crucial as the training itself. Individuals can ensure they're giving their bodies the best chance to recuperate, grow, and achieve optimal performance by incorporating these strategies.

Sleep's Role in Muscle Growth--Hormonal Regulation

Growth Hormone Release During Sleep

- **The Anabolic Window:** Sleep is often referred to as the body's natural anabolic state. During the deep stages of sleep, particularly during the rapid eye movement (REM) phase, there's a surge in the release of growth hormone. This hormone plays a pivotal role in tissue growth and muscle repair.

- **Recovery and Repair:** The growth hormone not only aids in muscle development but also helps in the regeneration of cells, the synthesis of proteins, and the repair of micro-tears that occur in muscle fibers during intense workouts.

- **Optimal Sleep Duration:** For maximal growth hormone release, getting between 7 to 9 hours of sleep for adults is typically recommended. Shortchanging sleep can significantly reduce the duration of the REM phase, thereby limiting the release of growth hormones.

Impact of Sleep on Testosterone Levels

- **Testosterone and Muscle Growth:** Testosterone is important in muscle growth, strength gains, and bone density. It also helps in fat metabolism, to reduce fat mass.

- **Sleep and Testosterone Production:** A significant portion of daily testosterone release in men occurs during sleep. Chronic sleep deprivation can lead to a drop in testosterone levels, which can impede muscle growth and reduce overall energy levels.

- **Quality Over Quantity:** It's not just the duration of sleep that matters. The quality of sleep is equally crucial. Disrupted sleep patterns or frequent awakenings during the night can hamper the optimal release of testosterone.

Role of Melatonin in Sleep Regulation

- **The Sleep Hormone:** Melatonin, often termed the 'sleep hormone', is produced by the pineal gland in the brain. Its primary function is to regulate the sleep-wake cycle, signaling the body when it's time to wind down and rest.

- **Melatonin and Muscle Recovery:** Recent studies suggest that melatonin might have antioxidant properties, which can aid in muscle recovery. By neutralizing free radicals produced during intense workouts, melatonin can potentially reduce muscle damage and inflammation.

- **Natural Production:** The production of melatonin is influenced by light. As it gets dark, melatonin levels rise, signaling the body to prepare for sleep. Exposure to artificial light, especially blue light from screens, can disrupt this natural flow, potentially affecting sleep quality and muscle recovery.

In conclusion, sleep is not just a passive state of rest. It's an active, intricate process governed by hormones, each playing its part in ensuring optimal muscle growth and overall well-being. Recognizing the profound impact of sleep on muscle growth underscores the importance of prioritizing rest in any fitness regimen.

Muscle Repair and Protein Synthesis

Increased Blood Flow During Sleep

The Restorative Phase: Sleep is a time when the body shifts its focus from daily activities to restoration and repair. One of the physiological changes that occur during sleep is an increase in blood flow to the muscles. This enhanced blood flow ensures that muscles receive an ample supply of oxygen and nutrients, which are vital for repair and growth.

Nutrient Delivery: As the heart rate slows and breathing becomes deep, the circulatory system efficiently delivers essential amino acids (the building blocks of protein) to muscle tissues. These amino acids repairs muscle fibers that have been damaged during workouts.

Detoxification Process: Increased blood flow also aids in the removal of metabolic waste products from muscle tissues. By flushing out substances like lactic acid, the muscles are better prepared for the next physical activity.

Role of Cytokines in Muscle Repair

- **Signaling Molecules:** Cytokines are a group of proteins that play a pivotal role in cell signaling, especially when it comes to inflammation and immune responses. During sleep, there's a release of specific cytokines that aid in muscle repair and recovery.

- **Anti-inflammatory Response:** Some cytokines, such as interleukin-6 (IL-6) and tumor necrosis factor-alpha (TNF-alpha), have been shown to increase during muscle repair. These cytokines help modulate inflammation, ensuring that it's beneficial (helping repair) rather than chronic and detrimental.

- **Immune Boost:** Apart from muscle repair, cytokines also bolster the immune system. A strong immune response ensures that potential infections or pathogens don't impede the muscle recovery process.

Importance of Uninterrupted Sleep

- **Deep Sleep and Recovery:** The most profound muscle repair and protein synthesis occur during the deep stages of sleep. Disruptions or frequent awakenings can limit the time spent in this restorative phase, potentially hampering muscle recovery.

- **Hormonal Harmony:** Uninterrupted sleep ensures a balanced release of the growth hormone and testosterone, both of which are crucial for muscle growth. Fragmented sleep can disrupt this hormonal balance, affecting muscle repair.

- **Mental Restoration:** It's not just the body that benefits from uninterrupted sleep. The mind, too, undergoes a process of rejuvenation. A well-rested mind ensures better focus during workouts, optimal technique, and a reduced risk of injuries.

In essence, while we often prioritize our waking hours for muscle building, the real magic happens when we close our eyes and drift into sleep. It's a time of profound repair, growth, and rejuvenation, making sleep an indispensable ally in the quest for muscle growth and overall well-being.

Neural Recovery and Performance

Restoration of Cognitive Function

- **Brain Detoxification:** During sleep, the brain undergoes a cleansing process where cerebrospinal fluid washes away harmful waste products that accumulate during waking hours. This "brain detox" is essential for maintaining cognitive health and ensuring optimal brain function.

- **Memory Consolidation:** Sleep plays a pivotal role in the consolidation of memories. It means better retention of workout routines, techniques, and strategies for athletes and fitness enthusiasts. The brain ensures that learning is solidified and readily accessible for future use by consolidating information from the day.

- **Mental Clarity and Decision Making:** A good night's sleep enhances mental clarity, focus, and decision-making skills. This is crucial for athletes who need to make split-second decisions during competitions or for anyone engaging in complex exercises that require precision and concentration.

Importance of Sleep in Motor Skills

- **Skill Enhancement:** Sleep is when the brain processes and refines motor skills. The neural pathways involved in these actions are strengthened, leading to better execution and performance.

- **Muscle Memory:** The term "muscle memory" is a bit of a misnomer, as it's the brain that remembers, not the muscles. During sleep, the brain repeatedly "replays" the motor actions of the day, further ingraining these patterns and making them more automatic over time.

- **Learning New Techniques:** For those learning new exercises or sports techniques, sleep can accelerate the learning curve. The brain optimizes the neural pathways associated with these new skills, making them easier to perform with each subsequent attempt.

Impact on Muscular Coordination

- **Synchronized Movement:** Proper muscular coordination is essential for efficient movement and peak performance. Sleep ensures that the neural networks governing coordinated movement are in top shape, allowing for fluid and synchronized muscle actions.

- **Reduction in Injury Risk:** Fatigue, often exacerbated by poor sleep, can lead to sluggish reactions and uncoordinated movements. This lack of coordination increases the risk of injuries, from minor strains to more severe mishaps.

- **Optimal Neuro-muscular Communication:** Sleep enhances the communication between the nervous system and muscles. This improved neuromuscular junction communication ensures that muscle contractions are timely, forceful, and precise, leading to better performance and reduced energy wastage.

In summary, while sleep's role in physical recovery is often emphasized, its impact on neural recovery and performance is equally vital. From refining motor skills to ensuring peak muscular coordination, sleep is a linchpin in the holistic development and performance of an athlete or fitness enthusiast.

- **Neurotransmitters Throughout the Brain.** This ensures that brain cells are adequately nourished and function optimally.

- **Supporting Brain Health:** By efficiently removing waste products and delivering vital nutrients, the glymphatic system plays a pivotal role in maintaining overall brain health, cognitive function, and mental clarity.

Replenishment of Glycogen Stores

- **Energy Reservoir:** Glycogen, stored primarily in the liver and muscles, acts as the body's primary energy reservoir. During periods of activity, glycogen is broken down to provide glucose, which strengthens our cells. Sleep is a crucial period when these glycogen stores are replenished, ensuring that the body has adequate energy reserves for the following day.

- **Supporting Muscle Recovery:** For athletes and those engaged in regular physical activity, the replenishment of muscle glycogen is particularly vital. Adequate glycogen ensures that muscles have the necessary energy for contraction, repair, and growth.

- **Optimizing Metabolic Function:** A consistent sleep pattern ensures that glycogen synthesis, regulated by various hormones and enzymes, occurs at an optimal rate. This not only supports physical activity but also maintains overall metabolic health.

Removal of Metabolic Waste Products

- **Cellular Clean-Up:** As cells function, they produce waste products. Accumulation of these by-products can be harmful and hinder cellular operations. Sleep provides the body with an opportunity to efficiently process and remove these waste products.

- **Lactic Acid Clearance:** Intense physical activity can lead to the accumulation of lactic acid in the muscles, contributing to muscle fatigue and soreness. During sleep, the body works to clear out excess lactic acid, aiding in muscle recovery and reducing post-exercise discomfort.

- **Promotion of Cellular Health:** By ensuring the timely removal of waste products, sleep supports cellular health and function. This is crucial for every bodily system, from the immune system to the muscular system, ensuring optimal health and performance.

In essence, sleep is not just a passive state of rest. It's an active period of restoration, repair, and rejuvenation. From the intricate workings of the glymphatic system to the replenishment of vital energy stores, sleep plays a central role in maintaining cellular health and overall vitality.

Strategies for Enhancing Sleep Quality

Establishing a Consistent Sleep Schedule

- **Biological Clock Alignment:** Our bodies operate on a circadian rhythm, an internal clock that regulates sleep-wake cycles. By going to bed and waking up at the same time every day, even on weekends, we can align with this natural tool, making it easier to fall asleep and wake up refreshed.

- **Regulating Sleep Hormones:** Consistency in sleep timings helps regulate the release of melatonin, the sleep hormone. This ensures that we feel sleepy at the right time and wake up alert.

- **Avoiding Sleep Debt:** By maintaining a regular sleep schedule, we can avoid accumulating sleep debt, which can lead to chronic fatigue and other health issues.

Creating a Sleep-Friendly Environment

- **Optimal Room Temperature:** A slightly cooler room, typically around 65°F (18°C), is considered ideal for sleep. It supports the body's natural dip in temperature during the night, promoting deeper sleep.

- **Darkness Matters:** Our sleep cycle is influenced by light. Using blackout curtains or eye masks can create a dark environment, signaling to the body that it's time to rest.

- **Quietude:** Minimizing noise disruptions with earplugs, white noise machines, or soundproofing can lead to uninterrupted sleep.

- **Comfortable Bedding:** Investing in a comfortable mattress and pillows can make a significant difference in sleep quality.

Limiting Blue Light Exposure

- **Digital Devices and Sleep:** Smartphones, tablets, computers, and TVs emit blue light, which can suppress melatonin production, making it harder to fall asleep.

- **Night Mode:** Many devices now offer a 'night mode' setting that reduces blue light emission in the evenings.

- **Digital Detox:** It's beneficial to have a digital curfew, avoiding screens for at least an hour before bedtime.

Relaxation Routines Before Sleep

- **Mindfulness and Meditation:** Engaging in mindfulness practices or meditation can calm the mind, preparing it for rest.

- **Reading:** Reading a physical book (as opposed to a digital screen) can be a relaxing pre-sleep ritual for many.

- **Warm Baths:** A warm bath can relax muscles and promote feelings of drowsiness.

- **Deep Breathing:** Techniques like the 4-7-8 breathing method can activate the body's relaxation response, aiding in sleep onset.

Dietary Considerations

- **Limiting Caffeine:** Consuming caffeine in the latter half of the day can interfere with sleep. It's advisable to limit coffee, tea, or other caffeinated beverages after mid-afternoon.

- **Avoiding Heavy Meals:** Eating a large or spicy meal before bedtime can cause discomfort and indigestion, disrupting sleep.

- **Alcohol and Sleep:** While alcohol might make you feel sleepy initially, it can interfere with the sleep cycle, leading to fragmented sleep.

- **Sleep-Promoting Foods:** Some foods, like turkey, almonds, and chamomile tea, contain nutrients that may promote sleep.

Incorporating these strategies can significantly enhance sleep quality, ensuring that the body and mind are well-rested and rejuvenated for the challenges of a new day.

Active Recovery and Rest Days

Benefits of Enhanced Blood Flow

- **Nutrient Delivery:** Active recovery exercises, such as light jogging or cycling, promote increased blood flow to the muscles. This enhanced circulation delivers essential nutrients that aid in the repair and rebuilding of muscle tissue.

- **Waste Removal:** Increased blood flow also facilitates the removal of metabolic waste products that accumulate during intense workouts. Muscles can recover more efficiently by clearing out these waste products.

- **Reduced Muscle Stiffness:** Gentle movement during active recovery can help alleviate muscle stiffness, ensuring better flexibility and range of motion in subsequent workouts.

Reduction of Muscle Soreness

- **Lactic Acid Dispersion:** Engaging in low-intensity activities helps disperse lactic acid, which can contribute to muscle soreness if allowed to accumulate.

- **Promotion of Muscle Healing:** Active recovery stimulates the body's natural healing processes, reducing the duration and intensity of muscle soreness post-workout.

- **Stretching and Mobility Work:** Incorporating stretching and mobility exercises during active recovery can further alleviate muscle tightness and soreness.

Mental Benefits of Active Recovery

- **Psychological Reset:** Active recovery provides a mental break from intense training, allowing individuals to recharge mentally, and reducing the risk of burnout.

- **Mood Enhancement:** Light physical activity can stimulate the release of endorphins, the body's natural mood boosters, promoting feelings of well-being and relaxation.

- **Maintaining Routine:** For many, exercise is a crucial part of their daily routine. Active recovery allows individuals to stay active without the intensity, ensuring consistency in their fitness habits.

Cross-Training Opportunities

- **Skill Development:** Active recovery days offer an opportunity to engage in different activities, allowing individuals to develop new skills or hobbies.

- **Reduced Risk of Overuse Injuries:** By diversifying activities, athletes can give specific muscle groups a break, reducing the risk of overuse injuries.

- **Enhanced Overall Fitness:** Engaging in different forms of exercise, such as swimming or yoga, can enhance overall fitness by challenging the body in new ways.

Therefore, active recovery is not about being inactive but rather about engaging in low-intensity activities that promote recovery and overall well-being. It's a balanced approach that ensures both the body and mind are rejuvenated and ready for more intense training sessions ahead.

Rest Days

Importance in Muscle Repair and Growth

- **Deep Tissue Repair:** While active recovery focuses on light activities, rest days involve minimal physical exertion, allowing muscles to undergo deep tissue repair. This is crucial after particularly strenuous workouts where muscle fibers experience significant wear and tear.

- **Muscle Hypertrophy:** Rest days are when muscle growth predominantly happens. After workouts, muscles are essentially "broken down", and it's during rest that they rebuild stronger and larger, a process known as hypertrophy.

- **Optimal Nutrient Utilization:** With adequate rest, the body can effectively utilize nutrients like proteins for muscle repair and carbohydrates for replenishing glycogen stores, ensuring muscles are ready for subsequent workouts.

Role in Central Nervous System (CNS) Recovery

- **Neural Fatigue Management:** Intense workouts, especially strength training, place a significant load on the CNS. Rest days allow the CNS to recover from this neural fatigue, ensuring optimal muscle performance in future sessions.

- **Prevention of Burnout:** Overloading the CNS without adequate rest can lead to burnout, characterized by prolonged fatigue, decreased performance, and increased susceptibility to injuries. Rest days are crucial in preventing this.

- **Enhanced Neuroplasticity:** Rest days can also promote neuroplasticity, the brain's ability to reorganize and form new neural connections, which is essential for learning new movements and skills.

Maintenance of Hormonal Balance

- **Cortisol Regulation:** Chronic training without adequate rest can lead to elevated cortisol levels, a stress hormone that can hinder muscle growth and impair immune function. Rest days help regulate and normalize cortisol levels.

- **Testosterone and Growth Hormone Balance:** Both are vital for muscle growth and recovery. Overtraining without sufficient rest can suppress their production, while rest days can ensure their optimal levels are maintained.

Mental Rejuvenation and Motivation

- **Psychological Break:** Rest days provide a necessary psychological break from the rigors of consistent training, allowing individuals to relax, reflect, and mentally prepare for upcoming challenges.

- **Prevention of Mental Burnout:** Just as the body can experience physical burnout, the mind can also become overwhelmed without adequate rest, leading to decreased motivation and enthusiasm for workouts.

- **Renewed Motivation:** A day off can often reignite the passion and drive for training, allowing individuals to return to their routines with renewed vigor and determination.

In summary, rest days are not just a break from physical activity; they are an integral component of any training regimen. They ensure that both the body and mind are optimally prepared and conditioned for the challenges of consistent training, promoting long-term health, growth, and performance.

Strategies for Effective Active Recovery and Rest Days

Planning Recovery Sessions

- **Structured Approach:** Just as workouts are planned, active recovery sessions should be structured. This ensures that they are effective and serve their purpose without becoming another strenuous workout.

- **Low-Intensity Activities:** Activities like walking, swimming, or cycling at a leisurely pace can be ideal. These activities enhance blood flow to muscles without placing undue stress on them.

- **Stretching and Mobility Work:** Incorporating dynamic stretches or yoga can help improve flexibility, alleviate muscle tightness, and enhance overall mobility.

- **Hydrotherapy:** Techniques like cold water immersion or contrast baths can help reduce muscle soreness and inflammation.

Emphasis on Sleep

- **Prioritize Sleep Duration:** Ensure you get 7-9 hours of sleep, especially after intense training days, to facilitate optimal muscle recovery.

- **Sleep Quality:** It's not just about the quantity but also the quality of sleep. Ensure a dark, quiet, and cool environment for uninterrupted rest.

- **Napping:** Short naps of 20-30 minutes during the day can also aid in recovery, especially if nighttime sleep is compromised.

Mindful Rest Techniques

- **Deep Breathing:** Engaging in deep breathing exercises can help reduce stress, lower cortisol levels, and promote relaxation.

- **Meditation:** Even a short 10-minute meditation session can help in mental relaxation, reducing anxiety, and promoting a sense of well-being.

- **Progressive Muscle Relaxation:** This technique involves tensing and then relaxing different muscle groups, which can help in alleviating muscle tension.

Nutritional Considerations

- **Hydration:** Drinking adequate water supports metabolic processes and helps in flushing out toxins.

- **Protein Intake:** Consuming protein-rich foods or shakes can aid in muscle repair and growth.

- **Micronutrients:** Vitamins and minerals, especially magnesium, zinc, and B vitamins, help in muscle recovery and should be incorporated into the diet.

- **Anti-inflammatory Foods:** Foods rich in omega-3 fatty acids, turmeric, and antioxidants can help reduce muscle inflammation and soreness.

Engaging in Mental Activities

- **Hobbies:** Engaging in non-fitness-related hobbies can be a great way to divert the mind and achieve a sense of accomplishment.

- **Reading:** Diving into a good book can be a perfect way to relax and take a mental break.

- **Nature Walks:** Spending time in nature, even if it's a short walk in a park, can have rejuvenating effects on the mind.

- **Social Connections:** Spending quality time with loved ones or friends can uplift spirits and provide emotional support.

Incorporating these strategies into active recovery and rest days ensures a holistic approach to recovery, addressing both physical and mental aspects. This comprehensive approach not only aids in muscle growth and performance but also promotes overall well-being and longevity in the fitness journey.

Stress, Recovery, and Overtraining

The Role of Stress in Muscle Growth

- **Eustress Versus Distress:** During exercise, not all stress is harmful. Eustress, or positive stress, is what we often aim for in training. It's the right amount of challenge that pushes the body to adapt and grow stronger. On the other hand, distress refers to excessive stress that can be detrimental to health and performance.

- **Mechanical and Metabolic Stress:** Mechanical stress refers to the physical strain placed on muscles during resistance training, leading to micro-tears. Metabolic stress, on the other hand, arises from exercises that deplete energy stores and increase metabolite accumulation in muscles.

- **Adaptive Response:** When muscles are exposed to stress, they undergo a process of adaptation to handle similar stress better in the future. This is the fundamental principle behind muscle growth and strength gains.

Physiological Responses to Training Stress

- **Inflammatory Response:** After a workout, the body initiates an inflammatory response to repair damaged muscle fibers. This is a natural and essential process, often manifesting as muscle soreness.

- **Hormonal Fluctuations:** Exercise stress triggers the release of various hormones. Cortisol, often termed the "stress hormone" increases post-exercise but is essential for regulating energy and inflammation. Growth hormone and testosterone, vital for muscle repair and growth, also see a surge post-exercise.

- **Neural Adaptations:** The nervous system also responds to training stress. Initially, strength gains are largely due to neural adaptations, as the body becomes more efficient at recruiting muscle fibers.

- **Energy Systems:** Depending on the type and intensity of exercise, different energy systems are stressed, leading to adaptations in how the body stores and utilizes energy.

Balancing Stress and Recovery

- **Importance of Balance:** While stress is essential for growth, continuous stress without adequate recovery can lead to overtraining and injuries. It's a delicate balance between pushing the body and allowing it to heal.

- **Listening to the Body:** It's crucial to align to one's body signals. Persistent fatigue, mood swings, or decreased performance can be signs that the balance is skewed.

- **Periodization:** This systematic approach to training varies the intensity and volume of workouts, ensuring that there are periods of high stress followed by adequate recovery.

- **Active Recovery:** Engaging in low-intensity activities on rest days can aid in recovery without adding significant stress.

Nevertheless, stress, when applied judiciously in the context of exercise, can be a potent catalyst for growth. However, striking balance is key, to ensure that the body is not pushed to its breaking point but is instead guided toward its peak potential.

Importance of Recovery

Role in Muscle Repair and Growth

- **The Repair Process:** When we exercise, especially during resistance training, micro-tears occur in our muscle fibers. However, it's a natural and essential part of muscle development. The real magic happens post-workout when the body begins its repair process. These fibers rebuild stronger and thicker, leading to muscle growth with adequate nutrients and rest.

- **Inflammation and Recovery:** During post-exercise, the body's inflammatory response is activated to heal the damaged muscle tissue. This inflammation is a double-edged sword. While necessary for signaling repair processes, prolonged inflammation without recovery can hinder muscle growth and lead to chronic issues.

- **Hormonal Role:** Recovery periods allow for the optimal release of anabolic hormones like testosterone and growth hormone, which play pivotal roles in muscle synthesis and repair.

Replenishment of Energy Stores

- **Glycogen Restoration:** Muscles store energy in the form of glycogen, which gets depleted during workouts. During recovery periods, especially when combined with appropriate nutrition, allow these glycogen stores to be replenished, ensuring that muscles have the energy needed for subsequent workouts.

- **ATP Regeneration:** ATP is the primary energy currency of cells. During exercise, ATP is rapidly consumed to enhance muscle contractions. Recovery periods allow for the regeneration of ATP, ensuring that the body is prepared for the next activity.

Restoration of Mental Focus and Motivation

- **Mental Fatigue:** Just as our muscles get tired, our brain, too, can experience fatigue, especially after intense or prolonged workouts. This mental fatigue can impact our motivation, focus, and even our perception of effort during subsequent workouts.

- **The Power of Rest:** Adequate recovery not only rejuvenates the body but also the mind. A well-rested individual is more likely to approach workouts with greater enthusiasm, clarity, and determination.

- **Psychological Reset:** Beyond the physical aspects, recovery provides a psychological reset. It offers a break, a moment to reflect, celebrate achievements, set new goals, and mentally prepare for upcoming challenges.

In summary, recovery is not merely the absence of training; it's an active and integral component of the fitness journey. It's the time when the body and mind heal, adapt, and grow, setting the stage for consistent progress and optimal performance. Without adequate recovery, even a well-designed training regimen can fall short of its potential.

Overtraining Syndrome

Symptoms and Impact on Health

- **Physical Symptoms:** Overtraining syndrome (OTS) manifests in various ways. Common physical symptoms include persistent fatigue, decreased performance despite intense training, increased susceptibility to injuries, prolonged recovery times, loss of appetite, and disturbed sleep patterns.

- **Mental and Emotional Symptoms:** Beyond the physical, OTS can have psychological repercussions. Affected individuals might experience mood swings, irritability, depression, loss of motivation, and decreased concentration. The joy and enthusiasm once associated with training can be replaced by a sense of dread.

- **Immune System Compromise:** Chronic overtraining can suppress the immune system, making athletes more susceptible to illnesses, especially upper respiratory tract infections.

- **Impact on Health:** Over time, if not addressed, OTS can lead to more severe health issues, including chronic fatigue syndrome, hormonal imbalances, and metabolic disorders.

Role of Hormonal Imbalances in Overtraining

- **Cortisol Overproduction:** One of the primary hormonal indicators of OTS is an increase in cortisol, the body's primary stress hormone. While cortisol plays a crucial role in various physiological processes, chronic elevation due to overtraining can lead to muscle breakdown, impaired recovery, and suppressed immune function.

- **Testosterone Decline:** Overtraining can lead to a decrease in testosterone levels, a hormone vital for muscle growth and repair. A reduced testosterone-to-cortisol ratio is often used as an indicator of OTS.

- **Impact on Sleep:** Elevated cortisol levels, especially in the evening, can disrupt the natural circadian, leading to sleep disturbances. Sleep is crucial for recovery and muscle growth, and its disruption can exacerbate the effects of overtraining.

Strategies to Recognize and Prevent Overtraining

- **Monitoring Training Load:** Keeping a detailed training log can help in tracking volume, intensity, and frequency. Any sudden or drastic increase in these parameters without adequate recovery can be a precursor to OTS.

- **Regular Check-ins:** Regular physical and mental check-ins can help in early detection. Monitoring resting heart rate, sleep quality, mood, and general energy levels can provide valuable insights.

- **Scheduled Rest and Deload Weeks:** Incorporating regular rest days and periodic deload weeks (reduced training volume or intensity) can prevent the accumulation of fatigue and stave off OTS.

- **Nutritional Considerations:** Ensuring adequate caloric intake, especially from quality protein and carbohydrates, can support recovery and reduce the risk of overtraining.

- **Active Recovery:** Engaging in low-intensity activities, like walking or light swimming, can enhance blood flow, aiding in recovery without adding significant training stress.

- **Seek Expert Guidance:** Working with a knowledgeable coach or sports scientist, especially for competitive athletes can help in designing a balanced training regimen that promotes growth while minimizing the risk of OTS.

In essence, while training hard is essential for progress, it's equally crucial to recognize the signs of overtraining and take proactive measures. Balancing exertion with recovery is the key to sustainable, long-term athletic success.

Strategies for Stress Management and Recovery

Incorporating Periodization in Training

- **Structured Approach:** Periodization involves breaking down training into specific cycles or phases, each with its own goals. This structured approach ensures that athletes are not constantly pushing their limits, reducing the risk of burnout and overtraining.

- **Varied Stimulus:** By changing the training focus periodically, from endurance to strength to power, the body is exposed to varied stimuli. This not only prevents adaptation and plateaus but also reduces the repetitive stress on specific muscle groups.

- **Scheduled Deloads:** Within periodized plans, deload weeks (reduced volume or intensity) are often incorporated to allow the body and mind a relative break, ensuring accumulated fatigue doesn't lead to overtraining.

Importance of Rest and Active Recovery

- **Rest Days:** These are days when no structured training is done, allowing muscles to repair and grow. It also provides the central nervous system a break from the stresses of intense training.

- **Active Recovery:** Engaging in low-intensity, low-impact activities like walking, cycling, or swimming can help increase blood flow, facilitating nutrient delivery to muscles and speeding up recovery.

Nutritional Strategies for Recovery

- **Post-Workout Nutrition:** Consuming a combination of proteins and carbohydrates post-workout can kickstart the recovery process. This combo helps in replenishing glycogen stores and initiating muscle protein synthesis.

- **Stay Hydrated:** Water plays a crucial role in almost every cellular process, including muscle recovery. Ensuring adequate hydration can aid in nutrient transport and waste product removal.

- **Micronutrients:** Vitamins and minerals, especially antioxidants like vitamins C and E, can combat oxidative stress induced by intense training, supporting recovery.

Sleep Optimization Techniques

- **Consistent Schedule:** Going to bed and waking up at the same time, even on weekends, can regulate the body's internal clock, improving sleep quality.

- **Sleep Environment:** A dark, quiet, and cool room can enhance sleep. Consider using blackout curtains, earplugs, or white noise machines if needed.

- **Limiting Screen Time:** The blue light emitted by phones and computers can interfere with melatonin production, a hormone responsible for sleep. It's beneficial to limit screen exposure to at least an hour before bedtime.

Stress Management Techniques

- **Mindfulness and Meditation:** These practices can help in centering the mind, reducing the feelings of stress, and improving the mind-muscle connection.

- **Deep Breathing Exercises:** Techniques like diaphragmatic breathing can activate the parasympathetic nervous system, promoting relaxation.

- **Hobbies and Downtime:** Engaging in non-training related activities that one enjoys can be a great way to divert the mind from daily stresses, promoting mental recovery.

In conclusion, while training is a significant component of muscle growth and athletic performance, recovery is equally, if not more, vital. By adopting a holistic approach that incorporates structured training, nutrition, sleep, and stress management, one can optimize muscle growth, prevent injuries, and ensure long-term athletic success.

Conclusion: Recovery and Muscle Growth

In the realm of muscle growth and athletic performance, the significance of training is often highlighted, but the pivotal role of recovery remains underemphasized. Chapter 10 delves deep into the multifaceted world of recovery, elucidating its paramount importance in the muscle-building journey.

From the intricate processes of muscle repair and growth to the prevention of overtraining, the initial sections underscored that recovery is not merely the absence of training but an active, essential process. Hormonal balance, often overlooked, plays a crucial role in muscle development, with sleep emerging as a key regulator. As we read through the chapter, it became evident that sleep is not just a passive state of rest but a dynamic period of repair, hormonal regulation, and neural recovery. The profound impact of a good night's sleep on muscle growth, neural function, and overall health cannot be overstated.

The chapter further illuminated the concept of active recovery and the importance of designated rest days. These aren't just breaks from training but are periods when the body undergoes significant repair, adaptation, and growth. The strategies provided offer a roadmap to maximize the benefits of these recovery periods, ensuring they're as productive as the training sessions themselves.

Lastly, the intricate relationship between stress, recovery, and overtraining was explored. While stress, in the right doses, can propel muscle growth, its chronic presence, without adequate recovery, can lead to the dreaded overtraining syndrome. The strategies delineated in the final sections provide a comprehensive approach to managing stress, optimizing recovery, and preventing overtraining.

In essence, Chapter 10 serves as a testament to the adage, "It's not about how hard you train, but how well you recover." As we transition to the subsequent chapters, let this be a reminder that in the quest for muscle growth and peak performance, recovery is not just a component—it's the cornerstone.

Next, we shall examine environmental adaptations, exploring how athletes adapt and thrive in extreme conditions, from scorching deserts to icy terrains and high-altitude peaks. We shall also see the body's physiological responses, the mind's resilience, and the strategies elite performers employ to conquer these challenges. Again, we will discover the secrets of training in heat, cold, and altitude, and learn from case studies of those who've faced these environments head-on. So, prepare to be enlightened on a whole new dimension of athletic performance and training!

CHAPTER 11

ADAPTATIONS TO HEAT, COLD, AND ALTITUDE

Training in different environmental conditions can have a significant impact on performance, muscle growth, and overall health. In this study, you'll discover that the environment is not just a backdrop for your training—it's an active participant that shapes your physiological and psychological responses. This chapter will also capture the physiological adaptations that occur when training in heat, cold, and altitude, providing practical guidelines and case studies to help you optimize your training in these conditions. Here's what you can expect:

- **Why Environment Matters**: We'll begin by exploring the fundamental reasons why training in different environments is not just a novel experience but a strategic approach to enhancing performance and health.

- **Physiological Adaptations**: One of the core focuses of this chapter will be the science behind how your body adapts to different environmental conditions. Whether it's the thermoregulatory demands of heat, the metabolic changes in cold, or the cardiovascular adjustments at altitude, understanding these mechanisms can empower you to train smarter.

- **Psychological Aspects**: Beyond the physical, we'll also examine the mental adaptations that occur. How does training in extreme environmental conditions affect your mental resilience, focus, and overall psychological well-being?

- **Practical Guidelines**: Armed with scientific insights, we'll transition into actionable advice. What are the best practices for training in these conditions? How can you modify your workout routines, nutritional intake, and recovery strategies to get the most out of your environment?

- **Case Studies**: To bring theory into practice, we'll share real-world case studies that illustrate the principles discussed. These will include accounts from athletes who have successfully adapted to extreme conditions, offering valuable lessons and insights.

- **Safety Considerations**: Last but not least, we'll discuss the essential safety measures you need to consider when training in extreme environments. From heatstroke prevention in hot climates to frostbite avoidance in the cold, safety is a paramount concern that will be thoroughly addressed.

By the end of this chapter, you'll have a clear understanding of how different environmental conditions can be leveraged to enhance your training, improve your performance, and boost your overall health. Whether you're a seasoned athlete or a fitness enthusiast, the knowledge and strategies presented here will equip you to take your training to new heights.

The Physiology of Heat Adaptation: Acclimatization and Training Strategies

What Happens During Heat Acclimatization

When you first start exercising in hot conditions, your body undergoes a series of physiological changes to help you cope with the increased heat stress. These changes are part of a process known as heat acclimatization. Here's what happens:

- **Sweat Mechanism**: Initially, you may find that you sweat more profusely. This is the body's primary cooling mechanism. As you become acclimatized, your sweat rate may actually decrease, but the sweat will be more effective at cooling you down because it will contain fewer electrolytes, conserving important minerals like sodium.

- **Cardiovascular Adaptations**: Your heart rate will likely be higher during your first few workouts in the heat. As you acclimatize, your cardiovascular system becomes more efficient, and your heart rate during exercise may decrease.

- **Blood Plasma Volume**: One of the most significant adaptations is an increase in blood plasma volume, which improves cardiovascular stability and can enhance endurance performance.

- **Core Temperature**: Initially, your core body temperature will rise more quickly during exercise in the heat. However, as you acclimatize, your body becomes more efficient at dissipating heat, and your core temperature will be better regulated.

- **Metabolic Changes**: Your metabolism may slow down slightly as your body tries to reduce internal heat production. This is usually a temporary change and reverses as you become more acclimatized.

Understanding these adaptations can help you train more effectively and safely in hot conditions. It's important to give your body time to adapt, which usually takes about 10-14 days of consistent heat exposure.

Training in the Heat

Exercising in hot conditions requires careful planning and execution to ensure safety and effectiveness. Here are some strategies and considerations:

- **Hydration**: Staying hydrated is crucial when training in the heat. Dehydration can lead to decreased performance and increased risk of heat-related illnesses. It's advisable to drink water before, during, and after your workout. Some athletes also opt for electrolyte drinks to replace lost minerals.

- **Clothing**: Wear lightweight, breathable, and moisture-wicking fabrics to help with sweat evaporation and cooling. Avoid dark colors that can absorb heat.

- **Time of Day**: If possible, train during the cooler parts of the day, such as early morning or late evening. This can help you avoid the peak heat times, reducing the risk of heat-related issues.

- **Acclimatization**: Start with shorter, less intense workouts and gradually increase the duration and intensity as your body adapts to the heat. This can take up to two weeks.

- **Rest and Recovery**: Take frequent breaks to rest and hydrate, especially if you're new to heat training. Listen to your body; if you feel dizzy, nauseous, or overly fatigued, it's important to stop exercising and seek shade and hydration.

- **Indoor Alternatives**: On extremely hot days, consider taking your workout indoors where you can control the climate. This can be a good way to maintain your training schedule without risking heat-related complications.

- **Monitoring**: Keep an eye on the weather forecast and be aware of the heat index, not just the temperature. The heat index takes into account humidity, which can affect your body's ability to cool itself.

    By taking these precautions and strategies into account, you can make your heat training both effective and safe. Always remember that the key to successful heat training is to respect the conditions and listen to your body.

Heat and Muscle Growth

Training in hot conditions can have unique effects on muscle growth and recovery. Here's how:

- **Increased Blood Flow**: The heat naturally dilates blood vessels, increasing blood flow to the muscles. This can enhance the delivery of nutrients and oxygen, potentially aiding in muscle growth and recovery.

- **Heat Shock Proteins (HSPs)**: Exposure to heat stress activates heat shock proteins, which have been shown to protect cells from damage and may aid in muscle recovery.

- **Protein Synthesis**: Some studies suggest that heat exposure can increase protein synthesis rates, although the evidence is not yet conclusive. If true, this could potentially accelerate muscle growth.

- **Hydration and Muscle Recovery**: Dehydration can impair muscle recovery. Since training in the heat increases the risk of dehydration, it's crucial to stay hydrated to support muscle growth and recovery.

- **Hormonal Responses**: Training in the heat can affect hormone levels, including cortisol, a stress hormone that can break down muscle tissue. Proper hydration and nutrition are essential to mitigate these effects.

- **Risk of Overtraining**: The added stress of heat can increase the risk of overtraining if not managed carefully. Overtraining can lead to muscle loss and increased recovery times.

- **Psychological Aspects**: Training in extreme conditions like heat can also build mental resilience, which can be beneficial in pushing through plateaus in both strength and hypertrophy.

Training in the heat even with some unique advantages for muscle growth also comes with risks that need to be carefully managed. Always consult with a healthcare provider before starting a new training regimen, especially one that involves extreme conditions like heat.

Cold Adaptation: How the Body Adjusts and Training Tips

Physiological Changes in Cold

When you train in cold conditions, your body undergoes several physiological adaptations to maintain core temperature and optimize performance. Here are some of the key changes:

- **Thermogenesis**: One of the first responses to cold exposure is thermogenesis, or heat production. Brown adipose tissue (BAI), also known as brown fat, plays a significant role in this process. It burns calories to generate heat and helps maintain core body temperature.

- **Shivering**: This involuntary muscle contraction is another mechanism the body uses to generate heat. While it's effective in the short term, shivering is not energy-efficient and can fatigue muscles if sustained over long periods.

- **Blood Redistribution**: To preserve core temperature, the body redirects blood flow away from the skin and extremities towards vital organs. This is known as vasoconstriction. While it helps maintain core temperature, it can also reduce muscle performance and increase the risk of frostbite in exposed skin.

- **Metabolic Rate**: Cold exposure can increase your basal metabolic rate (BMR) as your body works harder to maintain its core temperature. This can have implications for energy expenditure and caloric needs.

- **Hormonal Changes**: Cold exposure can lead to changes in hormone levels, including an increase in norepinephrine, which can have various effects such as increased alertness and reduced pain perception.

- **Oxygen Consumption**: Cold air is often denser than warm air, which can affect the respiratory system. Some people may experience increased oxygen consumption during cold-weather exercise, which can affect aerobic performance.

- **Immune Response**: There's some evidence to suggest that regular cold exposure can strengthen the immune system, although the mechanisms are not yet fully understood.

Understanding these physiological changes can help you adapt your training strategies to cold environments. For example, you may need to adjust your caloric intake to account for increased energy expenditure or take extra precautions to protect your extremities from reduced blood flow.

Training in Cold Environments

Training in cold conditions requires a unique approach to ensure both safety and effectiveness. Here are some in-depth strategies and considerations:

- **Warm-Up**: A thorough warm-up is even more crucial in cold conditions to prepare your muscles and cardiovascular system for exercise. Consider a longer warm-up period or even starting your warm-up indoors before heading out.

- **Nutrition**: Cold weather increases caloric burn due to the body's efforts to maintain core temperature. Make sure to consume enough calories to propel your workout and aid in recovery.

- **Footwear**: Choose shoes with good traction to prevent slips and falls on icy or snowy surfaces. Some athletes opt for specialized cold-weather footwear that provides extra insulation.

- **Skin Protection**: Cold wind and low temperatures can cause skin irritation or even frostbite. Use a skin barrier cream and lip balm, and cover as much skin as possible with clothing.

- **Breathing**: Cold air can be harsh on the respiratory system. Some athletes use a face mask or scarf to warm the air before it enters the lungs. This is especially important for those with asthma or other respiratory conditions.

- **Hydration**: It's easy to neglect hydration in colder weather because you might not feel as thirsty. However, you're still losing fluids through sweat and respiration, so keep hydrating.

- **Pacing**: Your body will fatigue more quickly in the cold, especially if you're not acclimated. Be mindful of your pacing and consider reducing the intensity or duration of your workout until you're more accustomed to the conditions.

- **Cool-Down**: Just as with the warm-up, a proper cool-down is essential to help your body transition back to a resting state. This is especially important in cold conditions to help prevent a rapid drop in core body temperature.

- **Post-Workout Nutrition**: Given the increased caloric expenditure, post-workout nutrition is crucial. Focus on a balanced meal that includes carbohydrates, protein, and fats to aid in recovery.

- **Monitoring Weather Conditions**: Always check the weather forecast before heading out and be prepared to adjust your plans. Pay attention to wind chill and precipitation, as both can significantly impact your safety and performance.

By taking these factors into account, you can make your cold-weather training both effective and safe. The key to successful training in the cold is preparation and adaptability. Always listen to your body and be willing to modify your workout plan as needed.

Cold and Recovery

The cold environment not only affects your training but also your recovery process. Here's how:

- **Reduced Inflammation**: Cold temperatures can reduce inflammation, which is why ice baths and cold packs are commonly used in recovery protocols. However, it's essential to balance this with the body's natural inflammatory response, which aids in healing.

- **Delayed Onset Muscle Soreness (DOMS)**: Cold exposure may help alleviate symptoms of DOMS by reducing muscle inflammation and improving blood circulation during the recovery phase.

- **Cryotherapy**: This is a more controlled form of cold exposure used to aid recovery. While the scientific evidence is still inconclusive, some athletes report benefits like reduced muscle soreness and improved mood.

- **Vasoconstriction and Vasodilation**: The cold induces vasoconstriction, reducing blood flow to the extremities. This can be followed by vasodilation, or increased blood flow, once you warm up. This cycle can help flush out metabolic waste products from the muscles.

- **Nutritional Needs**: As mentioned earlier, cold environments can increase caloric expenditure. This has implications for recovery nutrition, as you may need to consume more calories to adequately recover and prepare for your next training session.

- **Hydration**: Cold weather can suppress the thirst mechanism, leading to reduced fluid intake and potential dehydration. Proper hydration is crucial for recovery, so make sure to drink fluids even if you don't feel thirsty.

- **Sleep Quality**: Cold environments can affect sleep quality, which is a critical aspect of recovery. While some people find it easier to sleep in a cooler room, extreme cold can disrupt sleep patterns and impair recovery.

- **Psychological Recovery**: Training in harsh conditions can be mentally tasking. Make sure to include mental recovery strategies, such as mindfulness and relaxation techniques, to help you mentally recover from the added stress of cold-weather training.

Understanding how cold environments affect your recovery can help you make informed decisions about your post-workout routines. Whether it's adjusting your nutrition, incorporating cold-based recovery methods, or simply ensuring you stay hydrated, these considerations are crucial for optimizing your recovery in cold conditions.

Altitude Training: Benefits, Risks, and Practical Guidelines

Physiological Responses to Altitude

When you train at high altitudes, your body undergoes a series of physiological adaptations to cope with the reduced oxygen availability. Understanding these changes can help you adapt your training strategies. Here are some of the key physiological responses:

- **Hypoxia**: The most immediate challenge at high altitudes is hypoxia, or reduced oxygen levels. This triggers physiological responses aimed at improving the body's oxygen-carrying capacity.

- **Erythropoiesis**: One of the most significant adaptations is the stimulation of erythropoiesis, the production of red blood cells. This increases the blood's ability to carry oxygen, which can improve performance once you return to lower altitudes.

- **Hemoglobin Affinity**: At high altitudes, the affinity of hemoglobin for oxygen changes, allowing it to pick up and release oxygen more efficiently. This is a compensatory mechanism to mitigate the effects of hypoxia.

- **Respiratory Changes**: You may experience an increased respiratory rate as your body tries to take in more oxygen. While this is effective in the short term, it can lead to respiratory alkalosis, a condition where blood pH rises, if sustained over long periods.

- **Cardiovascular Adjustments**: Your heart rate and cardiac output may initially increase to pump more oxygenated blood to the tissues. However, these levels often normalize as you acclimate to the altitude.

- **Metabolic Shifts**: The body may shift from aerobic to anaerobic metabolism for energy production due to the limited availability of oxygen. This can affect endurance and lead to quicker fatigue.

- **Muscle Oxygen Saturation**: The reduced oxygen levels can lead to lower muscle oxygen saturation, affecting muscle function and potentially leading to quicker fatigue.

- **Endocrine Responses**: Altitude can affect various hormone levels, including cortisol and epinephrine, which can have implications for stress, metabolism, and recovery.

Understanding these physiological responses can help you adapt your training and recovery strategies when at high altitudes. It's crucial to monitor these changes and consult with healthcare providers to ensure you're adapting safely to the new environment.

High-Altitude Training: Strategies and Considerations

Training at high altitudes has been a popular strategy among elite athletes for decades. However, it comes with its own challenges and considerations. Here's what you need to know:

- **Live High, Train Low**: This is a common approach where athletes live at high altitudes to benefit from increased red blood cell production but train at lower altitudes where they can maintain higher training intensities. This strategy aims to get the best of both worlds.

- **Acclimatization Phase**: Before diving into your regular training regimen, spend at least two to three weeks acclimating to the altitude. During this phase, focus on lower-intensity workouts and gradually increase the volume and intensity as your body adapts.

- **Oxygen Saturation Monitoring**: Some athletes use pulse oximeters to monitor their oxygen saturation levels during workouts. This can help you adjust your training intensity in real-time to avoid overexertion.

- **Nutritional Adjustments**: At high altitudes, your metabolic rate may increase, requiring additional caloric intake. Also, consider increasing your iron intake to support increased erythropoiesis.

- **Hydration**: Due to lower air pressure and humidity, you may lose more fluids through respiration. Make sure to stay well-hydrated to support optimal performance and recovery.

- **Rest and Recovery**: The physiological stress of high-altitude training can extend recovery times. Make sure to incorporate more rest days or active recovery sessions into your training program.

- **Altitude Tents and Masks**: For those who can't train at high altitudes, simulated altitude devices like tents and masks can offer some of the benefits of high-altitude training. However, the effectiveness of these devices is still a subject of ongoing research.

- **Consulting Experts**: Due to the complex physiological responses to high-altitude training, it's advisable to consult with healthcare providers and sports scientists. They can help you tailor your training program and monitor your health markers.

You can optimize your training program to achieve your performance goals while minimizing risks by understanding the unique challenges and benefits of high-altitude training. Always remember that individual responses to altitude can vary, so it's crucial to listen to your body and make adjustments as needed.

Acclimatization to Altitude: A Step-by-Step Guide

Acclimatizing to high altitudes is a critical step for anyone planning to train or compete in such environments. The process involves a series of physiological adaptations that help your body cope with reduced oxygen levels. Here's a step-by-step guide to acclimatization:

- **Initial Exposure**: The first few days at high altitude are crucial. You may experience symptoms like headaches, fatigue, and shortness of breath. It's advisable to keep physical activity to a minimum during this period.

- **Gradual Increase in Activity**: After the initial exposure, start incorporating light physical activities like walking or jogging. Monitor your body's response closely and avoid overexertion.

- **Oxygen Saturation Monitoring**: Use a pulse oximeter to keep track of your oxygen saturation levels. If levels drop significantly during or after exercise, it's a sign that you need more time to acclimate.

- **Nutritional Support**: Increase your intake of iron-rich foods or supplements to support the production of hemoglobin, which is essential for oxygen transport. Also, stay well-hydrated to help with blood circulation.

- **Altitude-Specific Workouts**: As you acclimate, you can start incorporating workouts designed to exploit the benefits of high-altitude training, such as interval training with reduced oxygen. However, the intensity should still be lower than what you would do at sea level.

- **Rest and Recovery**: Given the added stress of training at altitude, make sure to allocate more time for rest and recovery. This includes both sleep and active recovery techniques like stretching and foam rolling.

- **Symptom Monitoring**: Keep an eye out for symptoms of altitude sickness, such as severe headaches, nausea, and extreme fatigue. If you experience any of these symptoms, consider descending to a lower altitude and seeking medical advice.

- **Time Frame**: It usually takes about two to three weeks for the body to fully acclimate to high altitudes. However, individual responses can vary, so listen to your body and adjust your acclimatization schedule accordingly.

- **Re-acclimatization**: If you leave the high-altitude environment for more than a few days, you'll likely need to go through a re-acclimatization process when you return. The length of this process depends on how long you were away and how well you maintained your fitness during that time.

By following these steps and monitoring your body's response, you can acclimate more effectively to high altitudes, allowing you to train and compete at your best while minimizing risks.

Periodization Strategies

Heat and Periodization: Integrating Thermal Stress into Training Cycles

Incorporating heat exposure into your periodized training plan can offer unique benefits but also requires careful planning. Here's how to integrate heat and periodization effectively:

- **Microcycle Adjustments**: During specific microcycles (typically a week), consider incorporating heat exposure sessions. These could be in the form of hot weather training, sauna sessions, or heated indoor workouts. The goal is to acclimate the body to heat stress gradually.

- **Mesocycle Planning**: In the broader mesocycle (several weeks to a few months), you should aim to align heat exposure with specific training goals. For example, if a mesocycle focuses on endurance, heat training can be particularly beneficial as it improves cardiovascular efficiency and sweat response.

- **Heat Acclimation Phases**: Just like altitude, heat acclimation should be phased in gradually. Consider a 1-2 week period where the primary focus is on getting accustomed to heat stress. This can be done before entering a more intense training phase.

- **Training Intensity**: Heat stress adds an extra layer of difficulty to workouts. Be prepared to adjust training intensity and volume during heat exposure sessions. Overexertion in hot conditions can lead to heat-related illnesses like heat exhaustion or heat stroke.

- **Hydration and Nutrition**: Heat exposure increases sweat rates, leading to higher fluid and electrolyte loss. Adjust your hydration and nutrition strategies to account for this additional stress.

- **Rest and Recovery**: Heat stress can prolong recovery times. Make sure to incorporate adequate rest days and consider using cooling strategies after workouts, such as cold water immersion, to speed up recovery.

- **Tapering and Peaking**: If you're planning to compete in hot conditions, align your tapering phase with the end of a heat acclimation cycle. This will ensure that you're both acclimated to the heat and at peak physical condition for the event.

- **Monitoring and Feedback**: Use metrics like core body temperature, heart rate, and perceived exertion to monitor your response to heat training. This data can help you make real-time adjustments to your training plan.

By thoughtfully integrating heat exposure into your periodized training plan, you can exploit the physiological benefits of heat acclimation while minimizing risks. As always, consult with healthcare providers and sports science experts to tailor your approach.

Cold and Periodization: Strategically Incorporating Cold Exposure into Training Cycles

Just as heat and altitude can be integrated into a periodized training plan, so can cold exposure. Here's how to do it effectively:

- **Microcycle Considerations**: You should designate specific sessions for cold exposure in a weekly training cycle. These could be outdoor workouts in cold weather or even controlled cold exposure like ice baths post-workout.

- **Mesocycle Alignment**: Over a longer training cycle (several weeks to months), align your cold exposure with specific training objectives. For instance, if you're focusing on strength, cold exposure can be used to aid in recovery and reduce inflammation.

- **Cold Acclimation Phases**: Similar to heat and altitude, it's beneficial to have a phase dedicated to acclimating to cold conditions. This could be a week or two where the focus is less on training intensity and more on getting accustomed to the cold.

- **Intensity and Volume Adjustments**: Cold conditions can affect your performance and perceived exertion. Be prepared to adjust your training intensity and volume accordingly during cold exposure sessions.

- **Nutritional Adjustments**: Cold environments can increase your metabolic rate, requiring additional caloric intake for both performance and recovery. Make sure to adjust your nutrition plan to meet these needs.

- **Hydration**: Cold weather can suppress the thirst mechanism, making it easy to neglect hydration. Ensure you're consuming enough fluids before, during, and after training.

- **Rest and Recovery**: Cold exposure, especially when not acclimated, can be stressful on the body, requiring longer recovery times. Make sure to incorporate adequate rest and active recovery sessions into your training plan.

- **Tapering and Peaking**: If you're preparing for an event in cold conditions, align your tapering phase with a period of cold acclimation. This ensures that you're at peak performance and fully acclimated to the cold environment.

- **Monitoring and Adaptation**: Keep track of key metrics like core body temperature, heart rate, and rate of perceived exertion (RPE) during cold exposure sessions. This data can help you adapt your training plan in real-time to optimize performance and safety.

You can harness the benefits of cold for recovery and performance while minimizing the risks associated with cold stress by carefully integrating cold exposure into your periodized training plan. As always, consult healthcare providers and sports science experts to channel your approach.

Altitude and Periodization: Synchronizing Altitude Training with Training Cycles

Incorporating altitude training into a periodized plan requires a nuanced approach to maximize benefits and minimize risks. Here's how to integrate altitude and periodization effectively:

- **Microcycle Planning**: Within your weekly training cycle, consider designating specific days for altitude training. These sessions should be carefully planned to align with your overall training objectives, whether they be endurance, strength, or speed.

- **Mesocycle Strategy**: Over a longer training cycle (several weeks to months), aim to synchronize your altitude training with specific phases of your periodization plan. For example, if you're in a hypertrophy phase, altitude training can be incorporated to potentially enhance red blood cell production and oxygen-carrying capacity.

- **Acclimatization Blocks**: Before going into high-intensity training at altitude, allocate a block of time (usually 2-3 weeks) for acclimatization. During this phase, the focus should be on moderate exercise and adaptation to the lower oxygen levels.

- **Training Intensity and Volume**: Altitude adds an extra layer of physiological stress, so be prepared to adjust your training intensity and volume. Overexertion at high altitudes can lead to altitude sickness and other health risks.

- **Nutritional Adjustments**: The metabolic demands at high altitudes may require an increase in caloric and micronutrient intake. Pay special attention to hydration as well, as the lower humidity can lead to quicker dehydration.

- **Rest and Recovery**: The stress of altitude training can extend recovery periods. Make sure to incorporate more rest days or lighter training days into your schedule to facilitate optimal recovery.

- **Tapering and Peaking**: If you're preparing for a competition at altitude, align your tapering phase with the end of an altitude acclimatization block. This ensures that you're both acclimated and at peak performance for the event.

- **Monitoring and Feedback**: Utilize metrics such as oxygen saturation, heart rate, and perceived exertion to gauge your body's response to altitude training. This data can inform real-time adjustments to your training plan.

By thoughtfully integrating altitude training into your periodized plan, you can exploit its unique physiological benefits while minimizing potential risks. As always, consult healthcare providers and sports science experts to tailor your altitude training strategy.

Case Studies on Training in Extreme Environments

Desert Ultra-Marathoners

The challenge of running an ultra-marathon in a desert environment is a unique test of human endurance and adaptability. The following case studies provide insights into how athletes prepare for and cope with such extreme conditions.

- **Preparation Phase**: Desert ultra-marathoners often undergo a rigorous training regimen that includes long-distance running, strength training, and heat acclimation. Some athletes even train in heat chambers to simulate desert conditions.

- **Nutritional Strategy**: Due to the extreme heat and physical exertion, these athletes require a specialized nutritional plan. This often includes high-calorie foods that are easy to digest, as well as electrolyte supplements to replace the salts lost through sweating.

- **Hydration Management**: Staying hydrated is a critical challenge. Athletes often carry hydration packs and have access to water stations along the route. Some also use oral rehydration solutions to maintain electrolyte balance.

- **Heat Acclimation**: Prior to the event, athletes spend time acclimating to the heat, either by training in similar environments or using heat adaptation techniques like hot baths or saunas.

- **Footwear and Gear**: Due to the sandy and often uneven terrain, choosing the right footwear is crucial. Many opt for shoes with extra grip and ankle support. Lightweight, moisture-wicking clothing is also essential.

- **Mental Toughness**: The psychological aspect of enduring extreme heat and fatigue is often cited as the most challenging part of the race. Athletes employ various mental strategies, such as visualization and mindfulness, to cope with physical and mental stress.

- **Race Strategy**: Pacing is crucial in desert ultra-marathons. Athletes often employ a run-walk strategy to conserve energy. They also take advantage of cooler temperatures during the early morning or late evening for more strenuous stretches.

- **Recovery**: Post-race recovery involves rehydration, nutrient replenishment, and active recovery techniques like stretching and foam rolling. Due to the extreme conditions, some athletes also undergo medical checks to assess their electrolyte levels and overall health.

- **Outcomes and Lessons**: Those who successfully complete a desert ultra-marathon often cite meticulous preparation, adaptability, and mental resilience as key factors. These case studies serve as valuable lessons for anyone looking to compete in extreme environments, offering insights into the strategies and mindset required for such extraordinary challenges.

Arctic Adventure Racers

Arctic adventure racing is a grueling sport that tests the limits of human endurance in some of the coldest environments on Earth. Here's how these athletes prepare for and adapt to the extreme cold:

- **Preparation Phase**: Training for an Arctic adventure race is a complex process that involves cardiovascular conditioning, strength training, and specific skills like navigation and survival techniques. Many racers also undergo cold exposure training to acclimate to the frigid temperatures they will face.

- **Nutritional Strategy**: The extreme cold increases metabolic demands, requiring a higher caloric intake. Athletes often rely on high-fat, high-protein diets to sustain energy levels and maintain body temperature.

- **Clothing and Gear**: Proper clothing is crucial for survival in Arctic conditions. Athletes use layered clothing systems designed for moisture-wicking, insulation, and wind resistance. Specialized gear like snowshoes, skis, and ice axes are also essential.

- **Cold Acclimation**: Prior to the race, athletes spend time acclimating to cold conditions. This can involve training in cold chambers, ice baths, or natural cold environments.

- **Mental Resilience**: The psychological toll of racing in extreme cold is significant. Athletes use mental conditioning techniques like mindfulness and positive visualization to prepare for the challenges ahead.

- **Race Strategy**: Pacing is even more critical in cold environments, where exhaustion can quickly lead to a drop in body temperature. Athletes often employ a conservative pacing strategy and take regular breaks to check their physical condition and equipment.

- **Health Monitoring**: During the race, athletes must constantly monitor for signs of frostbite, a drop in body temperature, and dehydration. Many races have medical checkpoints where athletes are assessed for these and other conditions.

- **Recovery**: Post-race recovery is a complex process that involves rehydration, nutritional replenishment, and warming the body to restore normal temperature. Athletes also undergo medical checks to assess any cold-related injuries or conditions.

- **Outcomes and Lessons**: Successfully completing an Arctic adventure race is a monumental achievement that requires meticulous preparation, adaptability, and mental toughness. These case studies provide a roadmap for athletes looking to compete in extreme cold, offering insights into the physiological adaptations and strategies required for such challenging endeavors.

High-Altitude Mountaineers

Scaling the world's highest peaks is an endeavor that pushes the boundaries of human physiology and mental fortitude. Here's a look at how high-altitude mountaineers prepare for and adapt to these extreme conditions:

- **Preparation Phase**: Training for high-altitude mountaineering is multifaceted, involving cardiovascular conditioning, strength training, and technical skills like rope work and crevasse rescue. Many mountaineers also engage in lower-altitude climbs to prepare for the unique challenges of high-altitude environments.

- **Nutritional Strategy**: At high altitudes, appetite can be suppressed, making nutrient-dense foods crucial. Many mountaineers rely on high-calorie, easy-to-digest foods and supplements to meet their energy needs.

- **Acclimatization**: A significant portion of the preparation involves acclimatizing to high altitudes. This is usually done in stages, with mountaineers spending time at various elevations to allow their bodies to adapt to the reduced oxygen levels.

- **Oxygen and Equipment**: Many high-altitude mountaineers use supplemental oxygen to help combat the effects of altitude sickness. The right equipment, including specialized clothing and climbing gear, is also vital for safety and performance.

- **Mental Resilience**: The psychological challenges of high-altitude mountaineering are immense, from coping with isolation to managing fear and uncertainty. Mental preparation techniques like meditation and visualization are often employed.

- **Climbing Strategy**: Due to the extreme conditions and unpredictable weather, a flexible climbing strategy is essential. Mountaineers must be prepared to adjust their plans based on real-time assessments of their own condition and external factors like weather.

- **Health Monitoring**: Regular health checks, including monitoring oxygen saturation levels and signs of altitude sickness, are crucial. Many expeditions include medical professionals skilled in high-altitude medicine.

- **Recovery**: After the climb, recovery involves not just physical rest but also careful monitoring for delayed onset of altitude-related illnesses. Nutritional replenishment and rehydration are also critical components of post-climb recovery.

- **Outcomes and Lessons**: Successfully summiting a high-altitude peak requires a combination of physical preparation, mental resilience, and the ability to adapt to rapidly changing conditions. These case studies offer invaluable insights into the strategies and mindset required for high-altitude endeavors, serving as a guide for future mountaineers.

Conclusion

Understanding how the body adapts to different environmental conditions can help you optimize your training and push your limits. Whether you're an athlete looking for a competitive edge or a fitness enthusiast seeking new challenges, training in heat, cold, or at altitude offers unique opportunities for growth and adaptation. As we conclude this comprehensive guide, let's examine some key takeaways and reflections:

- **Harnessing Environmental Factors**: One of the central themes of this book is the power of environmental factors as tools for training adaptation. Whether it's the heat of the desert, the cold of the Arctic, or the thin air of high altitudes, each environment offers a unique set of challenges and benefits that can be harnessed to improve performance and resilience.

- **Individualized Approach**: It's crucial to remember that everyone's body responds differently to environmental stressors. Therefore, an individualized approach to training, backed by scientific understanding and self-monitoring, is essential for optimal results.

- **The Role of Periodization**: As explored in various chapters, periodization isn't just for traditional athletic training; it's also crucial for preparing for extreme environments. Structured training cycles allow for targeted physiological adaptations and provide opportunities for recovery, reducing the risk of overtraining or injury.

- **Nutritional Strategies**: Adapting to extreme environments often requires specialized nutritional strategies. Whether it's higher caloric needs in the cold or electrolyte balance in the heat, understanding the nutritional demands of each environment is key to performance and safety.

- **Mental Resilience**: The psychological aspects of training in extreme conditions are often as challenging as the physical ones. Techniques like mindfulness, visualization, and positive self-talk are invaluable tools for building the mental toughness required to succeed.

- **Safety and Monitoring**: Regardless of the environment, safety should always be a top priority. This involves not only proper preparation and equipment but also real-time health monitoring to minimize risks and respond to potential issues as they arise.

- **Lifelong Learning**: The journey to mastering physical performance in extreme environments is ongoing. As research evolves and new techniques emerge, there will always be more to learn and ways to improve.

By taking a comprehensive, scientifically grounded approach to training in extreme environments, you can push the boundaries of what you thought possible, achieving new levels of performance and resilience. This book aims to be a foundational resource in that journey, providing the knowledge and strategies needed to face and overcome the challenges of the world's most demanding conditions.

CHAPTER 12

━◆━

CASE STUDIES

In this chapter, we examine muscle building through detailed accounts of various individuals' journeys. Each story offers a unique perspective, highlighting different approaches, challenges, and triumphs in the pursuit of muscle growth. Interestingly, readers can gain valuable insights, draw inspiration, and apply the lessons learned to their own fitness endeavors by exploring these real-life experiences. Below is a selection of compelling case studies.

Case Study 1: John's Transformation

John, a 30-year-old professional, embarked on a remarkable journey of transformation from being overweight and out of shape to achieving a muscular physique. His story is a testament to the power of determination, consistent effort, and a holistic approach to fitness. Let's delve into the details of John's inspiring transformation:

Mindset Shift and Igniting Change: For John, the catalyst for change came in the form of a mindset shift. He realized that his sedentary lifestyle and unhealthy habits were taking a toll on his physical and mental well-being. This realization ignited a deep desire for transformation and motivated him to take control of his health.

Challenges Faced: John encountered various challenges throughout his transformation journey. One of the major hurdles was overcoming years of unhealthy eating habits and sedentary behavior. He had to break free from his comfort zone and push through moments of doubt and temptation. Additionally, finding the time to exercise regularly amidst his demanding professional life posed a significant challenge.

Strategies Employed: To build muscle and shed excess body fat, John implemented a comprehensive and balanced approach to his fitness routine:

1. Nutrition: John adopted a healthy and sustainable eating plan. He focused on consuming nutrient-dense whole foods, including lean proteins, fruits, vegetables, whole grains, and healthy fats. He paid attention to portion control and made sure to fuel his body with the right balance of macronutrients.

2. Resistance Training: John incorporated regular strength training workouts into his routine. He followed a well-designed program that targeted different muscle groups and included exercises such as squats, deadlifts, bench presses, and rows. He gradually increased the intensity and weight lifted over time to stimulate muscle growth and strength development.

3. Cardiovascular Exercise: John recognized the importance of cardiovascular exercise for overall health and fat loss. He incorporated regular cardio sessions, such as running, cycling, or HIIT workouts, to increase his calorie burn and improve cardiovascular fitness.

4. Consistency and Progression: John maintained a consistent exercise routine, ensuring that he worked out several times a week. He gradually progressed his workouts by increasing weights, repetitions, or intensity to continually challenge his muscles and promote growth.

5. Accountability and Support: John sought support from a fitness coach and joined a community of like-minded individuals who provided motivation, guidance, and accountability. Having a support system helped him stay focused and committed to his goals.

Results and Lessons Learned: Through his dedication and adherence to his fitness plan, John achieved remarkable results. He transformed his physique, shedding excess body fat and building lean muscle mass. Beyond the physical changes, John also experienced increased energy levels, improved self-confidence, and enhanced mental well-being.

John's journey highlights several valuable lessons for those aspiring to achieve a similar transformation:

1. Mindset is Key: A shift in mindset is crucial to initiating change and staying committed to your goals. Believe in your ability to transform and embrace the journey.

2. Consistency is Essential: Consistent effort, both in nutrition and exercise, is vital for sustainable results. Small, daily actions compound over time to create significant change.

3. Embrace a Holistic Approach: Combine proper nutrition, resistance training, and cardiovascular exercise for optimal results. Take a comprehensive approach that addresses all aspects of your health and fitness.

4. Seek Support and Accountability: Surround yourself with a supportive network, whether it's a coach, workout partner, or an online community. They can provide guidance, motivation, and accountability along the way.

5. Celebrate Milestones: Recognize and celebrate your achievements, no matter how small. Each milestone reached is a stepping stone toward your ultimate goal.

John's transformation serves as an inspiration to anyone looking to make positive changes in their life. By adopting a holistic approach, staying consistent, and fostering a positive mindset, one can achieve remarkable transformations and unlock their full potential.

As we conclude this case study, it becomes evident that the pursuit of muscle building is a deeply personal and transformative journey. It requires commitment, discipline, and a willingness to adapt and learn along the way. Whether one's goal is to develop a competitive physique, enhance functional strength, or simply lead a healthier lifestyle, these case studies demonstrate that with the right mindset, knowledge, and dedication, remarkable transformations are within reach. Remember that every journey is unique, and results may vary. Stay committed, trust the process, and embrace the transformative power of your own personal fitness journey.

Case Study 2: Sarah's Bodybuilding Journey

Sarah, a dedicated bodybuilder in her early 40s, embarked on an inspiring journey towards competing in bodybuilding competitions. Her story showcases the incredible dedication, perseverance, and attention to detail required for high-level bodybuilding. Here's the details of Sarah's journey:

Passion Ignited and Goal Set: Sarah's passion for bodybuilding ignited when she witnessed the physical transformations and the incredible dedication of athletes in the sport. Inspired by their muscular physiques and disciplined lifestyles, she set a goal to compete in bodybuilding competitions and push her body to its limits.

Intense Training Regimen: Sarah committed herself to an intense training regimen designed to sculpt her physique and develop the muscle mass required for bodybuilding. Her workouts consisted of compound exercises, isolation exercises, and techniques to target specific muscle groups. She focused on progressive overload, gradually increasing the weights lifted and the intensity of her training sessions.

Meticulous Nutrition Planning: To support her training and achieve the desired muscle development, Sarah adopted a meticulously planned nutrition strategy. She calculated her macronutrient requirements, ensuring an adequate intake of proteins, carbohydrates, and fats. She prioritized whole, nutrient-dense foods and carefully timed her meals to optimize muscle growth and recovery.

Disciplined Lifestyle: Bodybuilding requires a disciplined lifestyle, and Sarah fully embraced it. She adhered to a strict schedule, ensuring she had sufficient time for training, meal preparation, rest, and recovery. She prioritized quality sleep to facilitate muscle repair and growth. She abstained from unhealthy habits and incorporated stress management techniques to maintain a positive mental state.

Attention to Detail: Sarah paid meticulous attention to every aspect of her bodybuilding journey. She tracked her progress, monitored her body composition, and adjusted her training and nutrition accordingly. She sought guidance from experienced coaches, who provided expertise and valuable feedback to optimize her physique and posing techniques.

Competition Preparation: As Sarah approached her first bodybuilding competition, her training and nutrition became even more focused and intense. She fine-tuned her posing routines, ensuring precision and grace on stage. She engaged in posing practice sessions to showcase her physique with confidence and poise.

Results and Lessons Learned: Sarah's dedication and commitment paid off as she stepped onto the competition stage, showcasing her already-developed physique and impressive muscles. Apart from gaining recognition, Sarah learned invaluable lessons throughout her journey:

1. Passion and Purpose: Pursuing a fitness goal propelled by passion and purpose provides the drive and motivation needed to overcome challenges and stay committed.

2. Consistency and Persistence: Consistency in training, nutrition, and lifestyle habits is essential for achieving significant results. Persistence through setbacks and obstacles is key to long-term success.

3. Attention to Detail: Paying close attention to every aspect of training, nutrition, and posing enhances performance and optimizes results.

4. Seek Guidance and Support: Engaging with experienced coaches and building a support system helps undergo the complexities of bodybuilding, provides valuable feedback, and keeps motivation high.

5. Embrace the Process: Embrace the journey and appreciate the personal growth and discipline required in bodybuilding. Celebrate milestones along the way and find joy in the daily progress.

Sarah's bodybuilding journey serves as a powerful example of how passion, commitment, and attention to detail can lead to extraordinary achievements. Her story inspires readers to pursue their own fitness goals with dedication, perseverance, and the understanding that transformation is possible at any age.

As we conclude this case study, remember that bodybuilding is a demanding sport that requires careful planning, discipline, and commitment. Find joy in the process, learn from each experience, and allow your passion for fitness to drive you towards achieving your goals.

Case Study 3: Emily's Functional Strength Quest

Emily, a 28-year-old fitness enthusiast, embarked on a captivating journey to develop functional strength through various training methods. Her story highlights the importance of versatility, adaptability, and continuous learning in achieving well-rounded strength and fitness. The details of Emily's inspiring quest are as follows:

Exploration of Different Disciplines: Emily recognized that functional strength encompassed more than just raw muscle power. Determined to enhance her overall athleticism and functional capabilities, she went into various disciplines, including calisthenics, weightlifting, and martial arts. This exploration allowed her to experience the unique benefits and challenges offered by each discipline.

Calisthenics and Bodyweight Training: Emily began her journey with calisthenics, focusing on bodyweight exercises to develop strength, mobility, and body control. She mastered fundamental movements such as push-ups, pull-ups, squats, and planks. Through consistent practice and progressive overload, she gradually increased the difficulty of her exercises, incorporating advanced variations like handstand push-ups and muscle-ups.

Weightlifting and Resistance Training: Recognizing the importance of external resistance for building strength, Emily ventured into weightlifting. She incorporated barbell squats, deadlifts, and bench presses into her routine to develop full-body strength and power. With proper form and progressive overload, she steadily increased the weights she lifted, challenging her muscles and stimulating growth.

Martial Arts and Functional Movement: To further enhance her functional strength, Emily explored martial arts disciplines such as Brazilian Jiu-Jitsu and Muay Thai. These disciplines provided opportunities to apply her strength and agility in practical and dynamic ways. The combination of striking, grappling, and footwork drills improved her overall coordination, speed, and functional movement patterns.

Versatility and Adaptability: Emily realized that true functional strength involves being adaptable to different physical challenges. She incorporated agility drills, plyometrics, and unconventional training tools such as kettlebells, medicine balls, and resistance bands into her workouts. This variety helped her develop versatility, agility, and the ability to perform well in a wide range of movements and activities.

Continuous Learning and Growth: Throughout her journey, Emily maintained a mindset of continuous learning and growth. She sought guidance from experienced coaches, attended workshops, and engaged in online communities to expand her knowledge and refine her techniques. This commitment to learning allowed her to constantly evolve and improve her functional strength.

Results and Lessons Learned: Emily's dedication and commitment to exploring various training methods and disciplines resulted in significant improvements in her functional strength and overall fitness. She experienced enhanced mobility, agility, and the ability to perform daily tasks with ease. Along her journey, she learned valuable lessons:

1. Versatility is Key: Developing functional strength requires a diverse range of exercises and training modalities. Embrace a variety of disciplines to challenge your body in different ways and develop well-rounded strength.

2. Adaptability Leads to Progress: Be adaptable in your training approach. Continuously challenge yourself with new exercises, equipment, and movement patterns to improve your functional capabilities.

3. Continuous Learning Enhances Growth: Seek knowledge and guidance from experts and peers. Attend workshops, engage in communities, and never stop learning. Embrace feedback and make adjustments where necessary to refine your techniques.

4. Patience and Persistence Pay Off: Building functional strength takes time and consistency. Embrace the process, stay patient, and remain persistent. Celebrate each milestone achieved along the way.

Emily's functional strength quest exemplifies the transformative power of versatility, adaptability, and continuous learning. Her story inspires readers to explore different training methods, challenge themselves in various disciplines, and embrace the journey of developing functional strength. Remember, functional strength goes beyond pure muscle size and promotes a well-rounded, capable body that can perform optimally in everyday activities and physical pursuits.

As we conclude this case study, embrace the versatility of your fitness journey. Explore different disciplines, be adaptable, and maintain a commitment to continuous growth. Develop functional strength that transcends the gym and enhances your overall physical abilities.

Case Study 4: Mike's Powerlifting Journey

Mike, a seasoned powerlifter in his mid-30s, shares his remarkable journey from being a recreational lifter to competing at national powerlifting championships. His story delves into the specific training protocols, periodization strategies, and mindset required to maximize strength gains and improve performance in the sport. Mike's journey highlights the importance of goal specificity, structured programming, and mental fortitude in the pursuit of strength and power. Below are the details of Mike's inspiring powerlifting journey:

From Recreational Lifting to Competitive Powerlifting: Mike's passion for lifting began as a recreational hobby. However, as he witnessed the incredible strength feats of competitive powerlifters, he set his sights on becoming a formidable athlete in the sport. This shift in mindset sparked his journey towards powerlifting excellence.

Goal Specificity and Structured Programming: To achieve his powerlifting goals, Mike understood the importance of goal specificity and structured programming. He set clear targets for his squat, bench press, and deadlift, focusing on increasing his one-repetition maximum (1RM) in each lift. With the guidance of a knowledgeable coach, Mike followed a meticulously designed training program designed to suit his strengths, weaknesses, and competition schedule.

Periodization and Progressive Overload: Mike embraced the principles of periodization and progressive overload to optimize his strength gains. His training program was structured into distinct phases, each targeting different aspects of strength development. He underwent cycles of higher volume and lower intensity, gradually building up to phases of higher intensity and lower volume as the competition neared. Mike stimulated his muscles to adapt and grow stronger by progressively increasing the weights he lifted over time.

Mental Fortitude and Mindset: In addition to physical training, Mike recognized the importance of mental fortitude and mindset in powerlifting. He developed mental resilience, focusing on positive self-talk, visualization, and confidence-building strategies. He learned to channel his energy and overcome challenges, such as lifting heavy weights and pushing through moments of doubt or fatigue.

Competition Preparation: As Mike prepared for the national powerlifting championships, his training intensified. He honed his technique, ensuring optimal form and maximizing his lifting efficiency. He practiced his lifts under competition conditions, visualizing success and mentally practicing each attempt. Mike also paid close attention to his nutrition, ensuring proper reinforcement and recovery to support his training and optimize performance on competition day.

Results and Lessons Learned: Mike's dedication, structured programming, and mental fortitude paid off as he competed at national powerlifting championships. He achieved personal bests, set new records, and experienced the thrill of competing at the highest level in the sport. Along his journey, Mike learned valuable lessons:

1. Goal Specificity Drives Progress: Clearly define your powerlifting goals and focus your training on specific lifts and performance targets. This provides direction and motivation throughout your journey.

2. Structured Programming Yields Results: Follow a well-designed training program that incorporates periodization, progressive overload, and tailored exercises to optimize strength gains and minimize the risk of injury.

3. Mental Fortitude Enhances Performance: Cultivate a positive mindset, practice visualization, and develop mental resilience. Powerlifting requires mental strength as much as physical strength.

4. Competition Prep is Crucial: Pay attention to the details of competition preparation. Adjust your technique, practice lifts under competition conditions, and prioritize nutrition and recovery for peak performance.

Mike's powerlifting journey serves as a testament to the transformative power of goal specificity, structured programming, and mental fortitude. His story inspires readers to set ambitious goals, embrace structured training, and cultivate a resilient mindset in their own pursuit of strength and power.

As we conclude this case study, remember that powerlifting is a demanding sport that requires dedication, discipline, and a commitment to continuous improvement. Harness your passion, train smart, and embrace the journey of becoming a stronger, more powerful version of yourself.

Case Study 5: Sophia's Sustainable Muscle Growth

Sophia, a busy working professional in her late 20s, embarked on a journey to achieve sustainable muscle growth while balancing the demands of her career and personal life. Her story serves as a testament to the power of time management, prioritization, and making informed choices regarding nutrition and training. Sophia's experience shows that with proper planning, consistency, and realistic expectations, muscle growth can be achieved even in the midst of a hectic lifestyle. Here are the details of Sophia's inspiring journey:

Time Management and Prioritization: Sophia recognized the importance of time management and prioritization to pursue her muscle growth goals effectively. She carefully evaluated her daily schedule, identifying pockets of time where she could dedicate herself to workouts and meal preparation. By making fitness a priority and aligning her schedule accordingly, Sophia ensured she had dedicated time for her training sessions and proper nutrition.

Informed Choices Regarding Nutrition: Sophia understood that nutrition played a vital role in supporting muscle growth. Despite her busy schedule, she made informed choices about her meals. She focused on consuming balanced meals rich in protein, carbohydrates, and healthy fats. Sophia incorporated lean sources of protein such as chicken, fish, and plant-based options, along with whole grains, fruits, and vegetables. She paid attention to portion sizes, ensuring she met her nutritional needs while maintaining a calorie balance suitable for her goals.

Consistency in Training: Sophia recognized the importance of consistency in her training regimen. She committed to a regular workout schedule, which included resistance training sessions targeting different muscle groups. She followed a structured program designed by a fitness professional, gradually increasing the weights and intensity over time. Sophia stayed consistent with her workouts, even on busy days, understanding that small, consistent efforts compound to produce significant results.

Realistic Expectations and Progress Tracking: Sophia approached her muscle growth journey with realistic expectations. She understood that sustainable progress takes time and that transformations don't happen overnight. Sophia tracked her progress by keeping a workout journal and measuring key indicators such as strength gains and body measurements. This allowed her to celebrate small victories and make informed adjustments to her training and nutrition as needed.

Efficient Training Techniques: Given her busy schedule, Sophia implemented efficient training techniques to optimize her workouts. She incorporated compound exercises that targeted multiple muscle groups simultaneously, maximizing her time in the gym. She also explored high-intensity interval training (HIIT) and circuit training, which provided effective workouts in shorter durations. These strategies allowed her to make the most of her limited time while still stimulating muscle growth.

Balancing Work, Life, and Fitness: Sophia recognized the importance of balancing her work, personal life, and fitness goals. She integrated physical activity into her daily routine, such as taking the stairs instead of the elevator and incorporating short bursts of activity during breaks. Sophia also sought support from her loved ones, explaining her fitness goals and enlisting their understanding and encouragement. Also, she managed to stay committed to her muscle growth journey without neglecting other aspects of her life by finding a balance and involving her support network.

Results and Lessons Learned: Through her consistent efforts, strategic planning, and realistic expectations, Sophia achieved sustainable muscle growth. She witnessed her strength and endurance improve, and her physique became more toned and defined. During the process, Sophia learned valuable lessons:

1. Prioritization and Time Management: Make fitness a priority and manage your time effectively to incorporate workouts and proper nutrition into your busy schedule.

2. Informed Nutrition Choices: Make informed choices about your nutrition, ensuring you consume balanced meals that support your muscle growth goals.

3. Consistency Trumps Perfection: Consistency in training and nutrition is key to sustainable progress. Stay committed, even on busy days, and understand that small consistent efforts lead to significant results over time.

4. Track Progress and Celebrate Milestones: Keep a workout journal and track your progress. Celebrate small victories along the way and make adjustments based on your results.

5. Balancing Work, Life, and Fitness: Find a balance that allows you to pursue your fitness goals while maintaining other aspects of your life. Involve your support network for understanding and encouragement.

Sophia's journey exemplifies that with proper planning, consistency, and realistic expectations, sustainable muscle growth is achievable even with a busy lifestyle. Her story inspires readers to prioritize their fitness goals, make informed choices, and find a balance that allows them to thrive both personally and physically.

As we conclude this case study, remember that sustainable muscle growth is a journey, and the key lies in consistency, informed choices, and finding a balance that suits your unique circumstances. Embrace the process, celebrate your progress, and enjoy the benefits of a stronger, healthier body.

Conclusion

These case studies showcase the diverse paths individuals have taken to achieve their muscle-building goals. By examining their unique journeys, readers can gain valuable insights into the importance of mindset, goal setting, nutrition, training methodologies, and maintaining a balanced lifestyle. Each story offers valuable lessons and practical takeaways that can be applied to individual circumstances and aspirations.

CONCLUSION

The Journey Beyond Muscle University

As we conclude our exploration into muscle growth and performance, it's crucial to pause and appreciate the comprehensive knowledge we've walked through together. From the intricacies of muscle anatomy to the profound strategies of training, recovery, and the pivotal mind-muscle connection, this guide has been a great tool that defines muscle growth.

Muscle development goes beyond the mere act of lifting weights or the consumption of protein-rich diets. It's a combination of physical, mental, and emotional elements, working in tandem. Our muscles, far from being mere anatomical structures, are deeply intertwined with our nervous system, hormonal balance, and even our psychological state. This holistic understanding is the cornerstone to unlocking unparalleled potential.

The multifaceted nature of our bodies, underscored by the significance of periodization, the rejuvenating role of sleep, the grounding essence of mindfulness, and the subtle yet profound impact of environmental factors, emphasizes a singular truth: Achieving optimal muscle growth demands a holistic approach. It's not merely about the weights; it's about the intention, technique, and holistic strategy surrounding each lift.

Every individual's journey to muscle growth is unique, and shaped by personal goals, challenges, and experiences. While this book offers a roadmap, the true adventure is deeply personal, filled with moments of self-discovery, boundary-pushing, and realization of one's potential.

As you progress in your fitness journey, remember that muscle growth is a harmonious pursuit for the mind and body. Embrace challenges as growth opportunities, savor your successes, learn from setbacks, and always prioritize progress over perfection. The path to peak performance is a dynamic one, filled with highs and lows, but with dedication, resilience, and the insights from this guide, it's a journey that promises unparalleled rewards.

MUSCLE UNIVERSITY

Thank you for allowing 'Muscle University' to be a beacon on your journey. Here's to a future of strength, growth, and boundless potential. As you continue to push boundaries and grow, always remember to be the best version of yourself, both inside and out.

To your strength and success,

Dr. Lee Doernte.

SCIENTIFIC REFERENCES SUPPORTING MUSCLE UNIVERSITY

1. Ahlborg, G., and P. Felig. Influence of glucose ingestion on the fuel-hormone response during prolonged exercise. J Appl Physiol 41:683-688. 1967.

2. Ahlborg, G., and P. Felig. Lactate and glucose exchange across the forearm, legs and splanchnic bed during and after prolonged leg exercise. J Clin Invest 69:45-54. 1982.

3. Albert, M. Eccentric Muscle Training in Sports and Orthopaedics. New York: Churchill Livingstone. 1995.

4. Allerheilegen, B., and R. Rogers. Plyometrics program design. Strength Cond 17(4):26-31. 1995.

5. American College of Sports Medicine. ACSM's Guidelines for Exercise Testing and Prescription, 7th ed. Baltimore: Williams & Wilkins. 2006.

6. American College of Sports Medicine. Exercise and physical activity for older adults. Med Sci Sports Exerc 30:992-1008. 1998.

7. American Orthopaedic Society for Sports Medicine. Proceedings of the Conference on Strength Training and the Prepubescent. Chicago: 1988.

8. Asmussen, E., and F. Bonde-Peterson. Storage of elastic energy in skeletal muscles in man. Acta Physiol Scand 91:385-392. 1974.

9. Åstrand, P., K. Rodahl, H.A. Dahl, and S.B. Strømme. Textbook of Work Physiology, 4th ed. Champaign, IL: Human Kinetics. 2003.

10. Aura, O., and J.T. Viitasalo. Biomechanical characteristics of jumping. Int J Sport Biomech 5(1):89-97. 1989.

11. Baechle, T.R., and B.R. Groves. Weight Training: Steps to Success, 2nd ed. Champaign, IL: Human Kinetics. 1998.

12. Baker, D., G. Wilson, and R. Carlyon. Periodization: The effect on strength of manipulating volume and intensity. J Strength Cond Res 8:235-242. 1994.

13. Barany, M., and C. Arus. Lactic acid production in intact muscle, as followed by 13C and 1H nuclear magnetic resonance. In: Human Muscle Power, N.L. Jones, N. McCartney, and A.J. McComas, eds. Champaign, IL: Human Kinetics. 1990. pp. 153-164.

14. Barnard, R.J., V.R. Edgerton, T. Furakawa, and J.B. Peter. Histochemical, biochemical and contractile properties of red, white and intermediate fibers. Am J Physiol 220:410-441. 1971.

15. Bean, R. M. (2017). The effects of depth jump implementation of sprint performance in collegiate and club sport athletes, Eastern Kentucky University.

16. Bean, R., Doernte, L., Lane, M. (2017). "Impact Kinetics of Depth Jumps with Varying Heights and the Relationships to Body Composition of Individuals."

17. Beck, K.C., and B.D. Johnson. Pulmonary adaptations to dynamic exercise. In: American College of Sports Medicine Resource Manual for Guidelines for Exercise Testing and Prescription, 3rd ed., J.L. Roitman, ed. Baltimore: Williams & Wilkins. 1998. pp. 305-313.

18. Bell, Z. W. (2017). The Effects Of Caffeine Supplementation When Manipulating The Time Of Ingestion Prior To Simulated Rugby Union Activity, Eastern Kentucky University.

19. Bergman, R.A., and A.K. Afifi. Atlas of Microscopic Anatomy. Philadelphia: Saunders. 1974.

20. Billeter, R., and H. Hoppeler. Muscular basis of strength. In: Strength and Power in Sport, P.V. Komi, ed. Boston: Blackwell Scientific. 1992. pp. 39-63.

21. Blanksby, B., and J. Gregor. Anthropometric, strength, and physiological changes in male and female swimmers with progressive resistance training. Aust J Sport Sci 1:3-6. 1981.

22. Bobbert, M.F. Drop jumping as a training method for jumping ability. Sports Med 9(1):7-22. 1990.

23. Bobbert, M.F., K.G.M. Gerritsen, M.C.A. Litjens, and A.J. Van Soest. Why is countermovement jump height greater than squat jump height? Med Sci Sports Exerc 28:1402-1412. 1996.

24. Bompa, T.A. Theory and Methodology of Training. Dubuque, IA: Kendall/Hunt. 1983.

25. Boobis, I., C. Williams, and S.N. Wooten. Influence of sprint training on muscle metabolism during brief maximal exercise in man. J Physiol 342:36P-37P. 1983.

26. Bosco, C., A. Ito, P.V. Komi, P. Luhtanen, P. Rahkila, H. Rusko, and J.T. Viitasalo. Neuromuscular function and mechanical efficiency of human leg extensor muscles during jumping exercises. Acta Physiol Scand 114:543-550. 1982.

27. Bosco, C., and P.V. Komi. Potentiation of the mechanical behavior of the human skeletal muscle through prestretching. Acta Physiol Scand 106:467-472. 1979.

28. Bosco, C., J.T. Viitasalo, P.V. Komi, and P. Luhtanen. Combined effect of elastic energy and myoelectrical potentiation during stretch shortening cycle exercise. Acta Physiol Scand 114:557-565. 1982.

29. Bosco, C., P.V. Komi, and A. Ito. Pre-stretch potentiation of human skeletal muscle during ballistic movement. Acta Physiol Scand 111:135-140. 1981.

30. Bridges, C.R., B.J. Clark, III, R.L. Hammond, and L.W. Stephenson. Skeletal muscle bioenergetics during frequency-dependent fatigue. Am J Physiol 29:C643-C651. 1991.

31. Brooks, G.A. Amino acid and protein metabolism during exercise and recovery. Med Sci Sports Exerc 19:S150-S156. 1987.

32. Brooks, G.A. The lactate shuttle during exercise and recovery. Med Sci Sports Exerc 18:360-368. 1986.

33. Brooks, G.A., K.E. Brauner, and R.G. Cassens. Glycogen synthesis and metabolism of lactic acid after exercise. Am J Physiol 224:1162-1186. 1973.

34. Brooks, G.A., T.D. Fahey, and K.M. Baldwin. Exercise Physiology: Human Bioenergetics and Its Application, 4th ed. New York: McGraw-Hill. 2005.

35. Burgomaster, K.A., G.J.F. Heigenhauser, and M.J. Gibala. Effect of short-term sprint interval training on human skeletal muscle carbohydrate metabolism during exercise and time-trial performance. J Appl Physiol 100:2041-2047. 2006.

36. Burgomaster, K.A., S.C. Hughes, G.J.F. Heigenhauser, S.N. Bradwell, and M.J. Gibala. Six sessions of sprint interval training increases muscle oxidative potential and cycle endurance capacity in humans. J Appl Physiol 98:1985-1990. 2005.

37. Campbell, W., M. Crim, V. Young, and W. Evans. Increased energy requirements and changes in body composition with resistance training in older adults. Am J Clin Nutr 60:167-175. 1994.

38. Campbell, W., M. Crim, V. Young, J. Joseph, and W. Evans. Effects of resistance training and dietary protein intake on protein metabolism in older adults. Am J Appl Physiol 268:E1143-E1153. 1995.

39. Carling, D. AMP-activated protein kinase: Balancing the scales. Biochimie 87(1):87-91. 2005.

40. Carnethon, M., M. Gulati, and P. Greenland. Prevalence and cardiovascular disease correlates of low cardiorespiratory fitness in adolescents and adults. JAMA 294:2981-2988. 2005.

41. Castro, M., D. McCann, J. Shaffrath, and W. Adams. Peak torque per unit cross-sectional area differs between strength-training and untrained adults. Med Sci Sports Exerc 27:397-403. 1995.

42. Cavagna, G.A. Storage and utilization of elastic energy in skeletal muscle. In: Exercise and Sport Science Reviews, vol. 5, R.S. Hutton, ed. Santa Barbara, CA: Journal Affiliates. 1977. pp. 80-129.

43. Cavagna, G.A., B. Dusman, and R. Margaria. Positive work done by a previously stretched muscle. J Appl Physiol 24:21-32. 1968.

44. Cavagna, G.A., F.P. Saibere, and R. Margaria. Effect of negative work on the amount of positive work performed by an isolated muscle. J Appl Physiol 20:157-158. 1965.

45. Centers for Disease Control and Prevention. Strength training among adults ≥65 years—United States, 2001. MMWR 53:1-4. 2004.

46. Cerretelli, P., D. Rennie, and D. Pendergast. Kinetics of metabolic transients during exercise. Int J Sports Med 55:178-180. 1980.

47. Cerretelli, P., G. Ambrosoli, and M. Fumagalli. Anaerobic recovery in man. Eur J Appl Physiol 34:141-148. 1975.

48. Charette, S., L. McEvoy, G. Pyka, C. Snow-Harter, D. Guido, R. Wiswell, and R. Marcus. Muscle hypertrophy response to resistance training in older women. J Appl Physiol 70:1912-1916. 1991.

49. Chargina, A., M. Stone, J. Piedmonte, H. O'Bryant, W.J. Kraemer, V. Gambetta, H. Newton, G. Palmeri, and D. Pfoff. Periodization roundtable. NSCA J 8(5):12-23. 1986.

50. Christmas, C., and R. Andersen. Exercise and older patients. Guidelines for the clinician. J Am Geriatr Soc 48:318-324. 2000.

51. Chu, D. Jumping Into Plyometrics, 2nd ed. Champaign, IL: Human Kinetics. 1998.

52. Chu, D., A. Faigenbaum, and J. Falkel. Progressive Plyometrics for Kids. Monterey, CA: Healthy Learning. 2006.

53. Chu, D., and L. Plummer. Jumping into plyometrics: The language of plyometrics. NSCA J 6(5):30-31. 1984.

54. Colliander, E., and P. Tesch. Bilateral eccentric and concentric torque of quadriceps and hamstrings in females and males. Eur J Appl Physiol 59:227-232. 1989.

55. Colliander, E., and P. Tesch. Responses to eccentric and concentric resistance training in females and males. Acta Physiol Scand 141:149-156. 1990.

56. Collopy, P., Lane, M., Doernte, L. Bean, R. and Owsley, Z. (2019). "Analyzing Fat Free Mass Index in Division IAA Football Players." Journal of Strength and Conditioning Research 33(2): e26-e27.

57. Constantin-Teodosiu, D., P.L. Greenhaff, D.B. McIntyre, J.M. Round, and D.A. Jones. Anaerobic energy production in human skeletal muscle in intense contraction: A comparison of 31P magnetic resonance spectroscopy and biochemical techniques. Exp Physiol 82:593-601. 1997.

58. Cramer, J.T. Creatine supplementation in endurance sports. In: Essentials of Creatine in Sports, J. Stout, J. Antonio, and D. Kalman, eds. New York: Springer. 2007.

59. Creer, A.R., M.D. Ricard, R.K. Conlee, G.L. Hoyt, and A.C. Parcell. Neural, metabolic, and performance adaptations to four weeks of high intensity sprint-interval training in trained cyclists. Int J Sports Med 25:92-98. 2004.

60. Cruse, J. L. (2018). The Acute Effects Of Alpha-Gpc On Hand Grip Strength, Jump Height, Power Output, Mood, And Reaction-Time In Recreationally Trained, College-Aged Individuals, Eastern Kentucky University.

61. Cureton, K., M. Collins, D. Hill, and F. McElhannon. Muscle hypertrophy in men and women. Med Sci Sports Exerc 20:338-344. 1988.

62. Davis, J.A., M.H. Frank, B.J. Whipp, and K. Wasserman. Anaerobic threshold alterations caused by endurance training in middle-aged men. J Appl Physiol 46:1039-1046. 1979.

63. De Vos, N., N. Singh, D. Ross, T. Stavrinos, R. Orr, and M. Singh. Optimal load for increasing muscle power during explosive resistance training in older adults. J Gerontol A Biol Sci Med Sci 60:638-647. 2005.

64. DiPrampero, P.E., L. Peeters, and R. Margaria. Alactic O2 debt and lactic acid production after exhausting exercise in man. J Appl Physiol 34:628-632. 1973.

65. Doernte, L. (2017). "Examination of Relationship Between Body Composition and Scoring Potential of Female Collegiate Soccer Players."

66. Doernte, L. (2018). Use Of Dual Energy X-Ray Absorptiometry Measurements To Evaluate Total Body Volume When Compared To Air Displacement Plethysmography For Evaluating Body Composition In A Four Compartment Model, Eastern Kentucky University.

67. Doernte, L. (2022). Effect of Metronome, Hospital Mattress, and Step Stool Usage on Chest Compression Rate and Depth During Cardiopulmonary Resuscitation (CPR): A Collection of Systematic Reviews and Meta-Analyses, ProQuest Dissertations & Theses Global.

68. Doernte, L. Lane, M. and Bean, R. (2017). "Relationship Between Preseason Football Injuries and Reinjuries, Body Weight Changes, Cumulative Stress, and Practice Times in Division I Athletes." Journal of Strength and Conditioning Research 31(S1-S81): S30.

69. Doernte, L., Lane, M., and Bean, R. (2017). "Relationships Between Injuries, re-injuries, Body Weight Change, and Time of Practice."

70. Drinkwater, B. Weight-bearing exercise and bone mass. Phys Med Rehabil Clin N Am 6:567-578. 1995.

71. Dudley, G.A., and R. Djamil. Incompatibility of endurance- and strength-training modes of exercise. J Appl Physiol 59(5):1446-1451. 1985.

72. Dudley, G.A., and R. Terjung. Influence of aerobic metabolism on IMP accumulation in fast-twitch muscle. Am J Physiol 248:C37-C42. 1985.

73. Dudley, G.A., and T.F. Murray. Energy for sport. NSCA J 3(3):14-15. 1982.

74. Dudley, G.A., R.T. Harris, M.R. Duvoisin, B.M. Hather, and P. Buchanan. Effect of voluntary versus artificial activation on the relation of muscle torque to speed. J Appl Physiol 69:2215-2221. 1990.

75. Dursenev, L., and L. Raeysky. Strength training for jumpers. Soviet Sports Rev 14(2):53-55. 1979.

76. Durstine, J.L., and P.G. Davis. Specificity of exercise training and testing. In: American College of Sports Medicine Resource Manual for Guidelines for Exercise Testing and Prescription, 3rd ed., J.L. Roitman, ed. Baltimore: Williams & Wilkins. 1998. pp. 472-479.

77. Edington, D.E., and V.R. Edgerton. The Biology of Physical Activity. Boston: Houghton Mifflin. 1976.

78. Enoka, R.M. Neuromechanical Basis of Kinesiology, 2nd ed. Champaign, IL: Human Kinetics. 1994.

79. Ericksson, B.O., P.D. Gollnick, and B. Saltin. Muscle metabolism and enzyme activities after training in boys 11-13 years old. Acta Physiol Scand 87:485-497. 1973.

80. Essen, B. Glycogen depletion of different fiber types in man during intermittent and continuous exercise. Acta Physiol Scand 103:446-455. 1978.

81. Evans, W. Exercise training guidelines for the elderly. Med Sci Sports Exerc 31:12-17. 1999.

82. Evans, W. What is sarcopenia? J Gerontol 50A:5-8. 1995.

83. Fabiato, A., and F. Fabiato. Effects of pH on the myofilaments and sarcoplasmic reticulum of skinned cells from cardiac and skeletal muscle. J Physiol 276:233-255. 1978.

84. Falk, B., and A. Eliakim. Resistance training, skeletal muscle and growth. Pediatr Endocrinol Rev 1:120-127. 2003.

85. Fiatarone, M., E. Marks, N. Ryan, C. Meredith, L. Lipsitz, and W. Evans. High-intensity strength training in nonagenarians: Effects on skeletal muscle. JAMA 263:3029-3034. 1990.

86. Fleck, S.J. Periodized strength training: A critical review. J Strength Cond Res 13(1):82-89. 1999.

87. Fleck, S.J., and W.J. Kraemer. Designing Resistance Training Programs, 3rd ed. Champaign, IL: Human Kinetics. 2003.

88. Fleck, S.J., and W.J. Kraemer. Resistance training: Exercise prescription. Phys Sportsmed 16:69-81. 1988.

89. Fowler, N.E., A. Lees, and T. Reilly. Changes in stature following plyometric drop-jump and pendulum exercises. Ergonomics 40:1279-1286. 1997.

90. Fowler, N.E., A. Lees, and T. Reilly. Spinal shrinkage in unloaded and loaded drop-jumping. Ergonomics 37:133-139. 1994.

91. Freund, H., and P. Gendry. Lactate kinetics after short strenuous exercise in man. Eur J Appl Physiol 39:123-135. 1978.

92. Frontera, W., C. Meredith, K. O'Reilly, H. Knuttgen, and W. Evans. Strength conditioning of older men: Skeletal muscle hypertrophy and improved function. J Appl Physiol 42:1038-1044. 1988.

93. Fuchs, F., Y. Reddy, and F.N. Briggs. The interaction of cations with calcium binding site of troponin. Biochim Biophys Acta 221:407-409. 1970.

94. Galvao, D., and D. Taaffe. Resistance training for the older adult.: Manipulating training variables to enhance muscle strength. J Strength Cond Res 27:48-54. 2005.

95. Gambetta, V. Plyometric training. Track Field Q Rev 80(4):56-57. 1978.

96. Garhammer, J. A comparison of maximal power outputs between elite male and female weightlifters in competition. Int J Sport Biomech 7:3-11. 1991.

97. Garhammer, J. A review of power output studies of Olympic and powerlifting: Methodology, performance prediction and evaluation tests. J Strength Cond Res 7:76-89. 1993.

98. Garhammer, J. Periodization of strength training for athletes. Track Tech 73:2398-2399. 1979.

99. Garrett, R.H., and C.M. Grisham. Biochemistry, 2nd ed. Fort Worth: Saunders College Publishing. 1999.

100. Gastin, P.B. Energy system interaction and relative contribution during maximal exercise. Sports Med 31(10):725-741. 2001.

101. Gollnick, P.D., and L. Hermansen. Significance of skeletal muscle oxidative enzyme enhancement with endurance training. Clin Physiol 2:1-12. 1982.

102. Gollnick, P.D., and W.M. Bayly. Biochemical training adaptations and maximal power. In: Human Muscle Power, N.L. Jones, N. McCartney, and A.J. McComas, eds. Champaign, IL: Human Kinetics. 1986. pp. 255-267.

103. Gollnick, P.D., R.B. Armstrong, B. Saltin, W. Saubert, and W.L. Sembrowich. Effect of training on enzyme activity and fiber composition of human muscle. J Appl Physiol 34:107-111. 1973.

104. Gollnick, P.D., R.B. Armstrong, W. Saubert, K. Piel, and B. Saltin. Enzyme activity and fibre composition in skeletal muscle of untrained and trained men. J Appl Physiol 33:312-319. 1972.

105. Gollnick, P.D., W.M. Bayly, and D.R. Hodgson. Exercise intensity, training diet and lactate concentration in muscle and blood. Med Sci Sports Exerc 18:334-340. 1986.

106. Grasberger, K. (2017). "Examination of body composition and performance metrics of division I collegiate baseball players."

107. Grassi, B. Delayed metabolic activation of oxidative phosphorylation in skeletal muscle at exercise onset. Med Sci Sports Exerc 37(9):1567-1573. 2005.

108. Häkkinen, K., A. Pakarinen, and M. Kallinen. Neuromuscular adaptations and serum hormones in women during short-term intensive strength training. Eur J Appl Physiol 64:106-111. 1992.

109. Häkkinen, K., A. Pakarinen, H. Kyrolainen, S. Cheng, D. Kim, and P. Komi. Neuromuscular adaptations and serum hormones in females during prolonged power training. Int J Sports Med 11:91-98. 1990.

110. Häkkinen, K., A. Pakarinen, P.V. Komi, T. Ryushi, and H. Kauhanen. Neuromuscular adaptations and hormone balance in strength athletes, physically active males and females during intensity strength training. In: Proceedings of the XII International Congress of Biomechanics, R.J. Gregor, R.F. Zernicke, and W. Whiting, eds. Champaign, IL: Human Kinetics. 1989. pp. 889-894.

111. Hamill, B. Relative safety of weight lifting and weight training. J Strength Cond Res 8:53-57. 1994.

112. Harris, R.C., R.H.T. Edwards, E. Hultman, L.O. Nordesjo, B. Nylind, and K. Sahlin. The time course of phosphocreatinine resynthesis during recovery of the quadriceps muscle in man. Pflugers Arch 97:392-397. 1976.

113. Harris, R.T., and G.A. Dudley. Factors limiting force during slow, shortening muscle actions in vivo. Acta Physiol Scand 152:63-71. 1994.

114. Hather, B.M., P.A. Tesch, P. Buchanan, and G.A. Dudley. Influence of eccentric actions on skeletal muscle adaptations to resistance. Acta Physiol Scand 143:177-185. 1991.

115. Henwood, T., and D. Taaffe. Improved physical performance in older adults undertaking a short-term programme of high-velocity resistance training. Gerontology 51:108-115. 2005.

116. Hermansen, L. Effect of metabolic changes on force generation in skeletal muscle during maximal exercise. In: Human Muscle Fatigue, R. Porter and J. Whelan, eds. London: Pittman Medical. 1981.

117. Hermansen, L., and I. Stenvold. Production and removal of lactate in man. Acta Physiol Scand 86:191-201. 1972.

118. Hewett, T.E., A.L. Stroupe, T.A. Nance, and F.R. Noyes. Plyometric training in female athletes. Am J Sports Med 24:765-773. 1996.

119. Hickson, R.C. Interference of strength development by simultaneously training for strength and endurance. Eur J Appl Physiol 215:255-263. 1980.

120. Hickson, R.C., B.A. Dvorak, E.M. Gorostiaga, T.T. Kurowski, and C. Foster. Potential for strength and endurance training to amplify endurance performance. J Appl Physiol 65(5):2285-2290. 1988.

121. Hickson, R.C., M.A. Rosenkoetter, and M.M. Brown. Strength training effects on aerobic power and short-term endurance. Med Sci Sports Exerc 12:336-339. 1980.

122. Hill, A.V. First and Last Experiments in Muscle Mechanics. Cambridge: Cambridge University Press. 1970.

123. Hill, A.V. Muscular exercise, lactic acid and the supply and utilization of oxygen. Proc Roy Soc Lond (Biol) 96:438. 1924.

124. Hirvonen, J., S. Ruhunen, H. Rusko, and M. Harkonen. Breakdown of high-energy phosphate compounds and lactate accumulation during short submaximal exercise. Eur J Appl Physiol 56:253-259. 1987.

125. Holloway, J. A summary chart: Age related changes in women and men and their possible improvement with training. J Strength Cond Res 12:126-128. 1998.

126. Housh, T.J., D.J. Housh, and H.A. DeVries. Applied Exercise and Sport Physiology, 2nd ed. Scottsdale, AZ: Holcomb Hathaway. 2006.

127. Hultman, E., and H. Sjoholm. Biochemical causes of fatigue. In: Human Muscle Power, N.L. Jones, N. McCartney, and A.J. McComas, eds. Champaign, IL: Human Kinetics. 1986. pp. 215-235.

128. Hultsmann, W.C. On the regulation of the supply of substrates for muscular activity. Bibl Nutr Diet 27:11-15. 1979.

129. Hunter, G.R., and M.I. Culpepper. Joint angle specificity of fixed mass versus hydraulic resistance knee flexion training. J Strength Cond Res 9(1):13-16. 1995.

130. Hunter, G.R., and M.I. Culpepper. Knee extension torque joint position relationships following isotonic fixed resistance and hydraulic resistance training. Athl Training 23(1):16-20. 1988.

131. Hunter, G.R., B.R. Newcomer, R.L. Weinsier, D.L. Karapondo, D.E. Larson-Meyer, D.R. Joanisse, and M.M. Bamman. Age is independently related to muscle metabolic capacity in premenopausal women. J Appl Physiol 93:70-76. 2002.

132. Hunter, G.R., J.P. McCarthy, and M.M. Bamman. Effects of resistance training on older adults. Sports Medicine 34(5):329-348. 2003.

133. Hunter, G.R., M.M. Bamman, D.E. Larson-Meyer, D.R. Joanisse, J.P. McCarthy, T.E. Blaudeau, and B.R. Newcomer. Inverse relationship between exercise economy and oxidative capacity in muscle. Eur J Appl Physiol 94:558-568. 2005.

134. Hurley, B.F., D.R. Seals, J.M. Hagberg, A.C. Goldberg, S.M. Ostrove, J.O. Holloszy, W.G. Wiest, and A.P. Goldberg. Strength training and lipoprotein lipid profiles: Increased HDL cholesterol in body builders versus powerlifters and effects of androgen use. JAMA 252:507-513. 1984.

135. Imamura, K., H. Ashida, T. Ishikawa, and M. Fujii. Human major psoas muscle and sacrospinalis muscle in relation to age: A study by computed tomography. J Gerontol 38:678-681. 1983.

136. Isaacs, J. P., Lane, M., Sciascia, A., Sabian, M., Doernte, L., and Bean, R. (2017). "Examination of Relationships Between Body Composition and In-Season Performance, by Player Position in Collegiate Softball Players."

137. Isaacs, J. P., Lane, M., Sciascia, A., Sabian, M., Doernte, L., and Bean, R. (2018). "Effects of Fire Gear on Predicted VO2 Max."

138. Isaacs, J. P., Lane, M., Sciascia, A., Sabian, M., Doernte, L., and Bean, R. (2018). "Heart Rate, Weight Loss, and RPE Response to Submaximal Walking Test."

139. Isaacs, J. Lane, M., Sciascia, A., Sabin, M. Bean, R. and Doernte, L. (2019). "Effects of Fire Gear on Predicted VO2max." Journal of Strength and Conditioning Research 33(2): e189-e190.

140. Jacobs, I. Blood lactate: Implications for training and sports performance. Sports Med 3:10-25. 1986.

141. Jacobs, I., P. Kaiser, and P. Tesch. Muscle strength and fatigue after selective glycogen depletion in human skeletal muscle fibers. Eur J Appl Physiol 46:47-53. 1981.

142. Jacobs, I., P.A. Tesch, O. Bar-Or, J. Karlsson, and R. Dotow. Lactate in human skeletal muscle after 10 and 30 s of supramaximal exercise. J Appl Physiol 55:365-367. 1983.

143. Jette, A., and L. Branch. The Framingham disability study: II. Physical disability among the aging. Am J Public Health 71:1211-1216. 1981.

144. Juel, C. Intracellular pH recovery and lactate efflux in mouse soleus muscles stimulated in vitro: The involvement of sodium/proton exchange and a lactate carrier. Acta Physiol Scand 132:363-371. 1988.

145. Karatzaferi, C., A. de Haan, R. Ferguson, W. van Mechelen, and A. Sargeant. Phosphocreatine and ATP content in human single muscle fibers before and after maximum dynamic exercise. Pflugers Arch 442:467-474. 2001.

146. Karlsson, J. Lactate and phosphagen concentrations in working muscle of man. Acta Physiol Scand 485:358-365. 1971.

147. Karlsson, J., L.O. Nordesjo, L. Jorfeldt, and B. Saltin. Muscle lactate, ATP and CP levels during exercise and after physical training in man. J Appl Physiol 33(2):194-203. 1972.

148. Kilani, H.A., S.S. Palmer, M.J. Adrian, and J.J. Gapsis. Block of the stretch reflex of vastus lateralis during vertical jump. Human Mvmt Sci 8:247-269. 1989.

149. Kindermann, W., G. Simon, and J. Keul. The significance of the aerobic-anaerobic transition for the determination of work load intensities during endurance training. Eur J Appl Physiol 42:25-34. 1979.

150. Klug, G.A., and G.F. Tibbits. The effect of activity on calcium mediated events in striated muscle. In: Exercise and Sport Science Reviews, vol. 16, K.B. Pandolf, ed. New York: Macmillan. 1988. pp. 1-60.

151. Komi, P.V. Training of muscle strength and power: Interaction of neuromotoric, hypertrophic, and mechanical factors. Int J Sports Med 7(suppl.):101-105. 1986.

152. Korchemny, R. Evaluation of sprinters. NSCA J 7(4):38-42. 1985.

153. Kraemer, W. Endocrine responses to resistance exercise. Med Sci Sports Exerc 20(suppl.):152-157. 1988.

154. Kraemer, W., A. Fry, P. Frykman, B. Conroy, and J. Hoffman. Resistance training and youth. Pediatr Exerc Sci 1:336-350. 1989.

155. Kraemer, W., K. Adams, E. Cafarelli, G. Didley, C. Dooly, M. Feigenbaum, S. Fleck, B. Franklin, R. Newtown, J. Potteiger, M. Stone, N. Ratamess, and T. Triplet-McBride. Progression models in resistance training for healthy adults. Med Sci Sports Exerc 34:364-380. 2002.

156. Kraemer, W., S. Mazzetti, B. Nindl, L. Gotshalk, J. Bush, J. Marx, K. Dohi, A. Gomez, M. Miles, S. Fleck, R. Newton, and K. Häkkinen. Effect of resistance training on women's strength/power and occupational performances. Med Sci Sports Exerc 33:1011-1025. 2001.

157. Kraemer, W.J. A series of studies: The physiological basis for strength training in American football: Fact over philosophy. J Strength Cond Res 11(3):131-142. 1997.

158. Kraemer, W.J., and L.P. Koziris. Muscle strength training: Techniques and considerations. Phys Ther Pract 2:54-68. 1992.

159. LaChance, P. Plyometric exercise. Strength Cond 17:16-23. 1995.

160. Lane, M., Doernte, L. Spears, A., Bean, R., and Moon, J. "Relationships Between Dual-Energy X-Ray Absorptiometry Bone Mineral Content and Bone Mineral Density and Standing and Sitting Bioimpedance Spectroscopy Variables in Healthy Men and Women." The FASEB Journal 32: 768.710-768.710.

161. Lane, M., Doernte, L. Spears, A., Bean, R., and Moon, J. (2018). "Effects of Body Position and Electrode Type on the Reliability of Bioimpedance Spectroscopy: 3356 Board# 225 June 2 9." Medicine & Science in Sports & Exercise 50(5S): 834.

162. Lane, M., Grassenberger, K., Doernte, L. Hartsell, R. Wagganer, J. and Barnes, J. (2019). "Body Composition and Body Composition Relative to Height in Collegiate Softball Players." Journal of Strength and Conditioning Research 33(2): e98.

163. Larry, J.A., and S.F. Schaal. Normal electrocardiograms. In: American College of Sports Medicine Resource Manual for Guidelines for Exercise Testing and Prescription, 3rd ed., J.L. Roitman, ed. Baltimore: Williams & Wilkins. 1998. pp. 397-401.

164. Layne, J., and M. Nelson. The effects of progressive resistance training on bone density: A review. Med Sci Sports Exerc 31:25-30. 1999.

165. Lehmann, M., and J. Keul. Free plasma catecholamines, heart rates, lactate levels, and oxygen uptake in competition weightlifters, cyclists, and untrained control subjects. Int J Sports Med 7:18-21. 1986.

166. Lexell, J., and D. Downham. What is the effect of ageing on Type II muscle fibers? J Neurol Sci 107:250-251. 1992.

167. Luhtanen, P., and P. Komi. Mechanical factors influencing running speed. In: Biomechanics VI-B, E. Asmussen, ed. Baltimore: University Park Press. 1978. pp. 23-29.

168. MacDougall, J.D., G.R. Ward, D.G. Sale, and J.R. Sutton. Biochemical adaptations of human skeletal muscle to heavy resistance training and immobilization. J Appl Physiol 43:700-703. 1977.

169. Mainwood, G., and J. Renaud. The effect of acid-base on fatigue of skeletal muscle. Can J Physiol Pharmacol 63:403-416. 1985.

170. Matveyev, L.P. Periodization of Sports Training. Moscow: Fisculturai Sport. 1966.

171. Mayhew, J., and P. Salm. Gender differences in anaerobic power tests. Eur J Appl Physiol 60:133-138. 1990.

172. Mazzeo, R.S., G.A. Brooks, D.A. Schoeller, and T.F. Budinger. Disposal of blood [1-13C] lactate in humans during rest and exercise. J Appl Physiol 60(10):232-241. 1986.

173. McArdle, W.D., F.I. Katch, and V.I. Katch. Exercise Physiology, 6th ed. Philadelphia: Williams & Wilkins. 2007.

174. McArdle, W.D., F.I. Katch, and V.L. Katch. Exercise Physiology: Energy, Nutrition, and Human Performance, 6th ed. Philadelphia: Lippincott, Williams & Wilkins. 2007.

175. McCartney, N. Acute responses to resistance training and safety. Med Sci Sports Exerc 31:31-37. 1999.

176. McCartney, N., L.L. Spriet, G.J.F. Heigenhauser, J.M. Kowalchuk, J.R. Sutton, and N.L. Jones. Muscle power and metabolism in maximal intermittent exercise. J Appl Physiol 60:1164-1169. 1986.

177. McComas, A.J. Skeletal Muscle: Form and Function. Champaign, IL: Human Kinetics. 1996.

178. Medboe, J.I., and S. Burgers. Effect of training on the anaerobic capacity. Med Sci Sports Exerc 22(4):501-507. 1991.

179. Meltzer, D. Age dependence of Olympic weightlifting ability. Med Sci Sports Exerc 26:1053-1067. 1994.

180. Metter, E., R. Conwit, J. Tobin, and J. Fozard. Age-associated loss of power and strength in the upper extremities in women and men. J Gerontol Biol Sci Med 52:B267-276. 1997.

181. Miller, A., J. MacDougall, M. Tarnopolsky, and D. Sale. Gender differences in strength and muscle fiber characteristics. Eur J Appl Physiol 66:254-262. 1992.

182. Moon, J. Lane, M., Doernte, L. Spears, A., and Bean, R. (2018). "Relationships Between Dual-Energy X-Ray Absorptiometry Fat and Lean Tissue Masses and Standing and Sitting Bioimpedance Spectroscopy Variables in Healthy Men and Women." The FASEB Journal 32: 910.912-910.912.

183. Moon, J. Lane, M., Doernte, L. Spears, A., and Bean, R. (2018). "Bioimpedance Spectroscopy Measurements Comparing Different Body Positions and Electrode Types in Men and Women: 1989 Board# 250 May 31 3: 30 PM-5: 00 PM." Medicine & Science in Sports & Exercise 50(5S): 482.

184. Murray, T.D., and J.M. Murray. Cardiovascular anatomy. In: American College of Sports Medicine Resource Manual for Guidelines for Exercise Testing and Prescription, 3rd ed., J.L. Roitman, ed. Baltimore: Williams & Wilkins. 1998. pp. 61-69.

185. National Strength and Conditioning Association. Strength training for female athletes. NSCA J 11:43-55, 29-36. 1989.

186. Newton, R.U., A.J. Murphy, B.J. Humphries, G.J. Wilson, W.J. Kraemer, and K. Häkkinen. Influence of load and stretch shortening cycle on the kinematics, kinetics and muscle activation that occurs during explosive upper-body movements. Eur J Appl Physiol 75:333-342. 1997.

187. Orr, R., N. de Vos, N. Singh, D. Ross, T. Stavrinos, and M. Fiatarone-Singh. Power training improves balance in healthy older adults. J Gerontol A Biol Sci Med Sci 61:78-85. 2006.

188. Otis, C., B. Drinkwater, and M. Johnson. American College of Sports Medicine: Position stand: The female athlete triad. Med Sci Sports Exerc 29:i-ix. 1997.

189. Ozmun, J., A. Mikesky, and P. Surburg. Neuromuscular adaptations following prepubescent strength training. Med Sci Sports Exerc 26:510-514. 1994.

190. Pauletto, B. Periodization-peaking. NSCA J 8(4):30-31. 1986.

191. Plisk, S.S., and M.H. Stone. Periodization strategies. NSCA J 25(6):19-37. 2003

192. Ploutz, L.L., R.L. Biro, P.A. Tesch, and G.A. Dudley. Effect of resistance training on muscle mass involvement in exercise. J Appl Physiol 76:1675-1681. 1994.

193. Poliquin, C. Five steps to increasing the effectiveness of your strength training program. NSCA J 10(3):34-39. 1988.

194. Poortmans, J.R. Protein turnover and amino acid oxidation during and after exercise. Med Sports Sci 17:130-147. 1984.

195. Radcliffe, J.C., and L.R. Osternig. Effects on performance of variable eccentric loads during depth jumps. J Sport Rehabil 4:31-41. 1995.

196. Robergs, R.A., F. Ghiasvand, and D. Parker. Biochemistry of exercise-induced metabolic acidosis. Am J Physiol Regul Integr Comp Physiol 287:R502-R516. 2004.

197. Rozenek, R., L. Rosenau, P. Rosenau, and M.H. Stone. The effect of intensity on heart rate and blood lactate response to resistance exercise. J Strength Cond Res 7(1):51-54. 1993.

198. Ryushi, T., K. Häkkinen, H. Kauhanen, and P. Komi. Muscle fiber characteristics, muscle cross sectional area and force production in strength athletes, physically active males and females. Scand Sports Sci 10:7-15. 1988.

199. Sahlin, K., M. Tonkonogy, and K. Soderlund. Energy supply and muscle fatigue in humans. Acta Physiol Scand 162:261-266. 1998.

200. Sant'Ana Pereira, J.A., A.J. Sargeant, A.C. Rademaker, A. de Haan, and W. van Mechelen. Myosin heavy chain isoform expression and high energy phosphate content in human muscle fibres at rest and post-exercise. J Physiol 496(Pt 2):583-588. 1996.

201. Selye, H. The Stress of Life. New York: McGraw-Hill. 1956.

202. Shephard, R. Exercise and training in women, part 1: Influence of gender on exercise and training response. Can J Appl Physiol 25:19-34. 2000.

203. Smerdu, V., I. Karsch-Mizrachi, M. Campione, L. Leinwand, and S. Schiaffino. Type IIx myosin heavy chain transcripts are expressed in type IIb fibers of human skeletal muscle. J Appl Physiol 267(6 Pt 1):C1723-1728. 1994.

204. Smith, S.A., S.J. Montain, R.P. Matott, G.P. Zientara, F.A. Jolesz, and R.A. Fielding. Creatine supplementation and age influence muscle metabolism during exercise. J Appl Physiol 85:1349-1356. 1998.

205. Stone, M.H., and H.S. O'Bryant. Weight Training: A Scientific Approach. Minneapolis: Burgess. 1987.

206. Stone, M.H., H.S. O'Bryant, and J. Garhammer. A hypothetical model for strength training. J Sports Med Phys Fitness (21):336, 342-351.1981.

207. Stone, M.H., H.S. O'Bryant, J. Garhammer, J. McMillan, and R. Rozenek. A theoretical model of strength training. NSCA J 4(4):36-40. 1982.

208. Stone, M.H., J. Potteiger, K.C. Pierce, C.M. Proulx, H.S. O'Bryant, and R.L. Johnson. Comparison of the effects of three different weight training programs on the 1RM squat: A preliminary study. Presented at National Strength and Conditioning Association Conference. Las Vegas, NV, June 1997.

209. Sutton, J. Hormonal and metabolic responses to exercise in subjects of high and low work capacities. Med Sci Sports 10:1-6. 1978.

210. Tanaka, K., Y. Matsuura, S. Kumagai, A. Matsuzuka, K. Hirakoba, and K. Asano. Relationships of anaerobic threshold and onset of blood lactate accumulation with endurance performance. Eur J Appl Physiol 52:51-56. 1983.

211. Taylor, D.J., P. Styles, P.M. Matthews, D.A. Arnold, D.G. Gadian, P. Bore, and G.K. Radda. Energetics of human muscle: Exercise induced ATP depletion. Magn Reson Med 3(1):44-54. 1986.

212. Tesch, P. Muscle fatigue in man, with special reference to lactate accumulation during short intense exercise. Acta Physiol Scand 480:1-40. 1980.

213. Tesch, P.A., L.L. Ploutz-Snyder, L. Ystrom, M.J. Castro, and G.A. Dudley. Skeletal muscle glycogen loss evoked by resistance exercise. J Strength Cond Res 12:67-73. 1998.

214. Thorstensson, P. Muscle strength, fiber types and enzymes in man. Acta Physiol Scand 102:443. 1976.

215. Thorstensson, P., B. Sjodin, and J. Karlsson. Actinomyosin ATPase, myokinase, CPK and LDH in human fast and slow twitch muscle fibres. Acta Physiol Scand 99:225-229. 1975.

216. Tschiene, P. The distinction of training structure in different stages of athlete's preparation. Paper presented at International Congress of Sport Sciences. Edmonton, AB, July 1979.

217. Vandervoot, A., and A. McComas. Contractile changes in opposing muscle of the human ankle joint with aging. J Appl Physiol 61:361-367. 1986.

218. VanHelder, W., M. Radomski, R. Goode, and K. Casey. Hormonal and metabolic response to three types of exercise of equal duration and external work output. Eur J Appl Physiol 54:337-342. 1985.

219. Vihko, V., A. Salmons, and J. Rontumaki. Oxidative and lysomal capacity in skeletal muscle. Acta Physiol Scand 104:74-81. 1978.

220. Walsh, B., M. Tonkonogi, K. Soderlund, E. Hultman, V. Saks, and K. Sahlin. The role of phosphorylcreatine and creatine in the regulation of mitochondrial respiration in human skeletal muscle. J Physiol 537(Pt 3):971-978. 2001.

221. Wathen, D. Periodization: Concepts and applications. In: Essentials of Strength Training and Conditioning, T.R. Baechle, ed. Champaign, IL: Human Kinetics. 1994.

222. Weir, J.P., and J.T. Cramer. Principles of musculoskeletal exercise programming. In: ACSM Resource Manual for Exercise Testing and Prescription, 5th ed., L.A. Kaminsky (senior ed.), S. Glass (section ed.). American College of Sports Medicine. Philadelphia: Lippincott, Williams & Wilkins. 2005. pp. 350-365.

223. Weltman, A., C. Janney, C. Rians, K. Strand, B. Berg, S. Tippet, J. b, Wise, B. Cahill, and F. Katch. The effects of hydraulic resistance strength training in pre-pubertal males. Med Sci Sports Exerc 18:629-638. 1986.

224. West, R. The female athlete: The triad of disordered eating, amenorrhoea and osteoporosis. Sports Med 26:63-71. 1998.

225. Westcott, W., and T. Baechle. Strength Training for Seniors. Champaign, IL: Human Kinetics. 1999.

226. Wilk, K.E., M.L. Voight, M.A. Keirns, V. Gambetta, J.R. Andrews, and C.J. Dillman. Stretch-shortening drills for the upper extremities: Theory and clinical applications. J Orthop Sports Phys Ther 17:225-239. 1993.

227. Williams, J.H., and G.A. Klug. Calcium exchange hypothesis of skeletal muscle: A brief review. Muscle Nerve 18:421-434. 1995.

228. Wilson, G.J., A.J. Murphy, and A. Giorgi. Weight and plyometric training: Effects on eccentric and concentric force production. Can J Appl Physiol 21:301-315. 1996.

229. Wilson, G.J., R.U. Newton, A.J. Murphy, and B.J. Humphries. The optimal training load for the development of dynamic athletic performance. Med Sci Sports Exerc 25:1279-1286. 1993.

230. Wilt, F. Plyometrics: What it is and how it works. Athl J 55(5):76, 89-90. 1975.

231. Withers, R.T., W.M. Sherman, D.G. Clark, P.C. Esselbach, S.R. Nolan, M.H. Mackay, and M. Brinkman. Muscle metabolism during 30, 60 and 90 s of maximal cycling on an airbraked ergometer. Eur J Appl Physiol 63:354-362. 1991.

232. Yarasheski, K., J. Zachwieja, and D. Bier. Acute effects of resistance exercise on muscle protein synthesis in young and elderly men and women. Am J Appl Physiol 265:210-214. 1993.

233. York, J., L.B. Oscai, and D.G. Penny. Alterations in skeletal muscle lactate dehydrogenase isozymes following exercise training. Biochem Biophys Res Commun 61:1387-1393. 1974.

Made in the USA
Coppell, TX
05 February 2024

28634667R00201